Caring for the Elderly in Japan and the US

In an era of changing demographics and values, this volume provides a cross-national and interdisciplinary perspective on the question of who cares for and about the elderly. The authors reflect on research studies, experimental programs and personal experience in Japan and the United States to explicitly compare how policies, practices and interpretations of elder care are evolving at the turn of the century.

This volume provides a broader picture of how elder care is defined at a time when aging is becoming increasingly defined as a social problem. It contextualizes its subject through a unique approach which brings together international experts from fields including anthropology, health economics, social work and psychology to examine the implications for elder care of demographic, social and economic change in both the US and Japan. Key issues which are addressed include:

- the role of gender in the assignment of caregiving duties;
- the impact of social change on reciprocal care and intergenerational justice;
- the influence of cultural assumptions on the shaping of policy through political process.

This book will be an invaluable resource to all students, teachers and researchers interested in health and welfare, applied social policy and gerontology.

Susan Orpett Long is Associate Professor of Anthropology at John Carroll University, USA. She has written extensively on welfare issues and social change in Japan.

Routledge Advances in Asia-Pacific Studies

1   Environment, Education and Society in the Asia-Pacific
Local traditions and global discourses
David Yencken, John Fien and Helen Sykes

2   Ageing in the Asia-Pacific Region
David R. Phillips

3   Gender Politics in the Asia-Pacific
Edited by Brenda S. A. Yeoh, Peggy Teo and Shirlena Huang

4   Caring for the Elderly in Japan and the US
Practices and policies
Susan Orpett Long

Caring for the Elderly in Japan and the US

Practices and policies

Susan Orpett Long

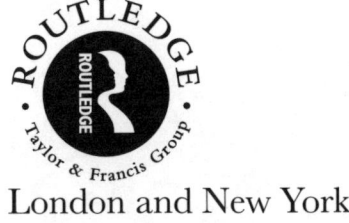

London and New York

First published 2000
by Routledge
11 New Fetter Lane, London EC4P 4EE

Simultaneously published in the USA and Canada
by Routledge
29 West 35th Street, New York, NY 10001

Routledge is an imprint of the Taylor & Francis Group

© 2000 Susan Orpett Long

Typeset in Baskerville by
HWA Text and Data Management, Tunbridge Wells
Printed and bound in Great Britain by
Biddles Ltd, Guildford and Kings Lynn

All rights reserved. No part of this book may be reprinted or reproduced or utilised in any form or by any electronic, mechanical, or other means, now known or hereafter invented, including photocopying and recording, or in any information storage or retrieval system, without permission in writing from the publishers.

British Library Cataloguing in Publication Data
A catalogue record for this book is available from the British Library

Library of Congress Cataloging in Publication Data
Caring for the elderly in Japan and the US – practices and policies [edited by] Susan Orpett Long.
    p.   cm.
   Includes bibliographical references.
   1. Aged–Care–United States.   2. Aged–Government policy–
United States.   3. Aged–Services for-United States.   4. Aged–Care
–Japan   5. Aged–Government policy–Japan.   6. Aged–Services for
–Japan.   I. Long, Susan Orpett
   HV1461.038   2000   99.38453
   362.6′0952–dc21   CIP

ISBN   0-415-22352-0

Contents

List of figures	*viii*
List of tables	*ix*
List of contributors	*x*
Acknowledgments	*xv*
List of abbreviations	*xvii*

Introduction   1
SUSAN ORPETT LONG

PART I
Assuring care: government policies and programs   17

1 Cultural meanings of "security" in aging policies   19
AKIKO HASHIMOTO

2 The socioeconomic context of Japanese social policy for aging   28
DAISAKU MAEDA

3 From the New Deal to the new millennium: bridging the gap in US aging and health policy   52
BRETT R. SOUTH AND DOUGLAS D. BRADHAM

4 Changing meanings of frail old people and the Japanese welfare state   82
JOHN CREIGHTON CAMPBELL

5 Critical issues in health care for the US elderly: beyond the millennium 98
DOUGLAS D. BRADHAM

PART II
Providing care: professional caregivers **119**

6 We live too short, and die too long: on Japanese and US physicians' caregiving practices and approaches to withholding life-sustaining treatments 121
MICHAEL D. FETTERS AND MARION DANIS

7 Difficult choices: policy and meaning in Japanese hospice practice 146
SUSAN ORPETT LONG AND SATOSHI CHIHARA

8 Policies and practices near the end of life in the US: the ambivalent pursuit of a good death 172
DAVID BARNARD

PART III
Assisting in care: non-profit organizations and volunteers **189**

9 The development of social welfare services in Japan 191
KIYOSHI ADACHI

10 The accountability dilemma: providing voluntary care for the elderly in the US and Japan 206
YUKO SUDA

PART IV
Coordinating and caring: family caregivers **229**

11 Variations in family caregiving in Japan and the US 231
RUTH CAMPBELL AND BERIT INGERSOLL-DAYTON

12 Recognizing the need for gender-responsive
    family caregiving policy: lessons from male
    caregivers   248
    PHYLLIS BRAUDY HARRIS AND SUSAN ORPETT LONG

PART V
Facilitating care of self   **273**

13 The creativity of the demented elderly:
    the use of psychological approaches in a
    Japanese outpatient clinic   275
    YUKIKO KUROKAWA

14 Visible lives: life stories and ritual in
    American nursing homes   289
    THU TRAM T. NGUYEN, JOAL M. HILL AND THOMAS R. COLE

15 Disclosure, decisions, and dementia in Japan:
    maximizing the continuity of self   303
    MASAHIKO SAITO

16 Concepts of personhood in Alzheimer's disease:
    considering Japanese notions of a relational self   318
    WILLIAM E. DEAL AND PETER J. WHITEHOUSE

17 Epilogue: downsizing the material self:
    late life and long involvements with things   334
    DAVID W. PLATH

    Glossary   *344*
    Index   *349*

Figures

3.1	Trends in US personal health care expenditure, 1960 to 2005	62
3.2	Comparions of health-to-GDP expenditures between the US and other OECD nations	63
3.3	Distribution of Medicare spending comparisons between 1980 and 1984	71
5.1	US elders' long-term care nexus and public policy options	99
5.2	US elderly age composition and fertility history of women	101
5.3	US elderly in the community with ADL limitations, by marital status 1990–2030	101
5.4	Living arrangements of US elderly, 1990–2030	101
5.5	Income of US elderly by marital status, 1990–2030	102
5.6	Who can afford nursing home care – percent of US elderly whose income is greater than 100 percent of nursing home costs	105
5.7	Who can afford LTC insurance – percent of US elderly who income is greater than 100 percent of LTC insurance costs	105
5.8	Annual expenditure shares of US elderly retirees	105
5.9	Compression of morbidity	112
5.10	Estimated number of persons and direct medical costs for persons with chronic conditions in the US, 1995–2050	113
5.11	Percent of US health care dollars by payer for acute versus chronic conditions, 1987	114
10.1	Accountability along with the order of relationships among key actors and stakeholders	207
15.1	Households with people aged over 65 in Japan	305
15.2	Households with people aged over 65 in Yamagata, Kagosima and Tokyo (1995)	310
15.3	Where patients with dementia receive care in Japan	305
15.4	Care providers for patients with dementia	305
15.5	Number of residents of nursing homes in Japan, 1975–1995	305

Tables

3.1	Milestones of US aging and health policy	53
5.1	Critical issues in health care for the US elderly	107
6.1	Demographics of participating physicians	128
6.2	Factors influencing decision-making	129
7.1	Staff members, Seirei Hospice	163
7.2	Structure of the hospice ward, Serei Hospice	163
7.3	Annual change in number of patients, Seirei Hospice	163
7.4	Distribution of patients according to gender and age, Seirei Hospice	164
7.5	Distribution of patients according to disease, Seirei Hospice	164
7.6	Distribution of patients according to religion, Seirei Hospice	164
7.7	Duration of hospice stay from the last admission to patient death, Seirei Hospice	165
7.8	Trends in duration of hospice stay, Serei Hospice	165
7.9	Trends of patients entering home hospice care at Serei Hospice	165
7.10	Average duration of home care in the case of patient death at Serei Hospice	165
7.11	A comparison between malignant neoplasms and other diseases in home care, Serei Hospice	166
10.1	Background information on organizations in study	209
10.2	Activities of 501(c)(3) organizations, US	226
13.1	Examples of themes of support group, Japan	284
13.2	Support Group Program, Japan	284

Contributors

Kiyoshi Adachi is associate professor of sociology at the School of Human and Environmental Studies, Kyushu University in Fukuoka, Japan. He completed his doctorate at the Graduate School of Sociology of Tokyo University in 1987. Recipient of an Abe Fellowship in 1994, he has published *The Sociology of Social Welfare Reform and Home Care Services in Japan* (Harvest Sha, Tokyo, 1998) and with coauthors James E. Lubben and Noriko Tsukada, "Expansion of Formalized In-home Services for Japan's Aged" in the *Journal of Aging and Social Policy* (1996).

David Barnard, Ph.D., is professor in the Department of Medicine and the Center for Bioethics and Health Law at the University of Pittsburgh. He is an authority on the integration of ethics and humanities into medical education, and on clinical and ethical aspects of palliative care. He is coauthor of *Crossing Over: Narratives of Palliative Care* (Oxford University Press, 2000).

Douglas Bradham, Dr.P.H., is associate professor of medicine at the University of Maryland, Baltimore, School of Medicine specializing in health economics, health services research and medical outcomes analysis. He is a recognized authority in cost analyses in clinical trials for chronic diseases, health economic policy for the elderly and health service for the elderly. He is the director of the Department of Veterans Affairs Health Services and Development Center at The Capital Network, located at the Baltimore Veterans Affairs Medical Center.

John Creighton Campbell, Ph.D., is professor of political science at the University of Michigan, specializing in Japanese politics, decision-making processes, and social policy. He is the author of *How Policies Change: The Japanese Government and the Aging Society* (Princeton University Press, 1992) and, with Naoki Ikegami, *The Art of Balance in Health Policy: Maintaining Japan's Low-Cost, Egalitarian System* (Cambridge University Press, 1998). He was the recipient of a 1997 Abe fellowship. He serves as the secretary-treasurer of the Association for Asian Studies.

List of contributors xi

Ruth Campbell, M.S.W., is associate director of social work and community programs for the University of Michigan Geriatrics Center and adjunct professor at the University of Michigan School of Social Work. Her publications include articles on peer counseling, writing groups, and long-term care in the United States. She has also written extensively on aging and caregiving in Japan, as well as cross-cultural comparisons of the elderly in both countries. She was a 1994 Abe fellow.

Satoshi Chihara, M.D., is a physician specializing in medical oncology and terminal care. Since 1982 he has been Medical Director of Seirei Hospice and from 1993 concurrently serves as vice president of Seirei Mikatahara General Hospital in Hamamatsu, Japan.

Thomas R. Cole, Ph.D., is professor and graduate program director at the Institute for Medical Humanities, University of Texas Medical Branch. He was trained as a cultural historian and helped develop the field of humanistic gerontology. His book, *The Journey of Life: A Cultural History of Aging in America*, (Cambridge University Press, 1992) was nominated for a Pulitzer Prize; he is senior editor of *Handbook of Humanities and Aging*, second edition, which will be published by Springer in fall, 1999.

Marion Danis, M.D., is trained in medicine and conducts research in medical ethics. She is head of the Section on Ethics and Health Policy in the Department of Clinical Bioethics at the National Institutes of Health. She has had a long-standing interest in finding approaches for balancing respect for patient treatment preferences and the need to distribute limited resources fairly.

William E. Deal, Ph.D., is Severance associate professor of the history of religions in the Department of Religion at Case Western Reserve University. He also serves as director of the Asian Studies Program. His research and publications focus on Japanese Buddhism and on biomedical ethics in Japan.

Michael D. Fetters, M.D., M.P.H., M.A., is a family physician and assistant professor in the Department of Family Medicine at the University of Michigan in Ann Arbor, Michigan. He is the founder and director of The University of Michigan Health System Japanese Family Health Program, an initiative that provides comprehensive, linguistically and culturally sensitive health care to the Japanese-speaking population of Southeast Michigan. He has published multiple articles about the interface of medical ethics and culture with a particular emphasis on Japan.

Phyllis Braudy Harris, Ph.D., is associate professor of sociology and director of the Aging Studies Program at John Carroll University, Cleveland, Ohio. Her research interests focus on the impact of dementing illness on family caregivers and diagnosed individuals, and the role gender plays in this process in both the United States and Japan. She is author of the book *Men Giving*

Care: Reflections of Husbands and Sons (with Joyce Bichler) (Garland Publishing, 1997), and has published extensively on the topic of male caregivers in leading gerontology journals, such as *The Gerontologist, The Journal of Aging Studies, The Journal of Cross-Cultural Gerontology* (with Susan O. Long), *The Journal of Clinical Geropsychology*, and *The Journal of Mental Health and Aging*.

Akiko Hashimoto is associate professor of sociology and Asian studies at the University of Pittsburgh. She is author of *The Gift of Generations: Japanese and American Perspectives on Aging and the Social Contract* (Cambridge University Press, 1996), and co-editor of *Family Support for the Elderly: The International Experience* (Oxford University Press, 1992). A 1996 Abe fellow, she is currently at work on a book on collective memories of World War II in Japan and Germany.

Joal Hill, J.D., M.P.H., research associate at the Park Ridge Center for the Study of Health, Faith, and Ethics, and a Ph.D. candidate at The Institute for Medical Humanities at the University of Texas Medical Branch, where her primary academic interests are clinical ethics, and literature and medicine. She was a fellow in bioethics at the Cleveland Clinic Foundation during the 1992–3 academic year, has twice been awarded a William Bennett Bean Scholarship, and in 1997 received the Medical Humanities Award at the National Student Research Forum for her paper on physician participation in capital punishment by lethal injection.

Berit Ingersoll-Dayton, M.S.W., Ph.D., received her doctorate in social work and psychology from the University of Michigan. She is currently a professor of social work at the University of Michigan. Her research interests focus on differences in social support and caregiving between genders and across cultures. She has written numerous journal articles and book chapters and has coauthored a book, *Balancing Work and Caregiving for Children, Adults, and Elders* (Sage Publications, 1993).

Yukiko Kurokawa, Ph.D., is chief researcher at Keiseikai Institute of Gerontology and works at Keiseikai outpatient clinic as a clinical psychologist. She received a Ph.D. from the University of Tokyo. She has recently edited *Oino Rinshō Shinri* (The Psychology of the Elderly), published by Nihon Hyōronsha in 1998.

Susan Orpett Long is associate professor of anthropology at John Carroll University. She is author of *Family Change and the Life Course* (Cornell University East Asia Papers, 1987) and editor of *Lives in Motion: Composing Circles of Self Community in Japan* (Cornell University East Asia Papers, 1999). She has published book chapters and articles on the topics of aging (with Phyllis Braudy Harris), health care, and gender in Japan. Her current research on bioethics and culture was supported by a 1995 Abe fellowship. She served as the founding coordinator of John Carroll University's East Asian Studies program from 1987–95.

Daisaku Maeda is professor of social welfare and director of the Social Work Research Institute, Faculty of Social Welfare at Rissho University in Tokyo. He was formerly professor at the Social Research Institute at the Japan College of Social Work and director of the Department of Sociology at the Tokyo Metropolitan Institute of Gerontology. He specializes in social gerontology, social welfare research, and gerontological social work and has served on a number of national and municipal advisory boards for welfare issues.

Thu Tram T. Nguyen is the Sealy Center on Aging pre-doctoral fellow, and a Ph.D. student at the Institute for Medical Humanities, University of Texas Medical Branch. Her interests are bioethics, the institutionalized elderly, and narrative. She received her Bachelor of Arts degree in the history of philosophy at Trinity University. Her newsletter piece, "Visual Biography: A Model for Individual and Family Developmental Tasks in Long-Term Care Facilities" was published in spring, 1998 *Dimensions Quarterly Newsletter* of the Mental Health and Aging Network of the American Society on Aging.

David W. Plath, Ph.D., retired from a position as professor of anthropology and Asian studies at the University of Illinois so that he could devote more time to producing documentary video programs. His most recent program, "Makiko's New World," was issued by the Media Production Group, which he heads, in the spring of 1999.

Masahiko Saito, M.D., Ph.D., was trained in psychiatry at the University of Tokyo and is currently director of Keiseikai Institute of Gerontology and vice director of Oume Keiyu Hospital, Tokyo, Japan. He specializes in clinical geriatric psychiatry, law and psychiatry, and medical ethics in psychiatry.

Brett South received a Bachelor's degree in biology and political science from the Utah State University of 1995. He has worked in the analytical support of health policy, focusing on the development of analytic tools to examine health care utilization and expenses. South is engaged in several studies of cost savings associated with new interventions in health promotion, peripheral arterial disease and obesity. He is currently the senior research analyst at the Veterans Affairs Capital Network Health Services Research and Development Center in Baltimore, Maryland. His graduate work centers on health policy analysis for public sector health care financing.

Yuko Suda, Ph.D., is currently program manager of Friedens Haus Senior Services and adjunct professor at St Louis University. She has received training in the disciplines of gerontology, health sociology and social statistical research. In 1994, she received an Abe Fellowship for comparative work on accountability in service organizations. Her book, tentatively titled, *Nàsu Saido Sutō in Sento Ruisu* [North Side Story in St Louis] will be published by Dai-ichi shorin, Tokyo. She is a founding member and former executive director (1989) of the Japan Networkers' Conference.

Peter J. Whitehouse, M.D., Ph.D., M.A., is professor of neurology, psychiatry, neuroscience, psychology, biomedical ethics, nursing and organizational behavior at Case Western Reserve University School of Medicine and the Alzheimer Center at University Hospitals of Cleveland. He received an M.D. and a Ph.D. in neuropsychology from The Johns Hopkins University, and a Master's degree in biomedical ethics in 1997 from Case Western Reserve University. His clinical focus is in geriatric and behavioral neurology with a special interest in dementia. His research has included work on the biology of Alzheimer's disease, international drug development, neuropsychology, health care systems, and ethics. His recent work includes cultural studies of science and information systems to support learning.

Acknowledgments

This volume represents two years of collegial discussions on the topic of "who cares?" We have reached, sometimes beyond a comfortable distance, to build bridges across academic disciplines, across the theory-practice divide, and across national boundaries. Our work has been enriched by our discussions.

This endeavor has been possible because of the support of the Abe Fellowship Program, which is administered by the Social Science Research Council in cooperation with the American Council of Learned Societies with funding provided by the Japan Center for Global Partnership. Six of the contributors (K. Adachi, J. Campbell, R. Campbell, A. Hashimoto, S. Long, and Y. Suda) have received Abe fellowships in support of their research. Many of the authors' ideas and chapter drafts grew out of participation in two workshops funded by the Abe Fellowship Program: "Aging Across Societies: Meaningful Life, Care, and Closure" held in Ann Arbor, Michigan April 11–13, 1997; and "Care and Meaning in Late Life: Culture, Policy, and Practice in Japan and the United States" held at Shonan International Village Conference Center in Hayama, Japan February 26 to March 1, 1998. Support for the editorial tasks of turning conference papers into a book came from a John Carroll University Summer Research Fellowship.

Numerous individuals contributed to making this volume a reality. Frank Baldwin and Takuya Toda of the Tokyo Abe Fellowship Office and Mary McDonnell of the Social Science Research Council were instrumental in organizing the two workshops and in providing assistance for the project. Albert I. Hermalin offered his support, ideas, and organizational skills for the Ann Arbor workshop which provided a stimulating set of background papers from which this project developed. All of the authors benefited greatly from the contributions and suggestions of Takako Sodei, Kei Ikeda, Glenda Roberts, and Shinya Hoshino who participated in the Hayama workshop. Kathleen Catanese has provided skilled and thoughtful research and editorial assistance for the project.

As editor, I am especially grateful to have had the opportunity to work with this group of scholars and practitioners who have collaborated to shape this book. Many of the authors have contributed beyond their chapters in less visible yet substantial ways, helping with the editorial work, clarifying background material, and providing moral support. They have been willing to share ideas, assist co-contributors, and stretch beyond their cultural and disciplinary assumptions.

I would also like to thank editors Victoria Smith and Craig Fowlie at Routledge for their assistance and advice, Yūzo Okamoto for first encouraging me two decades ago to study issues of elder care, the Horii family for their continuing instruction on Japanese society, and my family for their patience and support.

Abbreviations

AALL	American Association of Labor Legislation
AARP	American Association of Retired Persons
ADL	activities of daily living
AFDC	Aid to Families with Dependent Children
AIDS	acquired immune deficiency syndrome
AMA	American Medical Association
ARFM	aggressive risk factor management
COPD	chronic obstructive pulmonary disease
CT	computed tomography
CVD	cardiovascular disease
DHHS	Department of Health and Human Services
DI	Disability Insurance
DNR	do not resuscitate
DPAHC	durable power of attorney for health care
DRG	Diagnosis Related Groups
FFS	fee for service
FHA	Federal Housing Association
FMR	fair market rent
GDP	gross domestic product
GHQ	general headquarters
HAP	housing assistance payments
HCFA	Health Care Financing Administration
HI	Hospital Insurance
HMOs	health maintenance organizations
HUD	Housing and Urban Development
IADL	instrumental activities of daily living
ICU	intensive care unit
IRA	Individual Retirement Account
IRS	Internal Revenue Services
JSP	Japan Socialist Party
LDP	Liberal Democratic Party
LTC	long-term care
LTCI	Long-Term Care Insurance

MCCA	Medicare Catastrophic Coverage Act
MHW	Ministry of Health and Welfare
MRI	magnetic resonance imaging
MTA	Medical Trust Account
NCHS	National Center for Health Statistics
NIH	National Institutes of Health
NPO	nonprofit organization
OAA	Old Age Assistance
OAI	Old Age Insurance
OASDI	Old Age and Survivors Disability Insurance
OASI	Old Age Survivors Insurance
PAD	peripheral arterial disease
PHCEs	personal health care expenditures
POS	point of service
PPOs	preferred provider organizations
PPS	prospective payment system
RBRVS	Resource-Based Relative Value Scale
SNF	skilled nursing facility
SSI	Supplemental Security Income
SUPPORT	Study to Understand Prognoses and Preferences for Outcomes and Risks of Treatments
TEFRA	Tax Equity and Fiscal Responsibility Act
WAC	Wonderful Aging Club

Introduction

Susan Orpett Long

In English, the word "care" is highly ambiguous. Its interpretation in any particular linguistic situation may vary between the speaker and hearer, the writer and reader, the caregiver and the care recipient. Its meaning is shaded by social status, differently interpreted by men and women, by poor and wealthy, by personal experiences of dependency and of providing assistance to others, and by implicit understandings of how the universe, and human society in particular, operate. The term is also significantly different for scholars, administrators, and professionals depending on their disciplinary background.

This volume is concerned with the topic of elder care and its multiple meanings. It grows out of the support of the Abe Fellowship Program of the Social Science Research Council for work on contemporary issues surrounding medical care and social welfare for the elderly. Some of the contributors received funding for research presented here, and many participated in two conferences on elder care sponsored by the Abe program in 1997 and 1998.

We often, in the United States, hear the refrain, "Who cares?" In both Japan and the United States, people have come to fear that our families, our communities, and our nations do not care, or at least care enough, for the elderly. It has become commonplace to define aging as a social problem.

Once so defined, old age becomes stigmatized. Aging is viewed negatively, so that older people are motivated to adopt strategies to remain healthy and active participants in their society. Aging is considered an unavoidable problem requiring preparation, so that middle-aged people worry about caring for ill parents and wonder who will care for them when they themselves become frail. Governments and service agencies cope with questions of finances and ethics, struggling to make limited budgets stretch to meet needs which seem to grow endlessly greater. Professionals attempt to balance the needs of clients and family members with the constraints of time and costs; volunteers work to fill the holes in the floodgates. By various definitions, all of this is caring, yet these participants in caregiving rarely question the very categories of aging and crisis which are in the background of their efforts (Cohen, 1994).

Why then the sense that we do not care? The title of this volume points to the ambiguity of the word "care" in several ways. To provide a pension to pay for the physical needs of a wheelchair-bound elderly person is to care. To shop or cook or clean for a weak 95-year-old is to care. To offer art therapy for a demented older person is to care. Yet these actions do not add up to the full meaning of what we think "care" *should* be. Is providing care the equivalent of caring? The answer lies perhaps in the recognition that social changes, and their political response, have created new constellations of meanings. The definition of aging as a social problem is thus not an objective crisis of demography, but a crisis in the significance of biological aging, family relationships, and relations between individuals and the state. In the past, families might be expected to incorporate multiple meanings of care, the physical and the interpersonal. Providing nursing care, giving financial support, and maintaining the social meaning of the life of an old person converged historically in the family. As this has come to be challenged in government programs and private circumstances, some people have advocated a return to the era of family caregiving for the elderly. Yet to do so is to disregard the tremendous demographic and social changes that have led to more active and more independent lives for longer periods for many older adults, and to longer periods that the elderly live with debilitating illnesses that leave them dependent on others. It is also to ignore changes in the meaning of caregiving.

In our post-industrial societies, the various caregiving roles have become more specialized. Not only families, but government policies, private companies, nonprofit agencies, and the elderly themselves all have complementary responsibilities for various tasks of physically and socially supporting functionally impaired elderly citizens, depending on their specialized skills. Perhaps our fear that no one cares is accurate in the sense that in our rapidly changing world, it can no longer be expected that it is the sole responsibility of one family caregiver, or even the family as a whole, to care in all the meanings of the word.

The specialization of caregiving roles in recent decades has also led to the fragmentation of *research* on caregiving.[1] Most such work has been grounded in some limited aspect of caring, whether it be social policy, ethnographic description, or survey research. What is missing from the caregiving literature is a presentation of the large picture of how the pieces do and do not fit together to comprise a portrait of caregiving in the society at large.[2] This volume offers that wider view of societal caregiving by contextualizing elder care in two ways.

First, we have purposively constructed the book as an interdisciplinary endeavor. The authors come from the fields of anthropology, health economics, medical humanities, medicine, political science, psychology, public health, social work, and sociology. They bring with them varying notions of what "care" means. Each chapter not only represents specialized research in the author's discipline, but also explicitly addresses questions of the implication of his or her work for other realms of meaning: for policy, for practice, and for people. By doing so, the volume as a whole shows us the range of activities of caring, across the range of meanings of that term, in the society as a whole, allowing us to see the "big picture."

Secondly, caring is put into a wider context by the cross-national perspective of the volume. Japan and the United States have both experienced demographic, social, and economic changes[3] that present similar challenges to our societies and to our assumptions about what it means to care. Both have rapidly aging populations, have seen significant changes in the types of jobs and who holds them in the economy, have increased access to expanded quantities of information, and have evolved new ideas about authority and social relationships. Despite these common experiences, and a common willingness to treat the aging of society as a problem, there are differences in the ways Japanese and American societies respond to the challenges of elder care. By placing these responses side by side throughout this book, we provide a broader perspective on societal and individual choices that are framed by diverse cultural understandings. Each chapter in this volume is either comparative within itself, or is paired with another chapter so that together they point to the socially and politically negotiated ways in which issues are identified and resolutions found. This allows us to see that care cannot be understood apart from the understandings of the world which are shared to varying degrees among policy makers, professionals, volunteers, families, and the elderly themselves within a family, a community, or a nation. Our chapters raise questions about the assumptions people hold concerning the role of government and law, the nature of human relationships, the concept of service to society, and the rights and obligations to make decisions for oneself and others. All of these impact on decisions about late life care, but they are best understood when we look to another society which makes different assumptions than our own, challenging us to think more broadly about our own options and choices.

The following section presents background on the demographic and cultural changes that lie behind the definition of elder care as a social problem. We will then consider the stereotypes that Japanese and Americans have of aging in each other's countries, pointing to the need for more careful investigation of elder care in the two societies. The final section of this introduction will describe the organization of the volume and point to the ways that the chapters contribute to our understanding of the meanings of "care" in late life.

The parameters of the care "problem"

Three fundamental issues lie behind the definition of elder care as a social problem: changing demographics (the "aging of society"), decreased ability to count on historically assumed family caregivers to provide care, and the financing of services. In addition, there are challenges to commonly held assumptions about how things *should* work in old age: that there is a sharp dividing line between life and death that people "naturally" cross when they get old; that women (ideally related by blood or marriage) provide the best care (assuming that they combine the physical and emotional aspects of caring), and notions of intergenerational justice. In many ways, the experiences of Japan and the United States have been quite similar.

Population, life expectancy, and impairment

First, if we look at population statistics, we see that the populations of both Japan and the United States have been aging rapidly. In both countries, over 12 percent of the population is 65 years of age or older.[4] According to projections by the two governments, these proportions will continue to increase until they peak at 22 percent in 2050 in the US (93 million people) and 26 percent in 2025 in Japan (32.4 million people) (Hobbs, 1996; Kōseishō, 1996). These figures represent not only increased life expectancies,[5] but also decreased fertility rates.[6] With a smaller proportion of the population in the youngest age groups, the proportion of those in the older categories increases even without the increased life expectancy.

These figures alone might lead to a sense that there will be a problem concerning elder care. In addition, other statistics reveal a correlation of illness and frailty with the very oldest age cohorts. The need for assistance with daily activities is higher among the elderly than among younger people, and increases with age within the 65 and older group (Kōseishō 1997a; Hobbs, 1996). In the US, half of the community-dwelling very old (85 and older) need such assistance (Hobbs, 1996, pp. 3–18). Another survey found that 27 percent of non-institutionalized elderly in Japan who are 85 and over report health problems that interfere with daily activities (Kōseishō 1997a, p. 52).

Caregiver availability

These changes in the apparent need for elder care have been accompanied in both Japan and the United States by trends that suggest a decreased availability of family caregivers. Household size has decreased in both countries, shrinking in the US from 3.14 in 1970 to 2.65 in 1996. In Japan, household size has decreased from 3.45 to 2.85 over the same period (Kōseishō, 1997b). In both countries there has been an increase in the number and proportion of middle-aged women working outside of the home. In the US, 70.5 percent of women aged 15–64 were in the labor force in 1994 compared with 62.8 percent ten years earlier. The rates have increased in the same period from 57.2 percent to 62.1 percent in Japan (US Department of Commerce, 1997, p. 846). In both countries, jobs, company transfers, and job changes may require workers to relocate to other regions where they are unable to provide day-to-day care for elderly relatives.

Financing

In both countries, but especially in the United States, there has been widespread concern among government officials, politicians, and the media concerning the increasing costs of medical care and social welfare programs. As a proportion of gross domestic product, the US spent 9.2 percent and Japan spent 6.6 percent on health care in 1980. However, by 1995, the figures were

14.2 percent for the US and 7.2 percent for Japan (US Department of Commerce of the US, 1997, p. 835).[7]

Changing cultural assumptions

Behind these statistics presented in the previous sections concerning the need for, availability of, and costs of caregiving for the elderly, lie other changes which are more difficult to quantify. Citizens, government bureaucrats, and professionals alike have encountered challenges to their world views which impact on their attitudes toward late life care.

The process of dying

In both countries, dying (as well as living) has become increasingly medicalized. Definitions of life and death are less clear-cut in an era of high-tech medicine that includes intensive-care medicine and organ transplantation. In daily practice, the timing of death is now less often attributed to God or to nature and more often to physicians' interpretations of "objective" data or to patient directive. Dying a slow death has long been recognized as one pattern of dying as opposed, for example, to a sudden death from a heart attack. But the ability of modern medicine to control many infections, to support blood pressure, and to perform live-prolonging procedures have made protracted dying longer and have made us less certain of the dividing line between life and death. While all of life can be considered movement toward certain death, the increased frailty that often comes with very advanced age offers an extension of this ambiguity. What level of dependency on others constitutes an acceptable definition of "living" is a question that is increasingly asked as explicit rationing of health care surfaces as a potential solution to the financing dilemmas.

Gender and cultural notions of caregiving

Women have had most of the responsibility for the day-to-day activities of family caregiving in both the United States and Japan. This may be in part because both countries exhibit a degree of biological determinism in regarding women as "natural" nurturers. But in the broader economic picture, it also has to do with women's subordinate position in the labor market. In both countries, women are often considered dispensable workers in the labor force, and are given less training and lower remuneration than men. Women's workplace responsibilities are often regarded as less important than their responsibilities as nurturers in the home by both themselves and their employers. In the labor force of paid caregivers this gender bias is also evident. It is primarily women who work as nurses, aides, and home helpers to provide either residential or home care for the elderly (US Department of Commerce, 1977, p. 415 for US). Yet increased demand for caregiving services means that men may also need to be available to assist elderly relatives. In both countries, there is evidence of increased participation of men in paid and volunteer caregiving roles as the gender structure of the labor market has begun to change.

Intergenerational justice

Whether in family caregiving or social welfare policy, there exists a common basis of elder care in assumptions about intergenerational justice. Children will care for their elder parents in "exchange" for the care they received as children, and for the care they can expect to receive from their own children when they become old. The cohorts of young and middle-aged workers will finance pensions for the current elderly on the assumption that they will receive benefits when they retire. But with the growing proportion of elderly in the population and changed authority relations in the family and in society, the stability, sufficiency, and meaning of intergenerational support is increasingly questioned. Moves toward greater *intra*generational redistribution are proposed to solve "crises" in the health insurance system in Japan and in social security in the United States. The globalization of information, the role of the media in forming opinions and attitudes, and the increasing legalization of lives in both countries challenge notions of intergenerational justice. Diffuse sociocultural change as well as more narrowly focused citizens' movements have created demands for increased personal autonomy that challenge previously unquestioned relations of authority among generations, between spouses, between physician and patient, between social welfare worker and client, and between citizen and government.

Mutual misperceptions

Japan and the US have looked to each other's patterns of elder care through cultural lenses that color the view with ambivalence. Americans have been convinced that Japanese elderly enjoy the care and respect of their children and grandchildren living in large multigenerational families, and when the time arrives, accept a natural death surrounded by loving family. Images such as the AT&T advertisement several years ago for international calls showing a middle-aged Asian man on the telephone with a gray-haired elderly Asian woman draw from and reinforce the stereotype that the Japanese *care* for their elderly relatives. But as Tobin (1987) has pointed out, these images may be more about American fears than about Japanese behavior. He argues that the image provides reassurance to Americans that somewhere out there is an industrialized, modern "other" which has not abandoned its elderly. At the same time, America is not willing to make the commitments required to create such a society for itself and does not consider Japan a model for the future, in part because it does not know its reality. The reality is that most people over 65 in both societies are healthy and active. In reality, nursing homes in Japan have waiting lists. Family caregiving is seen as a burden in Japan by both givers and receivers of care, and the government has accepted responsibility for creating a new system to fund alternatives to family care. (See Chapter 2 by D. Maeda and Chapter 4 by J. Campbell, this volume.) Death in Japan is feared more often than calmly accepted, but as high suicide rates for the elderly suggest, perhaps it is not feared as much as becoming a burden on others.[8]

On the other hand, Japanese often believe that Americans abandon their older relatives to nursing homes and poverty. The only system that seems to operate in the United States is that of for-profit capitalism, and so Japanese gerontologists and government officials have looked to Scandinavia and Western Europe when they study policy alternatives. Yet practitioners have looked to the United States for models of volunteerism and end-of-life medical care in which stereotypes of altruism and autonomy predominate. But the reality is that Americans consider intergenerational bonds to be strong, families do provide the vast majority of elder care, and they do not take lightly the decision to institutionalize an elderly relative (see, for example, Bengston, Rosenthal, and Burton, 1994). Cost-containment practices have increased the burden on the elderly and their families in economic and social terms, and the US government increasingly entrusts the provision of health and welfare services to private and nonprofit corporations, to volunteers in the community, and to family caregivers of the ill who are discharged too rapidly from hospitals under "managed care" medicine. In an era in which most middle-aged women are active in the labor force, volunteers are increasingly the elderly themselves. In contrast to what many Japanese believe and despite vast media attention and educational efforts in the US, the majority of Americans have neither living wills nor hospice care when they face death.

People, practices, and policies

The chapters that follow all help to sort the images from the realities of late life care in Japan and the United States. The book is divided into five sections which focus on who is providing care: government policy; professional caregivers; nonprofit organizations and community programs; family; and the elderly themselves. Taken together, these present the broad spectrum of elder care in the two countries. Regardless of their focus, all of the authors reach beyond their usual research themes to consider the implications of that form of care for elder care policy, for practices of organizations and professionals, and for the people involved in giving and receiving care.

Assuring care: government policies and programs

The governments of both countries are involved in caregiving through the establishment of policy and the funding of programs. Research in policy studies in recent years has challenged previous assumptions of rational choice models, and advocated consideration of the relationship of policy to values and behaviors (see Coyle and Ellis, 1994; Estes, Linkins, and Binney, 1994; Stone, 1984, 1997; Yanow, 1996). March and Olsen note that " ... politics creates, confirms, or modifies interpretations of life … [R]itual, symbolic, and affirmative components of decisions are important aspects of the way institutions develop the common culture and vision that become primary mechanisms for effective action, control, and innovation" (1989, pp. 48–49). Policy is the social construction of a reality in which ambiguity provides flexibility and the potential for varying interpretations by those who implement it (Stone, 1984, 1997; Yanow, 1996). These interpretative approaches to policy ask about the creation and communication of shared and diverse meanings; the possibility of multiple meanings in policy and organizational actions; and the role of tacit knowledge in the communication of values, beliefs, and feelings (Yanow, 1996).

The chapters in Part I of this book point to the ways cultural assumptions influence the shaping of policy through political process, and the impact of these decisions on the way aging and elder care are viewed and practiced. Maeda's chapter demonstrates how conservative and progressive approaches to aging issues arise from different underlying assumptions. Japanese welfare policies result from political processes which refine these views in light of changing economic and social circumstances and varying interests, to shape Japanese policy. Campbell shows how government policy has shifted the public sense of problem regarding aging from demographics to caregiving, and by doing so has created a demand for new policies. The new Japanese long-term care insurance (*kaigo hoken*) represents the establishment of the welfare state in the area of elder care which radically redefines the roles of government, family, and individual.

These chapters on Japanese policy help American readers see the influence of cultural assumptions on their own practices. South and Bradham trace the gradual evolution of US policies *for* and policies that *affect* the elderly from the 1930s. They find that these incremental steps have improved the lives of many elderly people but that numerous contradictions and issues remain, embedded in political assumptions and process. Later, Bradham argues for the need for a preventive approach to illness as a way to both contain costs and to preserve independence and a sense of self.

Together these chapters support Hashimoto's conclusion to her comparative study of aging and the social contract in Japan and the United States, that fundamental beliefs and attitudes correspond to the approaches the two governments take in their policies.

> … the Japanese tend to expect more vulnerability in old age than the Americans, and seek security in maximizing the certainty of support rather than minimizing dependency. The Americans, by contrast, pursue a more open life course scenario than the Japanese, and tend to seek security by maximizing their autonomy. The premium placed on protection in Japan and on crisis intervention in the United States makes much sense in the context of these assumptions and preferences.
>
> (Hashimoto, 1996, p.184)

The new Japanese long-term care insurance, while its meanings are multiple and contested, thus arises out of common understandings of human society which contrast sharply with those of many Americans.

These chapters also point to differences in assumptions within the world of government and policy. Whereas built in to Japanese policies is an underlying dichotomy of welfare (which includes pensions) and medical services (see Bass, Morris, and Oka, 1996), American policy has allowed a more blurred distinction in the Medicaid program, but has placed great emphasis on housing which has been largely absent from Japanese policy concerns. The American framework might be divided into medical care, pensions (social security), and housing as its significant categories. These categories frame the questions and possible solutions that policies address. As Bradham's chapter exemplifies, American values emphasize maximizing choice and self-responsibility. He advocates a shift in assumptions of American policy to provide widespread support for self-care at earlier and healthier stages of life, focusing on prevention rather than the crisis intervention framework that has characterized American policy. Japanese policy, by contrast, begins with strong insistence on egalitarianism and government responsibility, but these values and assumptions may need to be challenged to achieve other goals such as financial solvency or community control of services. The process of creating definitions and finding solutions is never complete.[9]

Providing care: professional caregivers

Professional caregivers are a critical bridge between policy and programs on the one hand, and the elderly on the other. Their practices are necessarily shaped by policy, directly through funding and legal sanctions, and indirectly through the creation of common understandings of their roles. For patients and clients, their professional caregivers are the manifestation of policies, conveying government priorities to citizens through their practices. On the other hand, as professionals, these caregivers are expected to be responsive to the needs of patients or clients, and of their families. Whereas policy makers deal with aggregates, professional caregivers reinterpret concepts such as needs as they face individual cases. When services are inappropriate or inadequate, they may alter their practices, become advocates for individual clients, and/or become involved in movements for social change.

Part II of this volume focuses on professional caregivers. Fetters and Danis report on their investigation of the values Japanese and American physicians bring to their practices near the end of their patients' lives, and note the implications of physicians' decisions for policy. The chapters by Long and Chihara and by Barnard explore the relationship between hospice policy and practice in Japan and the United States respectively. In both countries, they find discrepancies between ideal hospice practice and the realities of hospice care due in part to funding decisions or regulations which limit the professionals' ability to carry out hospice philosophy. Although policies may be purposely ambiguous to accommodate conflicting interests (Stone, 1984; Yanow, 1996), in these cases, the ambiguity may additionally reflect broad cultural ambivalence about aging and dying.

Assisting in care: nonprofit organizations and volunteers

In the US and increasingly in Japan, the services established by policies are delivered to clients through non-governmental organizations. Like professional caregivers, the employees and volunteers in the nonprofit sector are in a structurally ambiguous position between policy and people, and they may experience conflict between their roles as service provider and as advocate.

In Part III, Adachi explores the relationship between Japanese government policy and the delayed creation of a nonprofit sector. The recent policy shift in Japan came about through the activism of local citizens searching for alternative approaches to elder care. Their challenge to the established paradigm of government responsibility and government control illustrates some of the issues of interpretive analysis introduced in Part I. Suda directly addresses the question of role conflict for volunteers and nonprofit organizations. She concludes that despite America's much longer experience with this mode of service provision, American policy and cultural expectations have maintained the stressful ambiguity of this form of care. The chapters in Part III importantly point out that in different cultural contexts, terms such as "volunteer" and "community welfare" may carry quite different meanings.

Coordinating and caring: family caregivers

In both countries, families provide the vast majority of hands-on care and coordination of services[10] for those of the elderly needing assistance (Doty, 1986). Most research on family caregiving has focused at the micro level, concerned with interpersonal relationships and caregiver burden. Recent studies are moving beyond the stress-and-coping model of caregiving (Pearlin *et al.*, 1990). As research on the elderly has begun to ask the elderly themselves about the meanings and practices of their lives (Gubrium, 1993; Kaufman, 1986; Myerhoff, 1978), there have been calls for a similar shift in caregiving research, away from standardized questionnaires of stress and toward the actual experience of caregivers. In this process, some researchers define "meaning" as attributing meaning to the caregiving experience as a coping mechanism that lessens the burden of caregiving (Noonan and Tennstedt, 1997). Others are discovering positive aspects of caregiving (Kinney and Stephens, 1989; Kramer, 1997; Miller and Lawton, 1997) that complement or substitute for a sense of burden.

A second trend in studies of family caregiving is a renewed attention to the influences of society and culture. Kahana *et al.* (1994) point out that society represents a critical context that facilitates or hinders caregiving by families, informal groups, or formal services. Social customs and sanctions, legal dimensions of caregiving and decision-making, and government policy are all factors that shape caregiving and receiving. Differing cultural backgrounds are among these wider social factors, leading to distinct social arrangements and understandings of key concepts (Fry, 1994; Hashimoto and Kendig, 1992; Sokolovsky, 1997). In the cases of Japan and the United States, research has suggested that the same words mean different things in the two countries: reciprocity (Akiyama, Antonucci, and Campbell, 1997); family (Campbell and Ingersoll-Dayton, this volume; Hashimoto and Kendig, 1992); old age (for example, whether it is commonly defined by social status such as labor force participation, or by chronological age; see Keith, 1992); and caregiver role (Keith, 1992; Long 1996).

The chapters of Part IV exemplify both of these trends. The authors attempt to achieve more open-ended and descriptive responses to questions about caregiving, resulting in more balanced views of the variety of caregiver experiences. They provide new understandings of motivations to take on and continue tasks. Yet through the comparative approach, they insist on consideration of the wider context and the variations within and between societies. Campbell and Ingersoll-Dayton report that the "who" and "how" of family caregiving vary greatly within each society and that practices are often inconsistent with our national cultural stereotypes. Questions of who constitutes "family" and of burden and dependency may, however, be framed differently in the two countries. Caregiving in the US "is usually a short-term, intermittent role, and one frequently combined with employment" (Moen, Robison, and Fields, 1994, S184). In Japan, co-residence may be the significant factor in defining the caregiving role. In the chapter by Harris and Long, the assumption of female caregiving as "natural" is challenged as men increasingly take on the responsibility for elder care in both countries. Both of these chapters in Part IV draw out implications for policy, stressing the need to be aware of unquestioned assumptions and of social change in creating programs and services. The meaning of experience cannot be predicted from surveys, nor can practice in individual cases be assumed by reference to cultural values.

Facilitating care of the self

Jaffe and Miller (1994) suggest that a problem with community surveys of caregiving is that they begin with the assumption that the elderly constitute a burden, and do not raise the question of meaning. Such research disregards the impact of societal and cultural factors on both caregiving and research interactions, and renders subjects' voices inaudible. There is a need to recognize the subjectivity and individuality of the experience of caregiving and to consider the meaning of care as facilitating continuity of self, whether that care is done by the self or others.

Part V of the book returns to the issue initially raised by Bradham in Part I: how can we best facilitate continuity of individual elderly selves? Bradham's answer is to alter the policy paradigm. In contrast, the chapters in this section by Kurokawa, Nguyen *et al.*, and Saito respond to this question by advocating particular programs and practices to assist in assuring that continuity. Kurokawa describes her work with dementia patients that offers opportunities for them to express creativity and thus a continued sense of self. Nguyen, Hill, and Cole have developed a program based on narrative and ritual to provide continuity in the lives of nursing home patients and to allow them to present themselves as whole persons rather than the frail physical beings they have become in late life. Saito explores problems with decision-making about elderly patients, advocating an approach that maximizes the continuity of their selves. These authors insist that policies and programs in both countries can and should do much more to insure care of *persons* rather than merely providing support for frail bodies viewed in isolation from the context of their life histories.

Because the experience of dementia challenges casual notions of "self," research in gerontology has paid particular attention to problematizing this concept. In this regard, the Japanese and American authors of this section come to different conclusions about what is needed for improving care for those with dementia due to different historical cultural assumptions in each society. Kurokawa and Saito argue that elderly people with dementia in Japan are often prematurely treated as incapable of autonomous decision-making and creative expression because of cultural assumptions regarding family caregiving. On the other hand, Nguyen *et al.* and Deal and Whitehouse see a need for care based not on the historical association of self with cognitive ability, but on continued integration of the person in family and community. Beginning from different problems, the Japanese and the American authors thus argue for shifting our concept of self in different directions, but all agree that the notion of continuity of self is critical to good care, and that we must expand our understanding of human aging to recognize both the autonomous and the social aspects of self.

The book concludes with an epilogue by David Plath, an eminent scholar of life course in Japan, who offers an alternative perspective. Reflecting on his own life course in light of his experiences in Japan and the US, he challenges us to reconsider our discussions of self and of care. He reminds us that humans are physical beings in a material world. Our definitions of selves are incomplete if we do not incorporate consideration of the body and its relationship to the material world. Aging and caregiving are readjustments and reinterpretations of this relationship, creating both continuities and discontinuities of self.

This volume, then, is designed to stimulate the reader to reconsider the multilayered meanings of care. It aspires to a more robust understanding of care and caring, from policy, cultural, and "on-the-ground" perspectives. It is our hope that this broad, integrated mosaic will illuminate care, caregiving, and meaning in late life.

Notes

1 For a discussion of the variety of theoretical approaches represented in gerontological research, see Marshall (1994).
2 Biegel and Blum (1990) lay out the spectrum of issues, but there does not seem to be any attempt to integrate the various levels of analysis.
3 See, for example, Noguchi and Wise (1994) for explicit descriptive comparison; however, they are not concerned with caregiving or with questions of meaning.
4 The 1997 figures for the US are 12.7 percent and for Japan 15.4 percent (US Department of Commerce, 1997, p. 832). We should note the arbitrary nature of the cut-off of the category of middle age at 65. The widespread use of this age in Japan seems to be relatively recent, since in the Chinese world view and in policies such as retirement age until very recently, other years, e.g. 55 and 60, were deemed significant. The age of 65 seems to have had little cultural significance until the need to make international comparisons.
5 76.0 in the US and 79.7 in Japan (US Department of Commerce, 1997, pp. 832–833).
6 2.06 in the US and 1.47 in Japan (US Department of Commerce, 1997, pp. 832–833).
7 See Ikegami and Campbell, 1996 for detailed analyses of differences in the two systems.
8 The rates for Japan (1993) were 16.6 per 10,000 for the entire population and 32.2 for those 65 and older. In the US (1991), the rates were 12.2 for the total population and 19.7 percent for the 65 and older population (World Health Organization, 1994). The rates for elderly Japanese women were higher than those for Japanese men and for American men and women, and this is often interpreted in Japan as an indication of their unwillingness to burden daughters-in-law with their care.
9 For descriptions of the Japanese care system, see Anbacken, 1997; Noguchi and Wise, 1994; and Bass, Morris, and Oka, 1996. For a discussion of US family policy, or lack thereof, see Hooyman and Kiyak, 1996.
10 Shanas and Sussman note that families can serve as a "buffer for elderly persons in [their] dealing with bureaucracies, examine the service options provided by organizations, effect the entry of the elderly person into the program of bureaucratic organizations, and facilitate the continuity of the relationship of the aged member with the bureaucracy" (1977, p. 216).

References

Akiyama, H., Antonucci, T.C., and Campbell, R. (1997). Exchange and reciprocity among two generations of Japanese and American women. In J. Sokolovsky (Ed.), *The cultural context of aging*. Westport, CT: Bergin & Garvey.
Anbacken, E.M. (1997). *Who cares? Culture, structure, and agency in caring for the elderly in Japan*. Stockholm: Stockholm East Asian Monographs, No. 9.
Bass, S.A., Morris, R., and Oka, M. (Eds). (1996). *Public policy and the old age revolution in Japan*. New York: Haworth Press, Inc.
Biegel, D.E., and Blum, A. (1990). Introduction. In *Aging and caregiving: Theory, research, and policy* (pp. 9–23). Newbury Park: Sage Publications.
Bengston, V., Rosenthal, C., and Burton, L. (1994). Paradoxes of families and aging. In R.H. Binstock and L.K. George (Eds), *Handbook of aging and the social sciences* (pp. 254–282). San Diego: Academic Press.
Cohen, L. (1994). Old age: Cultural and critical perspectives. *Annual Review of Anthropology* 23, 137–158.
Coyle, D.J., and Ellis, R.J. (1994). *Politics, policy, and culture*. Boulder: Westview Press.
Doty, P. (1986). Family care of the elderly: The role of public opinion. *Milbank Memorial Fund Quarterly 64*, 34–75.

Estes, C.L., Linkins, K.W., and Binney, E.A. (1994). The political economy of aging. In R.H. Binstock and L.K. George (Eds), *Handbook of aging and the social sciences* (pp. 346–361). San Diego: Academic Press..

Fry, C.L. (1994). Age, aging, and culture. In R.H. Binstock and L.K. George (Eds), *Handbook of aging and the social sciences* (pp. 118–136). San Diego: Academic Press.

Gubrium, J.F. (1993). *Speaking of life: Horizons of meaning for nursing home residents*. New York: Adine De Gruyter.

Hashimoto, A. (1996). *The gift of generations: Japanese and American perspectives on aging and the social contract*. Cambridge: Cambridge University Press.

Hashimoto, A., and Kendig, H.L. (1992). Aging in international perspective. In H.L. Kendig, A. Hashimoto, and L.C. Coppard (Eds), *Family support for the elderly: The international experience* (pp. 3–14). Oxford: Oxford University Press.

Hobbs, F.B. (1996). 65+ in the United States. Current Population Reports, Special Studies, P23–190. Washington, DC: US Department of Commerce, Economics and Statistics Administration, Bureau of the Census.

Hooyman, N., and Kiyak, H.A. (1996). *Social gerontology* (4th ed.). Boston: Allyn and Bacon.

Ikegami, N., and Campbell, J.C. (Eds). (1996). *Containing health care costs in Japan*. Ann Arbor: University of Michigan Press.

Jaffe, D.J., and Miller, E.M. (1994). Problematizing meaning. In J.F. Gubrium and A. Sankar (Eds), *Qualitative methods in aging research*. Thousand Oaks, CA: Sage Publications.

Kahana, E., Kahana, B., Johnson, J.R., Hammond, R.J., and Kercher, K. (1994). Developmental challenges and family caregiving. In E. Kahana, D.E. Biegel, and M.L. Wykle (Eds), *Family caregiving across the lifespan* (pp. 3–36). Thousand Oaks, CA: Sage Publications.

Kaufman, S.R. (1986). *The ageless self: Sources of meaning in late life*. Madison: University of Wisconsin Press.

Keith, J. (1992). Care-taking in cultural context: Anthropological queries. In H.L. Kendig, A. Hashimoto, and L.C. Coppard (Eds), *Family support for the elderly: The international experience* (pp. 15–30). Oxford: Oxford University Press.

Kinney, J.M., and Stephens, M.A.P. (1989). Hassles and uplifts of giving care to a family member with dementia. *Psychology and Aging, 4*, 402–408.

Kōseishō (Ministry of Health and Welfare). (1996). *Kōsei hakusho, Heisei 8 nenpan* (1996 Health and Welfare White Paper). Tˆokyo: Kōseishō.

Kōseishō (Ministry of Health and Welfare). (1997a). *Kokumin Eisei no Dōkō* (Trends in Public Health), *44*, 9. Tokyo: Kōsei Tōkei Kyōkai.

Kōseishō (Ministry of Health and Welfare). (1997b). *Kōsei hakusho, Heisei 9 nenpan* (1997 Health and Welfare White Paper). Tokyo: Kōseishō.

Kramer, B.J. (1997). Gain in the caregiving experience: Where are we? What next? *The Gerontologist, 37*, 2, 218–232.

Long, S.O. (1996). Nurturing and femininity: The ideal of caregiving in postwar Japan. In A. Imamura (Ed.), *Re-imaging Japanese women* (pp. 156–176). Berkeley: University of California Press.

March, J.G., and Olsen, J.P. (1989). *Rediscovering institutions: The organizational basis of politics*. New York: The Free Press.

Marshall, V.W. (1994). The state of theory in aging and the social sciences. In R.H. Binstock and L.K. George (Eds), *Handbook of aging and the social sciences* (pp. 12–30). San Diego: Academic Press.

Miller, B., and Lawton, M.P. (1997). Introduction: Finding balance in caregiver research. In Symposium: Positive aspects of caregiving. *The Gerontologist, 37*, 2, 216–217.

Moen, P., Robison, J., and Fields, V. (1994). Women's work and caregiving roles: A life course approach. *Journal of Gerontology: Social Sciences, 49*, 4, S176–186.

Myerhoff, B. (1978). *Number our days*. New York: Simon & Schuster.

Noguchi, Y., and Wise, D.A. (Eds). (1994). *Aging in the United States and Japan: Economic trends*. Chicago: University of Chicago Press.

Noonan, A.E., and Tennstedt, S.L. (1997). Meaning in caregiving and its contribution to caregiver well-being. *The Gerontologist, 37*, 6, 785–794.

Pearlin, L.I., Mullan, J., Semple, J., and Skate, M. (1990). Caregiving and the stress process: An overview of concepts and their measures. *The Gerontologist, 30*, 583–594.

Shanas, E., and Sussman, M.B. (1977). Family and bureaucracy: Comparative analyses and problematics. In E. Shanas and M.B. Sussman (Eds), *Family, bureaucracy, and the elderly* (pp. 215–225). Durham, NC: Duke University Press.

Sokolovsky, J. (Ed.). (1997). *The cultural context of aging* (2nd ed.) Westport, CT: Bergin & Garvey.

Stone, D. (1984). *The disabled state*. Philadelphia: Temple University Press.

Stone, D. (1997.) *Policy paradox: The art of political decision making*. New York: W.W. Norton & Co.

Tobin, J.J. (1987). The American idealization of old age in Japan. *The Gerontologist, 27*, 53–58.

US Bureau of the Census. (1996). *65+ in the United States, Special studies, P23-190*. Washington, DC: US Government Printing Office.

US Department of Commerce, Bureau of the Census. (1997). *The statistical abstract of the United States* (117th ed.). Washington, DC: US Department of Commerce, Bureau of the Census.

World Health Organization. (1994). *World health statitics annual, 1993*. Geneva: Organisation Mondiale de la Saute.

Yanow, D. (1996). *How does a policy mean? Interpreting policy and organizational actions*. Washington, DC: Georgetown University Press.

Part I
Assuring Care
Government policies and programs

1 Cultural meanings of "security" in aging policies

Akiko Hashimoto

Postindustrial societies today contend with a new population dynamics that has never before existed in their demographic history. As the number of older people grows, countries such as Japan and the United States must determine how to best organize themselves to provide for the needs of this population, while fostering the sense of social contract for the society as a whole. The constraints are real: fiscal and material resources are limited and must be shared in a way that is perceived to be just. These societies must therefore ultimately confront the fundamental question of who gets what, how, and why, to formulate their aging policies in the twenty-first century.

The reappraisal of fundamentals is important; after all, resource allocation hinges not only on fiscal and material constraints, but also on our values and interests – about who *ought* to help whom, and how we *ought* to organize such priorities. Ultimately, our preferences are subjective, based on cultural assumptions and ideals that are embedded in the political economy. Effective aging policies, therefore, require not just a technical evaluation of material costs and benefits of the social security system, but also a normative evaluation of the underlying values, choices, and preferences. In this chapter, my purpose is to explore just how such values and perceptions of security in old age compare in Japan and the United States, and then suggest how each affects social policy.

Cultural assumptions, as defined in this analysis, derive from our interpretations of the subjective experiences in this world, sedimented in our cultural memory. These assumptions are part of the internalized subjective knowledge that creates the symbolic universe, shared by the individuals in that culture (Berger and Luckmann, 1966). These assumptions constitute a *habitus*, a system of generative schemes that makes possible the thoughts, perceptions and actions that are inherent in the particular conditions of society (Bourdieu, 1990). Thus, cultural assumptions are part of a structure of dispositions conducive to particular preferences, and embrace their own logic of practice.

The notions of old-age security that we will discuss here are part of this internalized subjective knowledge. They derive from our perceptions and expectations about vulnerability at the end of life, and about the possibilities of help available in times of such need. The meanings of "security," then, are defined by these ideals, perceptions, and expectations of vulnerability and help (Hashimoto, 1996).

The cultural construction of old age security

Indeed, societies embrace different notions of "security," and refer to the different qualities of safety in everyday life. This security not only refers to physical safety, but also to safety in the generic sense, the feeling of being part of a social world that revolves around a familiar order with some predictability. It is a sense of fundamental trust that we understand that part of society which comprises our everyday world, and that we also have the ability to anticipate and encounter life's twists and turns with some measure of effectiveness. Such trust in the order of the world – ontological security – gives us the essential means to control our anxiety over what life has in store for us in a fundamental way (Giddens, 1984).

This security, broadly defined, is integral to our expectations about the quality of help we would like to receive in old age, and to our sense of control over possible future calamities. In a more concrete sense, security in old age refers to our sense that support and means of subsistence will be available in a particular way, given what we assume to be our future needs. In our US–Japan comparison, we can identify two *prototypes* of such old age security: the protective approach, and the contingency approach.

Structured security: the protective approach in Japan

The Japanese sense of security is based on a structure of *protection* that is geared toward promoting *certainty* and *predictability*. For many Japanese elderly, the concrete plan for old age derives from a preference for the security of knowing exactly when and from where support will come. A genuine sense of security in Japan, therefore, comes from an anticipation that help will be forthcoming from the elderly person's immediate environment as matters turn for the worse. The support system is therefore designed to protect and guarantee, rather than to promote autonomy and independence.

The relatively high rate of filial coresidence in Japan is one obvious example that attests to this fundamental ideal of long-term security. Even though primogeniture was abolished a half century ago, this residential pattern often continues to represent a cultural ideal and a common living arrangement that makes normative sense for many elderly.

Coresidence is preferred – even in its varied guises today – not only because of the obvious economic benefits of pooling financial resources and sharing the costs of living. It is preferred also because it offers a specific type of security that maximizes predictability. The three-generation household and its more recent variants (such as *nisedai setai*, where three generations live in two households housed in the same building or compound) are an entirely concrete and tangible informal social security system that establishes exactly who will do what for the elderly when they become frail, bedridden or otherwise acutely needy. The arrangement exacts that commitment from the coresident adult children even before such need arises – very early on in the family life cycle. As such, this arrangement creates certainty of knowledge about the definite availability of identifiable primary caregivers when need arises. This is what many Japanese consider "dependable" security.

The link between the preference for coresidence and the expectation of predictability is evident in the following remarks of Japanese elderly who were interviewed for my comparative study (Hashimoto, 1996):

> There used to be just the three of us here – me, my daughter and her husband. The younger ones lived out. Last summer, my grandson, his wife and the two children came back to live with us. They came back, because the little one goes to nursery school this year. He had to come back some time anyway. He's the eldest son.
> (Fuku Yoshino, aged 81, p. 76)

> I made up my mind long ago – what to do when my husband was gone. He used to say I should go with the one I liked. But the right thing was to be with the eldest son. This was all for the best. It's not done otherwise. It's not pleasant to mention [another option]. So, I never complained to anybody. I was going to go with my eldest son, unless something really bad happened. There are all kinds [of conflicts] when you have ten children.
> (Hiro Fukaya, aged 68, p.85–86)

> The younger ones used to live here upstairs, when they worked here. Then, my son was offered the shop over in Atsugi, so they moved. It's his own sushi shop now … So, after my wife died, I started to live alone. It never crossed my mind [to live in a nursing home]. Yes, when I can't manage anymore by myself in old age, my son in Atsugi is going to look after me. And my *o-yome-san* [daughter-in-law] is just a jewel. I genuinely have nothing at all to worry about. Yes, *eventually* – yes, I will move to Atsugi.
> (Fumihiko Sakuma, aged 66, p. 97)

As these examples illustrate, the premium is placed on certainty and predictability: the unwillingness to leave matters undecided and the unwillingness to leave help up to voluntary goodwill are also important characteristics of the Japanese sense of security in old age. Even when the timing of coresidence is postponed or delayed to adjust to geographically mobile children – such as in the Sakuma family above – this ideal of security often remains critical in many Japanese cases.

Diffused security: the contingency approach in the United States

Many Americans, by contrast, tend to embrace a structure of security that is geared toward promoting choice and autonomy. Characteristically, they take a *contingency* approach to old age security, which presupposes that individuals are self-sufficient until that critical point when they need to reach out to a variety of resources for help. The locus of action in this contingency approach is the receivers of help, not the givers of help as in the protective approach.

Help is customized according to individual need in the contingency approach, and the timing of intervention can vary from one person to another. For some, need may be precipitated by widowhood, and for others, by the onset of illness. Help is provided according to individual need, access and preferences, because the perception and recognition of need are individualized. As a general pattern, the American elderly tend to rely on their informal network for their emotional and some physical needs, while counting upon social security payments and other pension benefits for their financial independence. This *diffuse* helping network represents a preference for a particular kind of security that is different from the Japanese prototype: it privileges *autonomy* over certainty.

Children, relatives, friends and neighbors are all essential members of the resource network in this approach (Cantor, 1979); there is often a greater degree of triangulation of resources among Americans, extending beyond the older person's household. If the helping network can be spread widely, then the relative independence of the elderly person at the center of it can actually be enhanced. This extensive network therefore helps to safeguard autonomy for many of the elderly in the United States.

To put it differently, in this contingency approach, old age security is fully complete only when people can *choose* their own support from a range of options, because choice gives them a degree of control. It does not follow, then, that Americans are more carefree about old age than the Japanese, or that the Japanese children are more dutiful than Americans. The two approaches to security in old age differ because of different ideals and goals.

The link between the preference for autonomy and the expectation of open-ended choices in the American case is evident in remarks such as the following (Hashimoto, 1996):

> Years ago that's the way it used to be. Before you had those housing projects and social security. You had no choice. Either the poorhouse or go live with your daughter. Nowadays...very few people live with their children. They'd rather be in a place like this [public housing for the elderly] than go to a nursing home or live with their children ... they want to be independent – as long as they can take care of themselves. Because they've been that way all their lives – they don't want to be dependent on anybody.
> (Ernest McCarthy, aged 79, p.122)

> It's not a question of dislike or disliking their family style of living or anything else. It's just a matter of independence for ourselves. We would never want to feel that we're dependent on our children.
> (Ben Bloomfield, aged 66, p.138)

> I usually could depend, if anything happened, on my sisters. But my sisters, all of them are very old and not too happy themselves. And my adopted daughter Ellen, she has her own family, she lost her husband and [has] her own family to take care of. They don't have to ask me for nothing ... The only thing I can think of now – that's why I'm working – [is] trying not to put myself in the position that I have to call somebody because I can't pay my electrical bill, or can't pay my telephone bill.
>
> (Stella Richards, aged 72, pp.116–117)

The kind of network illustrated above seems more suited to a society which embraces household transitions as a necessary condition of changes in the family cycle. Since "leaving home" is a concomitant of adulthood (Bellah *et al.*, 1985), a shared expectation on the part of both parents and children, American individuals and couples tend to form extensive networks outside the household which promote *diffused security*. The filial orientation in Japan, on the other hand, is conducive to forming a concentrated network focused in coresident children, and promotes *structured security* inside the household.

The expectations of vulnerability

The two prototypes of security discussed here correspond to the distinct images of vulnerability in old age found in Japan and the United States. These different mental blueprints are indeed based on different visions of need in old age. Although much research has advanced our understanding of life course transitions, Gunhild Hagestad (1986) has pointed out that comparable work on life course trajectories, the "prospective view of life" based on cultural life scripts, has been limited. Perhaps the most well-known example, in the context of comparing Japanese and American societies, has been Ruth Benedict's arc of freedom describing the different levels of social constraints experienced through the life cycle ([1946]1967). The effort to etch the trajectories of need in later life from cultural life scripts has been sparse, and yet it is essential in understanding the fundamental expectations about what a support system *ought* to do.

Different life course trajectories affect our level of preparedness for need in old age, that is, our sense of urgency about what should be done, and who should do something about it. How we see the inevitability of frailty frames our blueprint for obtaining future help. If we think frailty *will* happen, then the utmost preparation for it is not only prudent but necessary. If, on the other hand, frailty is something that *might* be likely as a matter of probability, then plans for support require contingency measures, just in case. The logical choice of action regarding future care, therefore, depends on the forecast about the future and the calculation of risk for that future.

This trajectory of need also plays a role in assigning the responsibility (and blame) for the problem. If dire frailty must eventually happen to everyone, then an individual is absolved from the blame of being frail: no one can be responsible for preventing it. But when dire frailty is one of a number of possibilities occurring in later life, it is very much up to the individual to stay physically fit: each individual is responsible, after all, for preventing the worst possibility from occurring as best as she or he can.

Different trajectories of vulnerability, then, lead to different notions about when people are responsible and obliged to give help. In the *will need* scenario, the Japanese prototype, individuals are not necessarily expected to help themselves; caregivers must, therefore, be involved in planning support from an early stage. In the *might need* scenario, the American prototype, caregivers intervene only when individuals show that there are needs to be met. In the examples cited, Fumihiko's son has already built an extra bedroom that Fumihiko will use in the future, but Ernest's daughter is not responsible for making such advanced plans.

Therefore, expectations of frailty are based on distinct assumptions about the nature of growing old. Perceptions of need in old age vary in Japan and the United States, because the two societies tend to embrace different collective life scripts. Childhood, adulthood and old age signal different needs because expectations and priorities associated with each of these life stages are different. Cultural repositories have defined these specific relationships between age and need differently: both *will need* and *might need* scripts see childhood associated with high need and adulthood with low need, but follow different scenarios thereafter. In the *will need* script, a life course comes to a full circle in old age when need increases again to the level of childhood. In the *might need* script, increasing need in later life may or may not exceed beyond the threshold where self-sufficiency is diminished. Hence, the difference between Fumihiko and Ernest's plans is based on such different trajectories of need in later life, at the end of the life cycle.

The two life scripts mentioned here represent crude scenarios which, in reality, involve different probabilities and they both seem more or less plausible when tested by personal and collective experiences. Accordingly, people will modify the basic script in a way that is meaningful to their own subjective experiences. In this sense, the basic scripts are prototypes that conform to the general experience known to the collective, subject to individual revisions; such individual revisions vary, because people have different capabilities to translate ideas into action (Swidler 1986).

Life scripts, trajectories, and transitions

Of the two societies, life course trajectories and needs are more closely intertwined in Japan. Historically, Japanese life stages have been clearly defined, punctuated by age-related celebrations that were expressed as rites of passage. As Takie Lebra (1976) describes, these definitions are notable also for old age. David Plath (1980) also points to the importance of expressing models of maturity in age-specific terms. The fundamental assumption that the young and the old have distinct needs in different life stages by ascription was also noted. These life stages are often associated with different strengths and weaknesses according to age status, and imply that age differences are irrevocable. While this understanding endorses the inequities of health, wealth and other qualities according to life stages, it also reinforces the recognition that unequal needs according to age are legitimate and to be expected. Thus, increased need in old age can be recognized as a given part of the life script, assumed as a matter of course for each succeeding generation. As individuals, the elderly have different life circumstances, but as a collective group they are perceived as a seasoned but vulnerable population. This stronger consciousness of age differences in Japan – and of needs associated with specific life stages – is also confirmed in comparative surveys at the national level. The attitudinal survey of the Japan Prime Minister's Office's (*Rōjin Taisaku Shitsu*, 1982), for example, shows that the majority of the Japanese elderly think of themselves as unequal to the young, while the American elderly feel that they are equal to the young.

The American life script, on the other hand, offers a sequence of status transitions that presumes life stages to be distinct, but generally equal in their perceived merits and rewards. The young and old are inherently different, but the demarcation between life stages in adulthood is not always as clear-cut as it is in the Japanese life script. As Bernice Neugarten and colleagues (1968) suggest, age norms significantly define the shared time tables in American society; yet in comparative perspective, the American life script also seems to assume a great deal more individual variation so that age differences can at times even be revoked, such as taking part in marathons or remarrying at age 70. Sharon Kaufman (1986) has also noted that milestones between birth and death such as marriage, childbirth and divorce have become increasingly flexible and age-irrelevant, as preferences and choices of lifestyles override the traditional demands of age appropriateness. If aging cannot be entirely controlled, it is still individualized and assumed to be "manageable" in post-industrial America by individual effort. Age can be just a mindset; as the saying goes, "you are only as old as you feel." Given the ethnic variety and the country's relatively short unified past, the American sense of the life course is more abstract and unmolded than in Japan; it is therefore more amenable to individual adjustments. "Very" old age signals vulnerability and need, but it is not easily made part of a collective life script, because it is also expected to vary individually. The tension between the realities of the life cycle and the ideals of making a possible fresh start at any life stage creates an ambivalence in directly associating need with old age.

Implications for aging policy

Different visions of social relationships, life course, and security described in this chapter have important implications for organizing support systems in these societies. Our comparative analysis suggests that the hallmark of a "successful" aging policy for the Japanese is likely to be found in prudent planning; and for the Americans, in facilitating resilient independent living. An aging policy aligned to the protective approach – based on the *will need* trajectory – will therefore likely emphasize measures that forestall impending crises. Policies aligned to the contingency approach – based on the *might need* scenario – will likely emphasize measures to enhance individual control as calamities occur. These projections are based on observations that Japanese men and women tend to favor an approach that minimizes the impact of future crisis and need, by addressing them in advance – according to their later life's scenario – and that the American elderly tend to prefer an approach that maximizes flexibility, so as to customize helping arrangements to individual circumstances.

As population dynamics change in the next century, it is reasonable to expect that some of our needs and social relationships in old age will also be transformed. It is therefore likely that, in the long term, new definitions of old age security may also emerge. If aging policies are to succeed in providing genuine security, however, a fundamental assessment of such definitions, of the assumptions about vulnerability will also be essential.

Note

This chapter summarizes some ideas that I have elaborated in my *Gift of Generations: Japanese and American Perspectives on Aging and the Social Contract* (New York: Cambridge University Press, 1996). Here, I have concentrated specifically on the cultural constructions of security and vulnerability from that work. The names of Japanese and American interviewees cited in this chapter have been changed to protect their anonymity.

References

Bellah, R., Madsen, R., Sullivan, W., Swidler, A., and Tipton, S. (1985). *Habits of the heart: Individualism and commitment in American life*. Berkeley: University of California Press.

Benedict, R. (1967). *The chrysanthemum and the sword: Patterns of Japanese culture*. Cleveland: Meridian Books. (Original work published 1946.)

Berger, P., and Luckmann, T. (1966). *The social construction of reality: A treatise on the sociology of knowledge*. London: Penguin.

Bourdieu, P. (1990). *The logic of practice*. (R. Nice, Trans.). Stanford: Stanford University Press. (Original work published 1980.)

Cantor, M. (1979). Neighbors and friends: An overlooked resource in the informal support system. *Research on Aging, 1*, 434–463.

Giddens, A. (1984). *The constitution of society: Outline of the theory of structuration*. Berkeley: University of California Press.

Hagestad, G. (1986). The aging society as a context for family life. *Daedalus, 115*, 119–139.

Hashimoto, A. (1996). *The gift of generations: Japanese and American perspectives on aging and the social contract*. New York: Cambridge University Press.

Kaufman, S. (1986). *The ageless self: Sources of meaning in later life*. Madison: University of Wisconsin Press.

Lebra, T.S. (1976). *Japanese patterns of behavior*. Honolulu: University of Hawaii Press.

Neugarten, B.L., Moore, J.W., and Lowe, J. (1968). Age norms, age constraints, and adult socialization. In B. Neugarten (Ed.), *Middle age and aging* (pp. 22–28). Chicago: University of Chicago Press.

Plath, D. (Ed.). (1980). *Long engagements: Maturity in modern Japan*. Stanford: Stanford University Press.

Rōjin Taisaku Shitsu (Office for Elder Policy). (1982). *Rōjin no seikatsu to ishiki: Kokusai hikaku chōsa kekka hōkokusho* (The life and attitudes of the elderly: A report from an international comparative survey). Tokyo: Ministry of Finance Printing Bureau.

Swidler, A. (1986). Culture in action: Symbols and strategies. *American Sociological Review. 51*, 273–286.

2 The socioeconomic context of Japanese social policy for aging

Daisaku Maeda

The important events in the historical development of social policy for aging in the past fifty years in Japan can be interpreted as the outcomes of conflict between conservative and progress-oriented people. The conservatives want to preserve the traditional East Asian family system as long as possible with a minimum of public expenditure for social security and social services. In contrast, progressives place supreme importance on the building of a welfare state and a welfare society as an ultimate national goal. They desire to renovate our social system completely so as to realize a society in which women are liberated from the traditionally imposed burden of caring for impaired aged parents-in-law in their own homes, and thus create gender equality.

A parallel conflict is that between those who believe that a free market system with the least public intervention for redistribution of the national wealth is the best mechanism for the development of the nation as a whole and those who believe that a modified market economy with a much heavier emphasis on social security, public health, and social services is the soundest and most reliable way to attain the national goal of building a true welfare society.

These conflicts represent differing values that have been brought to the policy-making process and have been played out against a backdrop of the rapid and profound social and economic changes over the past fifty years in Japan since the end of the Second World War. In addition to the rapid aging of the population, industrialization and urbanization have had a serious impact on the lives of people in urban as well as rural areas. In parallel with this rapid economic development, access to higher education, especially that for women, spread very fast in Japan. These days, almost all girls enter senior high schools and nearly half (46.8 percent) of female graduates of senior high schools enter higher education institutions, mostly four-year regular colleges (Monbushō, 1997). Many women who graduate from institutions of higher education obtain full-time professional jobs as nurses, teachers, various kinds of technicians, and the like. Moreover, the influence of western modern culture, especially that of the philosophy of individual dignity that almost inevitably accompanies the advancement of higher education, has had further profound impact on the traditional East Asian value system that has placed total responsibility on the family regarding the care of aging parents. Until very recently many conservative Japanese people insisted that the care of aging parents should be done in their own homes by family members themselves. Even the assistance of public home helpers should not be utilized. It should be pointed out here that in most cases the person who actually takes care of aging parents is the spouse of the son (daughter-in-law) who is, legally speaking, not obliged to do so. In many cases, these daughters-in-law have been forced to sacrifice almost totally their own lives in their middle age. These traditional expectations regarding the care of aging parents are now changing very rapidly among educated men and women. These social changes have played a significant role in developments in Japan's care service system for the elderly.

Overview of prewar policy for aging

This paper focuses on Japanese aging policies and their changes after the end of the Second World War. It seems, however, that for those who are not familiar with the history of Japanese social services for the elderly, a brief discussion on prewar policy will be helpful before starting the discussion on the postwar era.

Before the Meiji Restoration (–1868)

Social efforts for the welfare of the elderly in Japan can be traced back to charitable work by Buddhist temples. Since in ancient times Buddhism was in effect the national religion in Japan, it might be said that at that time the state was providing relief to poor elderly people. In feudal times, however, societal efforts for relief almost disappeared because of incessant wars between feudal lords throughout Japan.

Approximately four hundred years ago, the Age of Civil Wars came to an end when Japan was unified once again by the Tokugawa regime. Owing to the peace and prosperity of the Tokugawa era, many Buddhist temples were engaged in charity as one of the most important parts of their activities. Older people were the main recipients, as the Tokugawa regime placed a special emphasis on the virtue of respect for the elderly. It should be pointed out, however, that relief was the responsibility of neither the central regime nor of the local feudal lords. In other words, in the Tokugawa era, relief was essentially a charity to be performed by Buddhist temples or charitable individual people, though some feudal lords immortalized their names with their sincere relief efforts.

From the Meiji Restoration to the end of the Second World War (1868–1945)

In 1874, the new Meiji government issued the famous administrative order called *Jutsukyū Kisoku* (Relief Order) of 1874, which stipulated that frail elderly people of 70 years or more who had no relatives to support them could be given public relief. Other targets of public relief were orphans and severely impaired people. The amount of money given as relief was very small, sufficient only to maintain a bare existence. Furthermore, this order did not cover indoor relief (institutional care). Thus, indoor relief to poor children and older people had to be provided by the private charity of organizations or individuals. What the government did was only to give these almshouses a partial grant which covered a very small proportion of actual expenses. This limited Relief Order was in effect for more than 60 years until 1932, when a new Public Relief Law (*Kyūgo Hō*) was put into practice. The number of homes for the aged throughout Japan, then, was only 85 (Zenkoku Yōrōjigyō Kyōkai, 1933).

The new public relief law (*Kyūgo Hō*) stipulated that the national government should take responsibility of relief for the poor. Eligibility for relief was eased a little in comparison with the previous order, though it was still very limited from the standpoint of modern social welfare philosophy. This law lowered the age limit for relief from 70 to 65. In addition, indoor relief was approved as a legitimate form of providing assistance. The number of relief institutions was, however, still seriously short of the actual needs. As a result, many older beggars could be seen wandering here and there throughout Japan, while a huge amount of money was ungrudgingly spent for the expansion of military forces.

Japan's entrance into the Second World War in 1941 caused a devastating effect on the lives of Japanese people, especially on the lives of older people without children on whom to depend, of orphans, and of the disabled. During the war with China in the 1930s, the Japanese economy continued to expand. However, after entrance into the Second World War, all resources were poured into war efforts. Because of the shortages of food, clothing, and above all, money allocated to services for these people, the death rate among the institutionalized, especially older people, was extremely high. Such miserable conditions continued until the end of the war in 1945.

From military state to welfare state: changing national goals after the end of the Second World War (1945–)

Realization of a modern public assistance system

The defeat of Japan in the Second World War caused a thorough eradication of prewar ultra-nationalism and militarism. Instead, peace, democracy, human rights, and social welfare became the nation's goals. Just one year after the end of the war the old public relief law (*Kyōgo Hō*) was abolished, and a completely new public assistance law (*Seikatsu Hogo Hō*, literally translated as the "Livelihood Protection Law") was enacted in accordance with modern social welfare philosophy, though it did not recognize the legal right of people to ask for the provision of public assistance. Five years later, in 1950, that Livelihood Protection Law was abolished, and a new Livelihood Protection Law enacted. This is the present Japanese public assistance law, which recognizes the legal right of people to ask for the provision of assistance, and the right of appeal to upper administrative offices and also to the court when the applicant thinks that the decision of the local welfare office is not adequate in light of his/her needs. Due to this law, the living conditions of poor older people were significantly improved. One of the most significant effects of the new law was that older beggars who had been so commonly seen everywhere in prewar days almost disappeared.

The significance of the modern public assistance system was far more important at the time it was enacted approximately fifty years ago than can be imagined at present. It should be remembered that fifty years ago Japan had a public pension system which only covered government officials and the employees of a very limited number of industrial firms. Nor was there a universal public health insurance system at that time. It can rightfully be said that, without the role played by the Livelihood Protection Laws of 1946 and 1950 in the field of medical assistance, low-income Japanese people would have suffered much more severely from the societal confusion after the war.

Expansion of coverage of the public pension system

Another important step for the construction of the welfare state was the establishment of a public retirement pension system with universal coverage to secure minimum income after retirement for all senior citizens. Actually the first step in this direction, though very limited in its scope, was taken in 1941, before the end of the Second World War, in the form of a law for the establishment of public retirement pension insurance for people employed in mining, manufacturing, and other industries important to the war effort. Three years later in 1944, one year before the end of the Second World War, this law was revised so as to expand its coverage. The main goal of the 1941 and 1944 laws was to raise the morale of the employees of key industries, and thereby contribute to the national effort to win a victory in the war. It is to be noted, however, that this law also aimed at collecting money in the form of insurance contributions to the public retirement pension fund (when the Japanese public retirement pension system was started, it adopted a so-called "fund-based method"), which the government wanted to use to finance the huge military expenses needed to continue the war. Whatever its goals may have been, the 1941 law was the predecessor of the present National Retirement Pension Insurance Program for the Employees of Private Firms (Kōsei Nenkin Hoken).

In 1954, almost a decade after the end of the Second World War, the 1944 law was revised so as to cover almost all employees working for private enterprises, including those which have only a very small number of employees. The most important socioeconomic background for the expansion of coverage of the public retirement pension system was that the Japanese economy at that time was beset by widespread strikes. Policy makers could not help but do something to ease tension between management and labor, and management agreed, though reluctantly, to bear the heavy financial burden of paying one-half of pension insurance contributions.

The national government had another reason to be eager to realize wider coverage for the public retirement pension system. In addition to easing management-labor tension, it would be able to collect a huge amount of money from working people as contributions to the public retirement pension fund. The government could then invest these funds for the expansion and improvement of such basic social infrastructure as railways, airports, highways, and the like that are indispensable for the fast and steady development of a national economy.

Social changes and their impact on the lives of the elderly after the mid-1950s

Japan underwent rapid economic development and urbanization from the mid-1950s. According to the national census of 1950 the proportion of the population engaged in primary industries was approximately 48 percent. The national census done 35 years later in 1985 showed that this proportion was reduced to approximately 10 percent. The impact of change was so profound that it is sometimes referred to as the "second industrial revolution." Naturally, this exerted a very strong influence on social security and on health and social welfare services in general. Such rapid industrialization and urbanization greatly affected the lives of Japanese older people through a number of changes in the social and economic structure of Japan. I shall discuss some of the important changes below before considering the next stage of the development of aging policy in Japan.

Aging of the population

Because of improvements in the general standard of living as well as in medical sciences, since the early 1950s the number of very old people, aged 80 years or above, increased significantly. The growth of the elderly has meant an increase in the demand for various forms of care services. This increased demand is accelerated by the decreased capability of family caretakers, because the more advanced age of dependent older parents means that the age of their caretaking children has become higher. In many cases, children themselves are already elderly and their own health is not adequate to provide needed care.

Migration of younger people from rural to urban areas

The reduction in the agricultural population during the decades following the war brought about a great migration from rural to urban industrialized areas. As a result, even in rural areas, the proportion of older people living alone or only with a spouse increased significantly, though the proportion of such older people in rural areas is still much lower than in urban areas, unlike in other industrialized countries in East Asia, namely Taiwan and South Korea.

Dispersion of industrial areas

In addition to the great migration of the younger generation from rural to urban areas, the development of manufacturing industry led to a dispersion of industrial areas since the early 1960s. A large number of young people were forced to move to other industrial areas to find jobs. Thus, those people who were born and raised in urban locations often have found it difficult to obtain a job in the same urban area where their older parents live. This is one factor in the increase in the proportion of older people living alone or only with their spouse in urban as well as rural areas.

Increase in geographic mobility

Industrialization has brought about much greater geographical mobility of working people in general. In industrialized societies, people change their jobs much more frequently than before. Even when they remain in the same firm, employees are often forced to move to other industrial areas for various reasons. In such cases aging parents often prefer to remain at the original residence rather than move to an unknown place with the child's family in order to continue to live together. Besides, in Japan's industrialized areas, housing for workers is, generally speaking, not spacious enough for three generations to live together.

Increase of working middle-aged women

Another conspicuous change is the growing number of working women. Because of the shortage of male workers, many married, middle-aged women who were once the most dependable caretakers of dependent older parents are now working outside their homes. In addition, the number of married women who are engaged in full-time professional jobs has been increasing significantly. These women seldom quit their jobs to take care of their aging parents as those with part-time and/or unskilled jobs frequently do.

Awakening of a sense of selfhood

The awakening of a sense of selfhood among the general public aroused by higher education, higher living standards, and the cultural influence of western industrialized countries has also played a very important role with regard to the change in living arrangements of the elderly in Japan. For example, these days an increasing number of both older and younger generations prefer to live separately from each other just for the sake of personal independence and freedom.

Decrease in the number of children

The number of children in Japan has decreased rapidly since 1950. As a result, people with fewer children are now gradually entering the aged population. Obviously, when old people have fewer children, their chances of depending on them in old age are reduced. This factor will make the need for services for old people, both community and institutional, more acute in the near future.

Development of social policies for the elderly since the 1960s

Universal coverage of public pension insurance and public health insurance

Public pension insurance

The rapid and profound social changes discussed above drew attention to the need for a universal public retirement pension insurance system and also a public health insurance system. Through the efforts of university scholars, unions, and self-help organizations, the social movement for a universal public retirement pension was exposed and endorsed by the national media. In response to this growing social movement, a national advisory council on the issue was created, and the Ministry of Health and Welfare took initiative by drafting new laws and revisions.

When Japan's rapid economic development started in the middle of the 1950s, the public retirement pension insurance system only covered the employed people of private firms employing more than five people and engaged in major industries, such as mining, manufacturing, transportation, and the like. The employees of minor industries, such as retail shops, hospitals, and social welfare services, were not covered. However, as discussed in the previous section, coverage was greatly expanded in 1954 so as to cover all the workers employed by firms with five or more employees. Soon after the 1954 revision, the need for the expansion of coverage to self-employed people was pointed out by many progressive leaders of society who were committed to impartiality in public benefits among different categories of people. Therefore, the national government soon began preparations for a new public retirement pension program for self-employed people. The universal public retirement pension insurance coverage came into being with the National Retirement Pension Insurance Law for Self-Employed People (*Kokumin Nenkin Hō*) which was enacted in 1959 and put into practice in 1961. At present, after a number of revisions to broaden the coverage, all employees of private corporations of any type are covered by the public retirement insurance system for employed people. Those who are employed by firms run by individuals are covered by the public retirement pension system for the self-employed.

Here it should be noted that the Public Retirement Pension Insurance Law for Self-Employed People (*Kokumin Nenkin Hō*) did not enjoy smooth passage through the National Diet. Almost all influential labor unions at that time ran active campaigns against the passage of this bill. The main reason was that the benefits in the new retirement pension insurance program were very low compared to those provided by the programs for employed people. This was because the insurance contributions were to be paid only by the insured people in the case of the program for self-employed people, while in the case of the programs for employed people, the employers pay one half of the contributions.

Furthermore, the average income of self-employed people in Japan was (and still is) significantly lower than that of employed people. Therefore, the amount of contribution self-employed people could afford to pay was thought to be much smaller than the amount employed people could afford. In addition, because of the difficulty in adopting an income-proportional method in the calculation of the amount of contribution (it is very difficult to know the exact amount of income of self-employed people in Japan), both the contribution and the benefit were set at an equal amount for all insured regardless of the amount of their income. (Needless to say the amount of benefit is to be determined by the length of time the insured has paid contribution to the fund.) This means that the burden of contributions was felt more severely by lower-income people than those with higher incomes, while for those who had a good amount of income, the retirement pension insurance meant much less than for the average self-employed person.

Labor unions were also antagonistic to the proposed law from the Marxist viewpoint that prevailed among labor leaders at that time. According to their view, the national government's real intention was to collect more money by siphoning this off from the people in the form of contributions to the public retirement pension funds, most of which was to be invested for the strengthening and improvement of basic infrastructure needed for the rapid development of the national economy. The aim of this policy was, in their view, solely to increase the profit of capitalists. In other words, the labor unions regarded the proposed revision as a means to give more money to the rich on the pretext of promoting the well-being of the poor.

In spite of the strong campaign by labor unions, the bill was approved by the National Diet because the conservative party at that time had a majority in both houses. The labor unions later changed their attitude, and at least stopped their antagonistic activities against the new system. It should be noted, however, that recently some of the points raised by labor unions at that time have proved at least partially valid. At present, this program is facing a very difficult situation, which I will discuss later in the section dealing with the recent renovation of the public retirement pension insurance system.

Public health insurance

Before the 1960s the public health insurance system covered employees and their dependents only. Though Japan had had public health insurance programs for self-employed people since 1938, they were not compulsory. Each local government decided whether to take up this program or not and, consequently, quite a large number of local governments did not put it into practice.

Universal coverage of public health insurance became a reality with the National Health Insurance Law for the Self-Employed (*Kokumin Kenkō Hoken Hō*) which was enacted in 1958 and fully implemented in 1961. As in the case of the public pension system, the main impetus for the realization of universal coverage was the goal of impartiality in public benefits among various categories of people. However, unlike the pension system, the national government received unanimous support for this proposal, from management organizations to labor unions, because this system was to be run without any reserve fund. It was to be administered in a so-called "pay-as-you-go" manner.

This public health insurance program, too, is presently facing difficulties. Because the premium is very high compared to the program for the employed (because there are no contributions from employers, which in the case of the programs for employed is one-half of the total of contributions), a significant proportion of the insured are exempted from the payment of contributions. There are also not a few people who do not pay contributions for various reasons. This is because, unlike in the programs for employed people where contributions are deducted from their salaries every month by the employer and paid to the programs, it is not an easy task to collect contributions from the self-employed. The national government has been very lenient about allowing people to receive needed medical benefits regardless of whether or not they have made the required payments because medical care has in Japan come to be regarded as a basic human right. At any rate, the enormous financial deficit of this system is being compensated by the national government with general revenues.

In addition to this problem, the National Health Insurance System for the Self-Employed (*Kokumin Kenkō Hoken Seido*) had another serious drawback which has its roots in the structure of the total public health insurance system of the nation. That is, it had to cover a much larger proportion of the retired, because when the employed workers retired, most of them left the program for the employed, and joined the one for the self-employed. (Some stayed with the programs for the employed as dependents of their children who worked as employees). To deal with this fundamental shortcoming of the program for the self-employed, the national government took drastic action in 1982 with the enactment of the Health Care for the Elderly Law (*Rōjin Hoken Hō*), which I will discuss later in more detail.

Development of public services for the elderly after 1960

By 1960, Japan managed to succeed in meeting the basic needs of her citizens. At the same time, the basic legislative and administrative framework needed for protecting and promoting basic human rights had been put into place, i.e., the Livelihood Protection Law (1950), Child Welfare Law (1947), and the Law for the Welfare of Handicapped People (1949), universal coverage of public health insurance (1961), and universal coverage of public retirement pension insurance (1961).

Subsequently, the national government began to pay more attention to the social and humanistic aspects of the life of the people, and started to develop various public services to meet such needs, including the needs of the elderly for health, social, cultural, and recreational services. The efforts of the national government to develop public services for the elderly before the 1980s were designed to catch up with those of the other industrialized countries of Western Europe and North America. Except for several unique actions, Japan followed the paths which other industrialized countries had trailblazed for the promotion of the well-being of the elderly. We shall touch briefly on those developments which seem important in light of the purpose of this book.

Enactment of the Welfare for the Elderly Law (Rōjin Fukushi Hō)

In 1963, the national government enacted the Welfare for the Elderly Law. This law has two characteristics. First, it is a basic law which stipulates several basic principles to which all the other laws as well as governmental and voluntary actions related to the life of the elderly should conform. At the same time it is a law which regulates welfare services for the elderly, including institutional services, community care services, recreational services, and the like. When this law was enacted, it did not start any new program; in other words, this law was only a compilation of existing services at that time.

Why, then, was this law enacted? It was to ameliorate partiality in public benefits among different vulnerable groups of people, i.e., children, the physically disabled, and older people. As referred to earlier in this paper, Japan enacted welfare laws for children and the physically handicapped around the year 1950. These two welfare laws proved to be very contributory toward promoting the well-being of these two groups of people. Especially because of these welfare laws, all the services for children and the physically handicapped were separated from the public assistance system, except for public assistance in the form of cash payments to those who lived in the community. Accordingly, the assets test was completely abolished, and, in addition, a fee scale based on the amount of income was introduced, so as to enable anyone to receive needed services regardless of their income. Besides this, the procedures for income testing were simplified to a great extent. By these actions, families with children or physically handicapped people who needed public services could apply for them without any sense of the shame which almost always accompanies the reception of public assistance.

One of the most important factors that contributed to the enactment of the Welfare for the Elderly Law was social action promoted by the National Association of Welfare Institutions for the Elderly. Its leaders wanted to relieve the institutionalized elderly and their families of the sense of shame that accompanies public assistance. They also wanted to draw public attention to the importance of welfare services for the elderly, and to raise their level to that of the western industrialized countries as soon as possible. It is also to be noted that Japan was one of the leading countries in the world to enact a special law for the welfare of the elderly. As intended by the leaders of the National Association of Welfare Institutions for the Elderly, the very existence of this law played a significant role in the development of various public health and welfare service for the elderly thereafter.

Tax deduction programs

The income-tax deduction program for those people supporting parents aged 70 and over was started in 1972, and a similar deduction program for local income tax was started in the following year. The purpose of these tax deduction programs was to stimulate and promote traditional family support and the care of aging parents, especially those who were frail and impaired, in their own homes.

It seems to me that another reason for these programs was the serious shortage of public care services, necessitating that the national government do something to show that it recognized the important contribution of the family to the care of the frail and impaired elderly. Whether these programs have been and are really playing an important role in the preservation of traditional family care is doubtful, since the amount of the deduction is much smaller than the actual cost of caring for frail and impaired aging parents in their homes. It is actually a small token of appreciation shown by the society to caring families who are thereby saving public money.

Development of old people's clubs

When the national government enacted the Welfare for the Elderly Law in 1963, the legislature requested that local governments make every possible effort to provide needed help to old people's clubs and other organizations that work for the well-being of the elderly. Along with the enactment of this law, the national government started a subsidy program for the establishment and operational expenses of old people's clubs. In 1996, there were more than 133,000 such old people's clubs throughout Japan, and about 8,800,000 people, approximately 34 percent of the population aged 60 and over, are members.

National support for the establishment of community centers for the elderly

In 1963, the national government started a subsidy program for the establishment of community welfare centers for the elderly. These centers are multipurpose senior citizens' centers designed to provide counseling, health, rehabilitational, cultural, and recreational services for the elderly. These centers also play an important educational role. They frequently hold a so-called "old people's college," which is a series of lectures for senior citizens.

National support for elderly education

The Ministry of Education started a national support for elderly education program in 1973, and now adult education courses for senior citizens are conducted at least once a year in almost all local communities.

Development of social policies for the elderly after 1980

Policy statement on the "society of longevity" (Chōju Shakai Taisaku Taikō)

The proportion of the elderly in Japan exceeded nine percent in the year 1980. Since then, although the proportion of the elderly in the population was still low compared to other industrialized countries, the impact of population aging became increasingly clear not only to those who were directly engaged in work for the elderly, but also to leaders in various areas of Japanese society. In addition, many people also became aware that Japan was to become one of the most aged countries in the world within 40 years, when the proportion of the elderly in our country will be far higher than the present percentage in the Scandinavian countries.

Thus, in the early 1980s, many national government bodies appointed advisory councils and instructed them to investigate policies to be adopted to prepare for the rapidly approaching highly aged society. Among them, the most important was the establishment in 1985 of the Sub-Cabinet on the Aging Society by the national government. In the following year, 1986, a Policy Statement on the National Long-Term Program to Cope with the "Society of Longevity" was adopted by the cabinet. The cabinet also decided that the progress of the National Long-Term Program should subsequently be evaluated regularly.

From the viewpoint of social gerontologists who are well-informed on social policies for the elderly in Western Europe and North America, the contents of this Policy Statement were not new. Moreover, the goals were described in very abstract terms. It should be stressed, however, that in spite of the lack of substantiality in its contents, the Statement played a very important role in the development of social policies for the elderly in Japan. Actually, even before its formal adoption, while it was still being formulated, it exerted a strong impact on the policies of various national government bodies.

Enactment of the Fundamental Law of Policies for the Aging Society (Kōrei Shakai Taisaku Kihon Hō).

In November 1995, approximately ten years after the promulgation of the Policy Statement on the Society of Longevity, the Fundamental Law on Policies for the Aging Society was enacted by the National Diet. The purpose of this law was to establish a more solid and powerful basis for national policies and programs for the aging society than the Policy Statement of 1986, which was only a kind of administrative guideline set by the national government, though actually it exerted a much stronger impact than expected.

In accordance with the law, in July 1996, the national cabinet adopted the Policy Statement on the Aging Society which was to replace the former one on the "society of longevity" promulgated ten years earlier. Actually, however, there is no substantial difference between the two.

Programs started since 1980

Enactment of the Health Care for the Elderly Law (Rōjin Hoken Hō)

In 1982, the Health Care for the Elderly Law (*Rōjin hoken Hō*) was enacted by the National Diet, and then put into practice early in 1983. The purpose of this law was twofold: first, to strengthen and expand the health and medical services for the elderly as stipulated in the chapter on health and medical services in the Welfare for the Elderly Law (*Rōjin Fukushi Hō*) of 1963. The second aim was to relieve the National Health Insurance System for the Self-Employed (*Kokumin Kenkō Hoken Seido*) from serious financial deficits resulting from a lack of coordination regarding payment of medical services for the elderly in the overall system of public health insurance.

Let us consider the first purpose. The earlier programs stipulated in the Welfare for the Elderly Law of 1963 were substantially expanded in many respects. One of the most significant revisions was the lowering of the age limit for health checks and preventive services; namely, the age limit was lowered from 60 to 40. According to the new law, every local government is required to provide health check screening regularly to all citizens aged 40 and over (for uterine and breast cancer, those aged 30 and over are covered). The health check services are to be given for only a moderate fee or free of charge for low-income people. This law intends to improve the health of our senior citizens in the next century.

The second purpose of this law was to reconstruct the basic financial structure of medical services for the elderly for the coming era of the highly aged society, and at the same time to relieve the National Health Insurance System for the Self-Employed (*Kokumin Kenkō Hoken Seido*) that had almost gone bankrupt. As already pointed out previously, due to the nature of the overall structure of Japan's public health insurance system, it was quite natural that the National Health Insurance System for the Self-Employed (*Kokumin Kenkō Hoken Seido*) failed to maintain a financial balance. Let me explain in more detail. When employed people retire, they often leave the insurance program for employed people to which they have belonged and join a program for self-employed people. (Some of them are insured as dependents under their children's programs.) Generally speaking, retirees have a much smaller income than the employed, and in addition, they tend to suffer from various illnesses much more frequently than the employed people. Therefore, the financial deficit of the National Health Insurance System for the Self-Employed had been not only growing larger every year, but its pace had even accelerated due to population aging.

Before the enactment of Health Care for the Elderly Law (*Rōjin hoken Hō*), this huge deficit was compensated with general revenues of the national government. While the system for self-employed people was suffering from huge deficits, the programs for employed people were enjoying huge surpluses. Many of these programs were spending this surplus on extra services for the insured, such as luxurious recreation centers at spas.

In order to correct this inequity in the sharing of the costs of medical services for the retirees that was anticipated to grow rapidly in accordance with the aging of the nation, the new law stipulated that every public health insurance program, including those for the self-employed and those for employees, should contribute to a pooled fund for medical services for the elderly according to the proportion of the participants aged 70 and over in each program. This meant a considerably heavier financial burden on the public health insurance programs for employees that had been enjoying huge surpluses. Therefore, at first, both management and labor were quite reluctant to accept this revision. However, due to public opinion, the new law was approved by the National Diet with only minor modifications.

The introduction of the new financial system for health and medical services for the elderly, however, did not touch the other fundamental shortcomings of the National Health Insurance System for the Self-Employed (*Kokumin Kenkō Hoken Seido*), i.e., a significantly higher amount of contribution compared to the programs for employees and a high proportion of people who do not pay contributions. Thus, the national government is still compensating the huge financial deficit of this system with general revenues. No proposal for improvement has so far been made by the national government.

Renovation of the public retirement pension insurance system

In 1985, the Japanese public pension insurance system was completely renovated. (The renovation was put into practice in April, 1986). The main purpose of this renovation was to restructure these programs so that they can function well even at the peak of the aging of our society, which will come around the year 2020. For this purpose, all the public retirement pension insurance programs were integrated into a comprehensive single system called the National Pension Insurance System (*Kokumin Nenkin Seido*), though fundamental structures of each of the preceding programs were maintained. The level of retirement benefits was considerably reduced, though serious consideration was given to the interests of those who had already retired. In light of the much longer average life span of women, the benefit to the widow of the insured husband without her own pension was increased to some extent.

The renovation of 1985 was, however, incomplete in light of the anticipated financial difficulty the public retirement insurance system will have to face in the future. One of the reasons was resistance from the management circle, or *zaikai*,[1] regarding a raise in the pensionable age for full retirement benefits of employed people. Management was concerned that if the pensionable age was raised, the mandatory retirement age (generally 60 years of age) also would have to be raised, leading to a significantly higher cost to management. However, it is self-evident that the pensionable age and mandatory retirement age must be jointly raised to avoid the anticipated financial deficit of the system. Because of this resistance from the management circle, the government did not propose to raise the pensionable age for full retirement benefit to the Diet at the time of the 1985 revision. Thus in 1994, a further revision of the public pension insurance system was proposed, the main purpose of which was to raise the pensionable age for full retirement benefits of employed people. This was approved in spite of opposition by both management and labor. As a result, the pensionable age for full retirement benefits is to be raised from 60 to 65 between the years 2001 and 2013. Between age 60 and 65, retired people will qualify for partial benefits, the amount of which will be determined in accordance with their income.

Another important problem of our National Pension Insurance System is the financial difficulties of the program for the self-employed, which I described briefly in the previous part of this chapter. Here, let me explain the problem in more detail. In 1997, 17.6 percent of those who are expected to contribute to this program are officially exempted from doing so, because their incomes were too small or they had no income. An additional 15 percent of the insured did not pay their contributions in 1995 (Kōsei Tōkei Kyōkai, 1997), probably because the burden of contribution is felt too heavily by low-income people. Due to the limited benefits of the program, others who can afford it participate in private pension programs, while neglecting their payment to the public program. Still others do not pay their contribution because they think that they have sufficient savings for life after retirement. Thus for a variety of reasons, more than 30 percent of the self-employed are not contributing to the mandatory program.

The huge financial deficit of the National Retirement Pension Insurance System for the Self-Employed is really one of the most difficult problems the national government is now facing. Therefore, in January 1998, the Minister of Health and Welfare asked the National Advisory Council on Public Retirement Pensions to discuss the matter and present their recommendations as early as possible.

National subsidy program for the establishment of geriatric health care facilities

In 1988, the national government started a subsidy program for the establishment of geriatric health care facilities (*rōjin hoken shisetsu*). The purpose of such institutions is to provide long-term institutional care for the elderly who are suffering from chronic diseases and need skilled care, but not hospitalization.

Before this subsidy program, because of the lack of public home care and institutional services and because of lenient health insurance regulations regarding long term hospitalization, many of these people had been hospitalized for long periods. Needless to say, this represented a waste of society's financial and manpower resources. Another purpose of these institutions is to improve services to such patients by caring for them in places that have more medical supervision than nursing homes (*tokubetsu yōgo rōjin hōmu*). That is, the Japanese nursing home is not a health care institution, but a social welfare institution. Therefore, the health and medical care provided in Japanese nursing homes is limited. The new geriatric health care facility is to fill the gap between hospitals and nursing homes.

Actually, however, the most important aim of this program is to accelerate the development of long-term care institutions as a whole by utilizing public health insurance funds. Previously, nursing homes were established and run with money from general revenues. As it is almost always difficult to expand general revenues, the development of nursing home services in Japan has not been able to keep pace with the rapidly expanding needs for long-term institutional care of the elderly. Many social gerontologists specializing in the long-term care of the elderly suggest that, in industrialized societies, the number of beds for long-term institutional care should be at least 4 percent of the population aged 65 and over, even when the home care and domiciliary services are well developed. This means that at the peak of population aging, i.e., around the year 2020, Japan will need to have approximately 1,200,000 such beds. However, there were only about 150,000 nursing home beds throughout Japan when this program started. It seems to me that, without the establishment of this new type of long-term care institution utilizing the money of the public health insurance programs, realization of this goal would be almost impossible. (The mechanism to finance the establishment and operation of geriatric health care facilities [*rōjin hoken shisetsu*] is to be transferred to the new public long-term care insurance system [*kaigo hoken*] from the year 2000, as will be discussed later in this chapter.)

The establishment of this new type of long-term care institution, geriatric health care facilities (*rōjin hoken shisetsu*), brought about a small but important change in our public elderly care service policy. That is, because the geriatric health care facility is not a social welfare institution but a health care institution, it can be utilized just as hospitals and clinics are. In other words, unlike nursing homes (*tokubetsu yōgo rōjin hōmu*), geriatric health care facilities can be utilized by any older person regardless of the amount of income or the availability of family care. The costs for geriatric health care facilities are the same for all users regardless of their income or their family's income in contrast with nursing homes which, as social welfare institutions, set fees according to a sliding scale. Furthermore, when it is possible for older people to receive decent care from family in their own homes, the local welfare office will not place them in nursing homes; in the case of geriatric health care facilities, there are no such limitations. However, in some areas where the supply of geriatric health care facility beds cannot meet the demand, clients have to wait, sometimes very long, before being actually admitted.[2]

The shift in thinking of institutional care as welfare to institutional care as an individual option did not attract the attention of the general public. But it seems to me that the establishment of geriatric health care facilities was actually the starting point of recent changes in the Japanese elderly care service policy with regard to the legal responsibility of the family.

National sheltered housing program

In 1987 our national government decided to start a national sheltered housing program for the elderly under the name "Silver Housing Project." Before the start of this program, the policy of the national government on housing for the elderly placed major emphasis on the provision of public housing that had limited consideration of structure or facilities for the weakened physical and mental capabilities of older residents. No attention was paid to needs for temporary care services during a short-term illness or emergency.

In light of the predicted sharp increase in the number of the elderly living alone or aged couples living by themselves in the community, it is quite clear that a special type of housing whose structure and facilities are purposefully designed to accommodate frail and/or impaired elderly people should be developed, so that such older people may continue to live independently in the community. This type of housing is also expected to have temporary care services for short-term illnesses. If we fail to supply such housing in sufficient quantity, the demand for institutional care services will unnecessarily expand, a trend which will be much costlier for society than providing such housing for the elderly. Moreover, to assist people to be as independent as possible is one of the most important goals for all human services.

However, due to serious shortage of public housing for middle-aged wage earners, and also due to a lack of awareness of these needs, the government did not allocate any funds for public sheltered housing programs for the elderly before 1987. The national government changed its mind because, owing to many years of efforts to build public housing for middle-aged wage earners, these needs seemed to be almost fulfilled as far as the quantity of such housing is concerned, and the Ministry of Construction had to find other outlets for the huge amounts of public money it had been spending. The needs of the elderly for a special type of housing seemed to them the most appropriate goal to attract the attention of society and thus continue to secure their share of the national budget.

Notwithstanding the importance of this program, its progress has been very slow. This is mainly due to the policy that, in principle, sheltered housing units for the elderly should be added to existing public housing complexes when they are rebuilt because of deterioration. I doubt that the national government can succeed in this manner to secure an adequate quantity of such housing before the coming of the highly aged society.

National registration system for trained careworkers (kaigo fukushi-shi)

In 1988 the National Registration System of Trained Careworkers was put into practice, and the first national examination was held in early 1989. The aim of this system was to improve the quality of careworkers, and therefore secure better services for frail and impaired people living in the community and also in various types of institutions.

An implicit but important reason that the national government started this program was to make preparations for the anticipated growth of private care service agencies. Until recently, the national government was reluctant to do anything for the development of care services by for-profit agencies. However, in order to accelerate the development of the supply of home help services, the national government changed its attitude. That is, it abolished most of the restrictive regulations and even took several measures to promote its development.

Without a registration system of trained careworkers, however, it will be very difficult for the government to control the quality of service provided by for-profit agencies. The government also hoped that the registration system would make a great contribution to the improvement of the quality of care services provided by public bodies and nonprofit agencies in the community and in institutional settings as well.

Recent trends and current issues

Restructuring of the administration of health and welfare services for the elderly

In the year 1990 we witnessed a significant development in our social policy for the elderly: a fundamental restructuring of the public health and welfare services for the elderly implemented through the revision of the Welfare for the Elderly Law, Health Care for the Elderly Law and several related laws and orders. The crux of the restructuring can be summarized in the following two points.

Decentralization

First, in the 1990 revision of the Welfare for the Elderly Law, the authority to admit an older person into a home for the aged or a nursing home was transferred from the prefectural to the local government. With this change, the local government has come to assume all responsibilities for public health and welfare services for the elderly, from long-term institutional care to preventive, promotive, and recreational services. As a result, there has been better coordination among the various care services in regard to both the maximum quality of life and efficiency.

Long-term planning

As a result of the revision of the two basic laws, that is, the Welfare of the Elderly Law and the Health Care for the Elderly Law, all local governments were required to make a long-term plan for the development of health and welfare services for the elderly, including institutional care services, community care services, and preventive, promotive, and recreational services. Before the end of fiscal year 1993, all local governments had completed these long-term plans.

Ten-Year Strategy to Promote Health and Welfare for the Elderly and the move toward the new system for "care security"

In 1990, Japan had another significant development in the services for the elderly. The Ten-Year Strategy to Promote Health Care and Welfare Services for the Elderly (*Kōreisha Hoken Fukushi Suishin Jukkanen Senryaku*, commonly called the "Gold Plan" – "*Gōrudo Puran*" in Japanese) was promulgated by the national government. According to this plan, the pace of the development of various public services for the elderly was to be greatly accelerated.

The reason for the Plan was that the existence of a gap between the pace of the aging of Japanese society and that of the development of various social policies for the elderly had become quite clear. In order to cope with the predicted gap between supply and demand, the national government planned to introduce a new "consumption tax." To persuade the public of the necessity of the new tax, it proposed the Gold Plan as a long-term plan to cope with the coming aging society, presenting it along with the necessary huge cost which could only be raised with a new tax system.

This Gold Plan had to face considerable revision only five years later in 1995. Let me explain in more detail along with the gradual but significant change in people's attitude toward the care of impaired older parents in their own homes.

Around the year 1990, the highly aged society of the twenty-first century had come to be quite visible to everyone, not only because of the chronological closeness but also because of the actual expansion of the needs of the impaired older people and their caring family members.

Although the quantity of services for the elderly had been increasing more rapidly than before, the gap between the needs and services became wider due to rapid expansion of the aging population, especially that of the very old. Newspapers and television companies took up stories of miserable conditions of these older people and their family caregivers and demanded that the national government take action quickly. Thus most middle-aged and older Japanese have come to realize that the burden of the care of impaired older people will be too heavy for the relatives to bear themselves in the coming twenty-first century. In other words, they had come to recognize the need for so-called *kaigo hoshō* (literally translated, "care security"), a social service system by which all the care of older people, including both institutional care and home care, are met publicly regardless of income.

In March 1994, the Advisory Group on the Welfare Vision in the Coming Highly Aged Society presented its report to the Ministry of Health and Welfare. This report proposed, among other things, the construction of a comprehensive public care service system. It also pointed out that the goals set by the 1990 Gold Plan mentioned above were not sufficient in light of the predicted future growth of the care needs of older people.

In September 1994, the National Advisory Council to the Minister of Social Security disclosed its second report on the "Future image of the social security system." Among other things, the report stressed the pressing need for the establishment of a comprehensive public care service system as an integral part of our social security system and proposed establishing a public long-term care insurance program as soon as possible.

In response to growing concern about the establishment of a public care service system, the national government took two important actions. One was the revision of the goals of 1990 Ten-Year Gold Plan, now called the Revised Gold Plan. The other was the creation of a special task force for the development of a comprehensive public care service within the Ministry of Health and Welfare.

The Revised Gold Plan was made public in December 1994. Below, let me briefly explain the contents of the Revised Ten-Year Gold Plan. Its goals were to be reached before the end of fiscal year 1999.

- The number of home helpers will be increased from 31,404 (1989) to 170,000 (the original goal was 100,000). When the goal is reached, the ratio between home helpers and the population aged 65 and over will be 1:127.6. In Sweden this ratio is roughly 1:50, and Japan's goal includes part-time workers. This means that Japan's level will still be far below the levels of other advanced countries of Western Europe.
- The number of day care centers for the elderly will be increased from 1,080 (1989) to 17,000 (the original goal was 10,000). When the goal is reached, Japan will have one such center for every 1,300 people aged 65 and over, or a typical medium-sized city of 100,000 population will have approximately 13 such centers.
- The number of beds for short-term stay service (respite care service) will be increased from 4,274 (1989) to 60,000 (the original goal was 50,000).
- The development of home nursing services for the elderly will be accelerated. The goal set by the Revised Ten-Year Gold Plan is 5,000 home nursing stations throughout Japan. This goal was newly added in the Revised Gold Plan (in 1989, the number of such centers was negligible).
- The number of beds for long-term institutional care will be increased from 189,830 (1989) to 570,000. This means that when the goal is attained in 1999, the proportion of institutionalized older people among those aged 65 and over will be 2.6 percent. This figure is far lower than those of countries in Western Europe and North America where the average

proportion is approximately 5 percent. Parenthetically speaking, however, the average length of stay of older people in hospital in Japan is much longer than in other advanced countries. Thus, the actual gap between the needs and the available resources in the year 1999 will be considerably narrower than pure numerical comparison would indicate.
- The number of qualified workers will be substantially increased through the strengthening of various training programs. That is, the number of qualified careworkers will be increased by 200,000, trained nurses by 100,000, and trained physical and occupational therapists by 15,000 before the end of 1999. This goal was not included in the original Gold Plan.

In addition to the numerical goals described above, the Revised Ten-Year Gold Plan is to promote the following services as quickly as possible:

- Development of round-the-clock visiting personal care services by home helpers
- Improvement of nursing home facilities so that they have more private rooms
- Strengthening of the family doctor system
- Development of individual care planning for older people needing community care service
- Development of meals-on-wheels service
- Improvement of personal care service in long-term care hospitals for aged patients
- Modernization of nursing homes through the provision of grants for mechanization
- Expansion of community-based rehabilitation services
- Improvement and development of services for demented older people, especially the expansion of group homes
- Expansion of educational facilities and in-service training programs for careworkers and social workers working for the welfare of the elderly
- Development of technical aid service systems, including the strengthening of research and development systems
- Utilization of voluntary and private (for-profit) services for the diversification of service resources and for flexibility of the service delivery system
- Expansion of specially designed public housing for the elderly
- Improvement of physical environments for the elderly and the disabled so that they may live pleasant lives safely in the community.

Epilogue: Future outlook

As described in this chapter, Japan has a wide variety of programs and services for the welfare of the elderly. Most of the important services, however, have yet to be fully developed. Especially in the field of long-term care services for both community and institutional care, the shortage of services is very serious. In order to cope with this situation, the national government promulgated the Ten-Year Gold Plan in 1990 and revised it in 1994. However, the problem is that the aging of the population will continue at an accelerated pace in the next century, and various needs of older people, especially needs for long-term care, will grow very rapidly.

In order to meet the expanding needs for long-term care and secure a decent level of care services for every senior citizen, we shall have to start another Ten-Year Gold Plan before the year 2000. The budget needed for it will be much greater than that for the present Revised Gold Plan. Thus, securing the necessary amount of revenue for the second Plan to be started soon is one of the most important issues facing the national government.

The response of the national government is the establishment of a public long-term care insurance program. In June 1996, the Ministry of Health and Welfare finished its first draft of such a program and presented it to the National Advisory Council on the Health and Welfare Services for the Elderly. After long, patient negotiations with a number of related government advisory councils, political parties, and representatives of local governments, the Ministry of Health and Welfare finalized its draft in November 1996, and presented it to the National Diet. The bill was approved in December 1997.

As the subsequent chapter by J. Campbell (Chapter 4) will discuss issues related to the Public Long-Term Care Insurance System in detail, I here describe only some of the most important points of the new system. The Public Long-Term Care Insurance System will begin in the year 2000. It will cover both community care and institutional care services for older and middle-aged people aged 40 and over. It is to be financed with insurance contributions (50 percent) and general revenue (50 percent).

Therefore, in order to cope with the predicted conspicuous increase needed in the amount of general revenue due to this system and other related expenditures in the coming highly aged society, the national government raised the rate of the consumption tax from 3 percent to 5 percent from April 1997.

One of the very conspicuous social phenomena leading to the realization of this new program was the social action taken by a number of progressive voluntary associations such as *Kaigo no Shakaika o Susumeru Ichimannin Shimin Iinkai* (Ten Thousand Citizens' Association for the Promotion of Socialization of the Care of the Elderly and the Impaired) and *Kōreika Shakai o Yokusuru Josei no Kai* (Women's Association for the Realization of Better Aging Society). Some women's groups supported the proposal for long-term care insurance because they believed that the new system would relieve Japanese women from the traditionally imposed burden of caring for impaired aging parents or parents-in-law in their own homes. Representatives of some of the important citizens' organizations, including the women's groups, were invited by the Ministry of Health and Welfare to serve as members of national advisory councils to the Ministry. In addition, these groups held a number of national conferences to promote public long-term care and actively lobbied the government to make their voices heard. In addition, almost all media clearly supported the Ministry of Health and Welfare proposal. Thus, the voices of conservatives, especially of those who would stick to traditional gender roles became gradually weaker, and in the final stage of public decision we hardly heard them except in regard to some minor technical points.

In closing, I want too stress once again the anticipated revolutionary impact of the public long-term care insurance on our traditional value system. Even today, not a small number of middle-aged professional women, such as veteran school teachers, quit their jobs to take care of their own or their husband's aging parents. When the new system is put into practice, however, Japanese people will change their attitude, and place primary responsibility for hands-on care on the public long-term care insurance program. This is because in the insurance system insurer must provide the contracted benefits as a right of the insured regardless of whether or not they have children to depend upon as caregivers. Thus, the obligation of children toward the care of aging parents will become much lighter than at present. The expected role of children, especially that of the daughters-in-law, will be to provide auxiliary care voluntarily when the services provided by the insurance do not seem sufficient for maintaining the life of aging parents at a desired level.

It seems to me that the public long-term care insurance represents a major shift toward the emancipation of women from the traditionally imposed role of caring for impaired aged parents and parents-in-law in their own homes, a movement that started half a century ago in the miserable social and economic conditions resulting from the tragic war against universal human values, freedom, democracy, and above all, equality of all citizens.

Notes

1 Literally translated, *zaikai* means "finance world." In Japan, there are three national organizations of owners and top managers of business corporations. These people exert their influence on the ruling party in Japan through these three national organizations. In addition, these organizations have representatives on various national advisory councils.
2 The shortage of long-term care beds, both in geriatric health care facilities and nursing homes, is very serious in large metropolitan areas, like Tokyo, Yokohama, Nagoya, Osaka, and so forth. The reasons are the very high price of land in these areas. Thus, legally, older people can utilize a geriatric health care facility freely now, but actually in large metropolitan areas, it is just a "painted rice-cake" (*ga-bei*), as the Japanese proverb says. By the way, if older people move to areas where the supply of long-term care beds are sufficient, they can utilize them freely. But most of the elderly want to age at the place where they spent their middle age. In this respect, the Japanese and American older people seem to differ greatly.

References

Kōsei Tōkei Kyōkai (Health and Welfare Statistics Association) (Ed.). (1997). *Hoken to nenkin no dōkō* (Trends in public health insurance and pension insurance systems) (pp. 194–195). Tokyo: Kōsei Tōkei Kyōkai.

Monbushō (Ministry of Education). (1997). *Gakkō kihon chōsa* (Report of Fundamental Survey on Schools). Tokyo: *Chōsa Tōkei Kikakuka* (Statistics and Planning Section), *Daijin Kanbō* (Minister's Secretariat), *Monbushō* (Ministry of Education).

Zenkoku Yōrōjigyō Kyōkai (National Association of Homes of the Aged). (1933). *Daiikkai zenkoku yōrōjigyō chōsa* (The first national survey on institutional care services for the aged). Reprinted in Y. Ogasawara (Ed.), *Rōjin mondai kenkyū kihon bunkenshū* (Basic historical sources for the study of the problems of the aged), Vol. 4. Tokyo: Ōzorasha Publishing Company, 1990.

3 From the New Deal to the new millennium

Bridging the gap in US aging and health policy

Brett R. South and Douglas D. Bradham

Setting the stage for US aging and health policy development

Major policy issues surrounding the elderly in America are best understood in the context of a gradual federal-state commitment toward the aging population. In America, social welfare policies were born out of incremental government efforts to extend cash assistance, retirement benefits, and health care for selected groups of the poor, the elderly and the medically needy. Beginning in the late 1800s America's elderly gained increased attention as a national concern. With new advances in economics, business practices, technology, science and medicine, a changing perception of the elderly and their potential social contributions emerged. When the declining functions of old age slowed the speed and accuracy demanded in the work place, older workers were discharged. As medical advances documented the physical effects of old age – chronic illness, mental confusion and loss of physical functioning, the aged were seen as incapacitated and enfeebled. American society's view of the elderly, which had once depicted them as healthy and full of moral wisdom and practicality, was reduced to a diminished regard for their potential social contributions. By the turn of the century, with the growing public acceptance of these social concerns, increased public attention was placed on the needs of the elderly (Achenbaum, 1978). As early as 1914, many states adopted social programs meant to serve the health care and social welfare needs of the elderly, but it was not until the great depression of the 1930s that the federal government assumed an active role in social welfare issues through Roosevelt's "New Deal" program.

Throughout this chapter our discussion of US aging and health policy centers on both an historical and a policy perspective. Viewed from an historical perspective, the single most important aspect of US aging policy is the tremendous expansion of these programs that has occurred over a relatively short period of time (see Table 3.1). Since the mid-1930s, a complex institutional framework meant to assist aged Americans has developed in the United States. Eighty years ago, no nationwide apparatus offered any direct means of old-age assistance, nor did any federal institution seek to improve the general welfare

Table 3.1 Milestones of US aging and health policy

Year	Legislation	Provisions
1798	Congress passes act to tax seamen for health care	Establishes the US Merchant Marine Hospital Service and introduces the concept of pre-paid medical care
1935	Social Security Act (PL 74-241)	Establishes the Old Age Insurance program (OAI) which provides the mechanism to fund the public assistance programs of income replacement and retirement benefits
1937	Housing Act of 1937	Establishes the low-rent public housing program and provides housing and farm labor subsidies
1939	Social Security Amendments of 1939	Expanded Social Security Coverage to include survivor's benefits OAI is renamed Old Age and Survivor's Insurance (OASI)
1950	Social Security Amendments of 1950	Establishes a new payroll tax schedule, a higher taxable wage base, allows cost of living increases, and creates new ceilings on Social Security Payment calculations
1956	Social Security Amendments of 1956	Establishes the Old Age and Survivor's Disability Insurance Program. Introduces Social Security benefit payments to the disabled and their survivors
1957	The Forand Bill (HR9467)	Calls for an increase in the Social Security OASI payroll tax to provide for up to 120 days of hospital, nursing and surgical services. Although no Congressional action is taken, the Forand Bill draws increasing public interest
1959	Housing Act of 1959	Establishes further housing assistance by providing direct loans and mortgage subsidies
1960	Kerr-Mills Bill	Extends the 1950 Social Security Amendments by providing matching federal funds to the states for provider payments
1961	King-Anderson Bill	Proposed revisions of the Forand Bill by the Kennedy Administration
1964	Food Stamp Act of 1964	Provides a voucher system or "coupons" for low-income elders or families to obtain a nutritionally adequate diet
1965	Johnson Hospital Care Bill	Proposed bill by the Johnson Administration. Allows coverage of sixty days of medical care instead of ninety days

Continued ...

Table 3.1 Milestones of US aging and health policy (continued)

Year	Legislation	Provisions
1965	AMA Eldercare Bill	Proposed bill by the American Medical Association calling for "voluntary" comprehensive medical insurance for those over sixty-five funded by matching federal-state funds
1965	Byrnes Bill	Proposed bill sponsored by representative John W. Byrnes calling for a "voluntary" comprehensive medical insurance for those over sixty-five financed by graduated income tax premiums
1965	The Health Insurance for the Aged Act (PL 89-97)	Compromise plan that emerges from the above three proposed bills. Establishes the programs of Medicare and Medicaid
1972	Social Security Amendments of 1972	Establishes the federal program Supplemental Security Income (SSI) which provides further public assistance for the aged, blind and disabled
1974	Housing and Community Development Act of 1974	Amends the Housing Acts of 1937 and 1959 by expanding federal assistance for housing subsidies
1982	Tax Equity and Fiscal Responsibility Act (TEFRA)	Establishes managed care capitated payment options under a prospective payment system. Introduces the Diagnosis Related Groups
1986	The Omnibus Reconciliation Act of 1986 (PL 99-509)	Expands availability of Medicaid assistance to the poor and elderly through "buy-in" agreements between the states and the federal government
1988	The Medicare Catastrophic Coverage Act of 1988 (MCCA)	Expands Medicare to cover all hospitalization costs after payment of an annual deductible, increases Medicaid buy-in provisions, adds spousal protections, creates the Pepper Commission, places caps on out-of-pocket physician costs, and covers prescription drugs
1989	Repeal of the 1988 Medicare Catastrophic Coverage Act	Repeals all provisions of the 1988 MCCA except the Medicaid buy-in provisions, spousal protections and the Pepper Commission.

or health care of America's elderly. Today, every elderly person is affected in some way by one or more programs providing an ever-expanding range of benefits. Public assistance[1] programs have now taken the place of the financial and health care arrangements of older persons that were at one time the responsibility of the family or the private individual. From a policy perspective, the needs of older persons are not generalizable. That is, they are not necessarily applicable to all who share only an approximate age factor. Older people do not universally experience the same degree of income or health problems nor require equivalent levels of government support. While a small percentage of the aged live comfortably in retirement communities, others require more substantial government funding than is currently available to provide simply a means of escape from poverty (Browne and Katz, 1983). Public perceptions of, and attitudes towards, welfare and public assistance programs have further complicated formulation of policy programs that balance the goals of policy makers. In America, government-sponsored programs of welfare and public assistance have traditionally been viewed as a privilege not to be abused, or as temporary aid to be used only during hard times. This attitude has helped shape nearly all social welfare legislation in the United States.

Elizabeth Kutza (1981) defines two broad categories that describe America's major aging and health policies – those that provide "universal" and those that provide "selective" benefit entitlement. Universal programs are those available to all older persons based on age, whereas selective programs are available to a limited number of older persons based on proven need. Universal programs are Old Age Survivors Insurance (OASI) (Social Security), Medicare, and the provisions provided under the Older Americans Act. Universal programs then, are those public assistance programs that are intended *for* the elderly. Selective programs are those public assistance programs that *affect* the elderly. Examples of selective programs are Supplemental Security Income, Medicaid, food stamps and housing subsidies. Much of this chapter will be devoted to the discussion of these policy categories, and their relationship with existing social welfare programs and cost-containment strategies.

Social security and the "New Deal"

With the great depression of the 1930's national interest in social welfare gained widespread public attention. The depression left millions destitute and brought with it new social welfare problems on a far greater scale than had ever before existed. Without means to provide themselves with adequate food, shelter and health care, many Americans found themselves at the mercy of state programs that profoundly lacked the means necessary to provide assistance to the poor, the homeless, the disabled, and the aged. Because of the many social welfare issues that emerged, the depression created both public pressures for some sort of economic security program and greater public willingness to accept remedial action taken by the federal government. The Social Security Act of 1935 (PL 74–271) was one of the most comprehensive social welfare bills ever passed by Congress. Enacted at the urgent requests of President Franklin D. Roosevelt as part of his "New Deal," the Social Security Act of 1935 forever changed the role of federal-state relations in establishing welfare policy and providing economic security in the US. By establishing a mandatory, nation-wide program of income security, the US government assumed an active and permanent responsibility for functions traditionally reserved for the family, local governments, and charitable institutions.[2]

The first major policy objective of the Social Security Act of 1935 was to create a system of income replacement programs designed to ensure that individuals had some source of income for essential expenses when their regular income was cut off by retirement, unemployment, disability, or the death of a working spouse. This objective was met by establishing the Old Age Assistance program (OAA), a federal-state unemployment insurance program for persons temporarily unable to find work. The OAA also provided a system of federal grants to the states for partial reimbursement of the costs of aid to the indigent elderly, or children with no form of financial support (Landers et al., 1989). The second objective of the Social Security Act was to provide a floor of protection for the most needy segment of the elderly population. This objective was met by establishing the Old Age Insurance (OAI) program, a federal retirement insurance plan financed by a payroll tax, for persons too old to work. OAI would function as a national pension system, under which prospective beneficiaries would pay a premium in the form of a mandatory payroll tax and would be compensated under specific conditions, in this case retirement. The income replacement programs of the Social Security Act, particularly unemployment insurance, also had the secondary function of stabilizing the national economy by keeping steady the purchasing power of different groups in good and bad economic times. These income replacement programs also established retirement as an option for all walks of life in America.

The Old Age Insurance program provided retirement benefits for the insured worker only. However, between 1935 and 1939, Congress increased Social Security benefits, made more people eligible for them, and placed greater emphasis on establishing an adequate retirement income. In 1939, benefits were expanded to include monthly payments to dependents of an insured retiree while he was living and to his survivors after his death. As result of these changes, the OAI program was renamed the Old Age and Survivors Insurance program or OASI. The 1939 amendments also introduced the concept of basing the amount of a worker's monthly Social Security payment on the worker's average monthly wage over his entire working career (Landers et al., 1989).

As the Social Security program began to mature it had a greater impact on society. By the late 1940s, there was a rapid increase in the number of beneficiaries and a corresponding rise in benefit payments. With the growing demand for program outlays, increased burdens were placed on the retirement system. By 1950, Congress found it necessary to overhaul and update the entire retirement program, including the establishment of a new payroll tax schedule and a higher taxable wage base and setting a higher earnings ceiling upon which initial calculations of Social Security payments were made. Compensations for cost of living increases were also included in the program at this time. In 1956, the need to support disabled persons caused Congress to establish a separate Disability Insurance (DI) trust fund, renaming the Social Security program Old Age and Survivors Disability Insurance (OASDI) (Lammers, 1983; Landers et al., 1989).

The 1950s and 1960s saw increases in economic prosperity and workers' wages increased at a relatively rapid rate compared with price increases.

Consequently, the Social Security program developed a large cushion of reserves from the payroll taxes on higher wage earners. During the late 1950s and 1960s, Congress continued to expand Social Security benefits through gradual efforts. By 1964 almost 90 percent of all employment in the nation was covered by the expanded OASDI program, and nearly 76 percent of the nation's aged were receiving Social Security benefits (Landers *et al.*, 1989). By the early 1960s, the OASDI program had become the most important entitlement program for the elderly and disabled. In 1961, President John F. Kennedy began to press for a federally funded health insurance program for the elderly. When the programs of Medicare and Medicaid were enacted in 1965, health insurance revenues were placed in a new Hospital Insurance (HI) trust fund separate from the DI and OASI trust funds. This separation became the foundation of America's reliance on health care as the principal policy mechanism to achieve aging policy goals.

Supplemental security income

Inflationary trends that emerged from increased federal deficits and federal social welfare programs established under President Lyndon B. Johnson's "Great Society" led Congress to propose a comprehensive overhaul of the Social Security System in 1972. The large trust fund reserves that had resulted from increased wage levels and payroll tax revenues of the 1950s and 1960s led Congress to make basic changes in the way Social Security benefit increases were calculated: future increases in Social Security benefits were tied to the consumer price index rather than on an ad hoc basis (Cochran *et al.*, 1996; Landers *et al.*, 1989). Indexing in this way was seen as a method of keeping benefit expenditures low by insulating the process of benefit calculation from the pressures of benefit-hungry constituents.

The 1972 legislation also made a revolutionary shift in the structure of Social Security by introducing a new program of assistance to the aged poor, the Supplemental Security Income (SSI) program, to guarantee that the annual income of an older or disabled person would not fall below a minimum level. This new program redirected responsibility for adult welfare categories (i.e., the aged, blind and disabled) from the states to the federal government. Unlike the Old Age Assistance program, the new program would be financed by the federal government from general tax revenues and would set uniform national eligibility standards. The 1972 amendments ended the multiplicity of eligibility requirements and benefit levels that had characterized the assistance programs formerly administered at the state and local levels. To qualify for SSI individuals must have attained the age of 65 or be blind or disabled. For the income test, an individual is eligible for SSI benefits if his or her income falls below $6,000 per year (or less than $9.012 for a couple) as of January 1, 1999 (Social Security Administration, 1999). Benefits provided under the program are direct monthly cash payments and are adjusted annually for cost-of-living increases (Kutza, 1981). Benefits, however, have proved insufficient, and most states supplement SSI with their own funds with little federal government involvement. Over 70 percent of all aged beneficiaries use SSI benefits to supplement Social Security benefits when they are below SSI standards (Cochran *et al.*, 1996).

Housing subsidies

Public involvement in housing assistance emerged almost in concert with Social Security legislation as both policy objectives were meant to provide relief for those most severely affected by the great depression of the 1930s. Various programs of housing assistance stretch as far back as 1937. Examples are public housing, rural and farm labor housing, rent and mortgage subsidies. All attempt to provide decent housing for the poor, the disabled and the elderly. There are two methods the federal government uses to help secure adequate housing for these groups. First, housing demand can be subsidized – that is, providing income support to offset housing expenses, or tax deductions. Second, housing suppliers can be subsidized so that they are able to sell or rent housing for less than the prevailing market price. Most federal housing programs for middle- and upper-income groups use demand subsidies in the form of tax deductions; where as programs for low-income persons work through supply subsidies. Given the low-income status of most older persons, the majority of housing benefitting the elderly involve supply subsidies. There are four programs of federal housing assistance that directly benefit the elderly: low-rent public housing, the section 202 direct loan program, the section 236 program intended for the lower-middle income groups, and the Department of Housing and Urban Development (HUD) Section 8 Program. All public housing programs are administered by the HUD and receive funding through annual budget appropriations.

Low-rent public housing

The low-rent public housing program authorized under the Housing Act of 1937, and amended by the Housing and Community Development Act of 1974, was intended to help low-income families obtain decent, safe, and sanitary housing. Units within public housing projects are rented to low-income families, elderly individuals aged 62 or older, or handicapped individuals who meet income limitations *and* who qualify for assistance by local requirements. Benefits are awarded in two forms: loans to housing authorities for rehabilitating, purchasing, leasing or constructing public housing projects, and reduced rentals for tenants. Rent levels take into account the tenant's ability to pay and the financial solvency of the housing project. By law, rents in these units may not exceed 25 percent of the family's income (Kutza, 1981; Keigher, 1991).

Supportive housing for the elderly

Federal construction loans are for housing projects that serve elderly and disabled families and individuals under Section 202 of the Housing Act of

1959, as amended by the Housing and Community Development Act of 1974. The Section 202 program increased the housing supply for moderate-income elderly and disabled individuals with incomes too high to qualify for public housing units but too low to obtain housing in the private market. Eligibility for Section 202 loans is limited to nonprofit corporations or cooperatives. Tenants are eligible for these units by virtue of age, disability and limited income. Section 202 loans are restricted to construction or substantial rehabilitation of housing for the elderly and disabled. Sponsors receiving the loans, which can be up to 100 percent of the mortgage, repay the government over a fifty-year period at 3-percent interest (Kutza, 1981; Keigher, 1991).

Mortgage subsidies

The Section 236 program provides private enterprise with additional means for developing quality rental and cooperative housing for low- and moderate-income persons by lowering the costs through interest reduction payments. Approved HUD Federal Housing Administration (FHA) lenders are eligible and must be willing to receive monthly interest-reduction payments on behalf of the project mortgagors. Eligible families or tenants must have an annual adjusted income not exceeding 80 percent of the area's median income. Tenants are expected to pay at least 25 percent of their income for rent but not more than the fair market price. In projects designed for the elderly, interest subsidies can be used to construct or rehabilitate community kitchens, common dining areas, and other shared facilities. Benefits paid under Section 236 are combinations of mortgage-insurance and mortgage-interest subsidies to suppliers of low-income housing (Kutza, 1981; Keigher, 1991).

Housing assistance payments program

The current Section 8 housing assistance payments (HAP) program provides two subsidy methods to help low-income families and private individuals meet housing costs. Under the Section 8 certificate program, HUD pays the difference between the housing units' actual rent and 30 percent of a tenant's adjusted income. Eligible households rent an existing unit that meets certain property standards and with rent not exceeding the fair market rent (FMR) for the area. The section 8 voucher system differs from other programs because it provides a shopping incentive to tenants. The dollar amount of the rental subsidy is fixed, but a family is free to rent a unit above or below the 30-percent income level (Keigher, 1991; US Department of Housing and Urban Development, 1998).

Homelessness and housing problems

Today millions of Americans, particularly single elderly persons and low-income families, live in substandard, dilapidated and overcrowded dwellings.

Enforcement of new housing codes designed to rehabilitate or to prevent deterioration of neighborhoods during the 1980s had the unintended consequence of reducing availability of single-room-occupancy apartments that formerly housed many of today's homeless and elderly singles. Public housing units have not replaced these units, nor have housing allowances or subsidies stimulated building or rehabilitation of low-cost units. Ironically, federal policy of income-tax deductibility for mortgage interest and home-loan guarantee programs provides more housing assistance to middle- and upper-income than to poor elderly people (Kutza, 1981). Therefore, much of the problem affecting housing in America is not simply due to a lack of housing stock, but rather to the lack of affordable low-cost housing.

In 1995, the Clinton administration targeted federal housing programs for reforms: making public housing safe and attractive by allowing police greater latitude in sweeping them for illegal guns and drugs; allowing tenants to purchase their own apartments; and replacing public housing with a system of rent vouchers. Despite concerns that low-income tenants pay more of their income for rent under a voucher system, housing vouchers have become an increasingly important means of providing low-income housing.

Food stamps

The Food Stamp Act of 1964 permits low-income households to purchase a nutritionally adequate diet through normal channels of trade. Eligibility for food stamps is determined by annual household income. To qualify for food stamps, annual household income must fall below the poverty line set annually by the Office of Management and Budget. During fiscal year 1997, 7 percent of all participants in the food stamp program were elderly. Benefits under this program take the form of coupons made available to eligible households. These coupons can be used to purchase any food (except alcoholic beverages and tobacco) in retail stores. Food stamps may also be used to purchase plants and seeds for use in home vegetable gardens, or to purchase meals prepared and delivered by meal delivery services. Benefits are keyed to the price of food, the cost of a decent diet, family size and income. Each month an eligible household receives an allotment of stamps, the number determined by the amount it would cost to purchase a "thrifty food plan" as determined by the Department of Agriculture for various family sizes (US Department of Agriculture, 1998). The food stamp program reveals basic assumptions about welfare and poverty in America, for it is rooted in the desire to see the poor adequately fed but also in a distrust of their spending habits.

The evolution of United States health and aging policy

While aging policy in the US appropriately focused first on the elderly's most crucial needs for income, housing and food, the movement toward health care concerns and their utility as a policy tool places health care policy squarely in the middle of aging policy development. This transition was largely a move to politically address the growing elderly special interest group and their concerns about health care needs in the 1960s. However, in order to frame our discussion of these incremental developments of aging policy through health care changes, we must review some historical aspects of the health industry in the US. Table 1 is useful in guiding this overview. The initial issue is government's involvement in a private industry – health care delivery. This concern had an historical precedent,[3] which became more important in the decades following the 1960s.

Overview of the United States health care system

As US health policies have evolved, objectives of policy makers have focused on providing equitable health care access to the elderly at reasonable cost to the individual and the nation, while at the same time ensuring the highest possible quality of health care.

The United States differs from other industrialized nations in that it does not have a national health insurance program to finance health care services for the entire population. Instead, the US health care system is a unique mixture of private insurance, public financing and direct out-of-pocket spending (Cochran et al., 1996). The US health care system is often described as a multiplicity of subsystems, each serving distinct populations in different ways, with little central planning or coordination among subsystems (Torrens, 1988). While each subsystem is independent, they all compete for the same resources within the same economy. Between individual subsystems, there is direct competition for facilities, personnel and available funds, or alternatively, each subsystem may function at a unique level separate from the others.

Financing structure has shaped the US health care system as it evolved. At the highest levels of clinicians (nurse practitioners, physician assistants, physicians, psychiatrists and dentists), fee-for-service (FFS) financing has traditionally been the rule.[4] Health insurance coverage has increased dramatically over the last two decades. Since the early 1970s there has been a shift in US health care policy prompting movement away from the traditional FFS system toward pre-paid risk-sharing health maintenance organizations (HMOs), and more recently, toward managed care systems.[5] In 1991, 99.1 percent of the elderly were covered by some form of health insurance. Of these, 68.3 percent had private health insurance, with 33.2 percent of all coverage provided by employer-related plans. In that same year, 96.0 percent of all elderly persons having health insurance were covered by government-sponsored programs (Health Insurance Association of America, 1992).

The decentralized nature of the American health care system and the direct competition that exists between subsystems creates a payment structure whereby medical care costs are paid through complicated arrangements among government agencies,[6] individuals and private insurers. Individuals pay for a variety of services directly, but they also pay indirectly by purchasing private health insurance. These insurance companies then reimburse providers for *covered* services, which vary widely according to the terms of particular policies. Most private insurance is purchased through or provided by employers, with the employers passing their costs on to employees in the form of lower wages (Cochran *et al.*, 1996; Torrens, 1988). Pooling risks through insurance or government programs assures stable financing of health care, limits the potential catastrophic expenses, and relieves the uncertainty of paying for unexpected health needs.

Since 1960, the share of overall gross domestic product (GDP) expenditures for health care has been increasing.[7] For example, from 1960 to 1994 national personal health care expenditures (PHCEs) increased from 4.7 percent to 12.4 percent respectively. This increase shows an average annual rate of change of 11.0 percent. Between 1960 and 1993, direct out-of-pocket patient spending was offset by increased shares paid by public and private third parties. In 1960, out-of-pocket patient spending was around 56 percent of all personal health care expenditures. By 1993, out-of-pocket patient spending had dropped to only 20 percent of all personal health care expenditures.

Health care and comparison with other nations

Health care systems in other industrialized nations tend toward greater organization and centralization, with less private, fee-for-service practice. There are two health care approaches used by other nations. In the first approach, the central government operates a national health service, as is the case in Canada or Great Britain. In the second approach, the central government mandates universal insurance coverage either through employer or private sources or provides government insurance for the poor or medically needy, as is the case in Sweden, Germany, France and Italy. Under national health care systems, privatization is minimal and health care providers work for the government. Under universal systems, the central government does not actually operate all

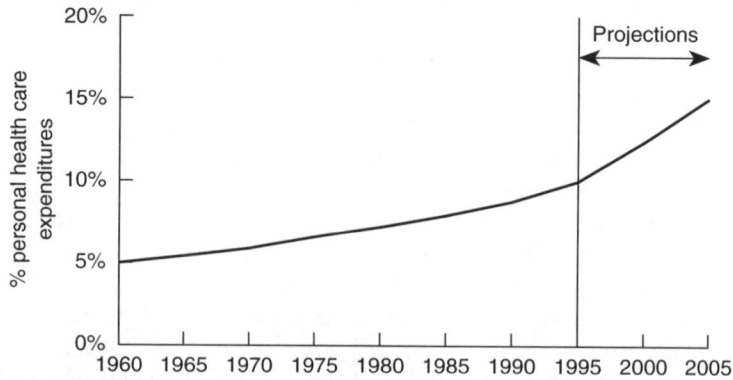

Figure 3.1 Trends in personal health care expenditures 1960 to 2005

Source: *Heatlh Care Financing Review, Statistical Supplement, 1996*, Fig. 1, p. 10. Baltimore: Health Care Financing Administration, Office of Research and Demonstrations.

health care programs, but exercises considerable influence over them (Cochran et al., 1996; Glaser, 1984).

There are other important differences between the US health care system and other nations' systems. Many of these differences involve health care payment structure as well as health insurance coverage. In the US, government-financed health care is primarily provided for only the poor and elderly. In contrast, many universal systems provide broader coverage. In these nations, the wealthy seek private health care in addition to, or as a replacement for, government programs (Cochran et al., 1996; Glaser, 1984). Additionally, in most nations, third-party payments (those amounts paid by public and private health care providers) cover a higher percentage of medical bills than in the US. Therefore, patients in other nations have fewer out-of-pocket expenses than Americans. In none of these countries are medical bills allowed to place a catastrophic or long-term burden on individuals or their families.

Although other nations have more extensive health care coverage, none have higher total cost than the US system. These comparisons (see Figure 3.2) show that Americans face the highest rate of increase in health care spending relative to GDP, as well as increases in health care inflation and overall spending patterns. Growth in the US health-to-GDP ratio continues to outpace that in other nations. In recent years, costs of health care have stabilized in other nations, while American costs continue to increase. At the same time, the US ranks behind other nations in outcome indicators of infant mortality and life expectancy. However, in terms of access to care, the US appears to be comparable to other nations (Anderson, 1997). Over the last 40 years, many nations have implemented programs to hold down health care costs. Compared with other nations, the US has achieved slow progress towards cost containment.

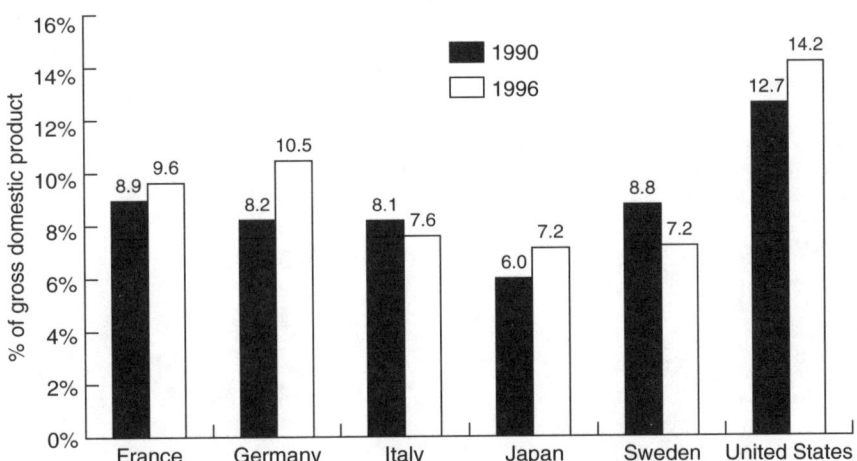

Figure 3.2 Comparisons of health-to-GDP expenditures between the US and other OECD nations

Source: Anderson, 1997, Exhibit 1

This is due in large part to the pluralistic debate that ensues over each modification, resulting in only incremental changes at the margin.

Health care policy through incremental progress

Although poverty among the aged had been substantially reduced with the implementation of Social Security, a large proportion of elders in the United States were still without adequate health insurance or easy access to health care as late as the 1960s. However, subtle linkages between Social Security and health policy provided important inroads for development of government-sponsored health insurance for the elderly. From 1935 on, bills calling for sweeping revisions of the Social Security Act were introduced regularly in Congress.[8] In 1950, Congress moved to help states provide medical assistance to welfare recipients through amendments to the Social Security law. Under this plan, benefits paid under the Old Age and Survivors Insurance (OASI) programs were directed at assisting elderly persons who had high health care costs and low incomes and thus could not afford the high premiums of commercial health insurance (Cochran *et al.*, 1996; Lammers, 1983; Landers *et al.*, 1989).

A compromise takes shape

It was not until the mid-1960s that the American public became involved in the health care debate. Following unsuccessful efforts to pass a hospital care bill in the early 1960s, President Lyndon B. Johnson introduced a proposal in 1965 which formed the basis of a successful compromise.[9] "Medicare" was created in 1965 as a federal program providing hospital and medical insurance coverage to persons who are entitled to Social Security in the form of cash benefits and health coverage. "Medicaid" was added to help the states pay the medical expenses of welfare recipients. It is important to note, however, that neither program was designed to change the organization or delivery of health care in America, but only to pay some of the bills and supply care to many not adequately served by private insurance and existing public health care programs.

Public financing of health care for the elderly becomes reality

As passed by Congress in 1965, the Health Insurance for the Aged Act (PL 89–97) added two new titles to the Social Security Act – XVIII (Medicare)[10] and XIX (Medicaid). Part A of Title XVIII (later known as Medicare Part A) provided persons over 65 with insurance to cover the costs of hospital and related care. Medicare Part A was financed by a Social Security trust fund to which employers and employees were required to contribute. The second part of Title XVIII (later known as Medicare Part B) called for a voluntary system of supplemental medical insurance covering doctors' fees and certain other health services. Title XIX, the Medicaid section of the bill, provided a program of federal matching grants to states that chose to make medical services available to welfare recipients and the medically needy (Lammers, 1983; Landers et al., 1989).

Medicare

Medicare consists of two parts: Hospital Insurance (HI), known as Part A, and Supplementary Medical Insurance (SMI), or Part B. Hospital Insurance (Part A) covers a broad range of hospital and post-hospital services[11] subject to some deductibles and coinsurance. Medicare does not cover outpatient prescription drugs nor long-term care, two ancillary services of profound importance for the elderly (Cochran et al., 1996). For any given benefit period, Part A beneficiaries must pay a deductible for hospital care set at the approximate cost of one day of hospital care. For the first 60 days of hospitalization, Medicare pays the entire cost of care. For hospitalization days 61–90 patients are required to make coinsurance[12] payments. There are also 60 additional days in lifetime reserve, called lifetime reserve days, that are available for use after 90 days of hospitalization. However, for lifetime reserve days, beneficiaries must make even higher coinsurance[13] payments.

Beneficiaries may also elect Part B coverage for physicians' services, which requires cost-sharing. Medicare does not pay for ordinary nursing home or routine home care, but it does pay the reasonable cost of hospice care for terminally ill patients. Medicare hospice expenditures have grown significantly from $1.4 billion in fiscal year 1994 to $1.9 billion in 1995, an increase of nearly 35.7 percent (Health Care Financing Administration [HCFA], 1998; National Center for Health Statistics [NCHS], 1997; US Department of Health and Human Services [DHHS], 1996).

Medicaid

Medicaid is a joint federal and state program administered by the states that finances health services primarily for individuals who are eligible for several federal welfare programs. Chief among these are Aid to Families with Dependent Children (AFDC) and SSI for the aged, blind, and disabled. Medicaid has no entitlement features. Recipients must prove their eligibility according to their income. Because many of the elderly (12.2 percent) are in poverty, they qualify for SSI, and subsequently for Medicaid (US Bureau of the Census, 1993).

Broad federal requirements and guidelines allow states flexibility in administration of their Medicaid programs. Covered benefits and provider payment mechanisms vary from state to state. These include: hospital, physician, laboratory and x-ray, skilled nursing facilities (SNF) services for persons at least age 21, home health, family planning, rural health clinic services, and health assessment services for children. States may determine the scope of services offered and provide other elective services including: prescription drugs, eyeglasses, intermediate care facilities, inpatient psychiatric care for the aged and persons under 21 years of age, physical therapy and dental care (US DHHS, 1996).

Medicaid operates as a "vendor" payment program; that is, payments are made directly to providers. Payment levels are subject to conditions that all state Medicaid plans and agencies must satisfy. First, payments must be sufficient to enlist enough providers in the plan to ensure that beneficiaries receive benefits equal to those covered by private insurance within the same geographic location. Second, participating providers must accept the Medicaid payment as payment in full. Third, payments made to providers must be consistent with the Health Care Financing Administration's efficiency, economic, and quality-of-care standards (US DHHS, 1996).

In 1986 Congress expanded the availability of Medicaid assistance to the poor and elderly population. States could extend full or partial Medicaid coverage to Medicare-eligible elders to help pay their Medicare premiums, deductibles, and copayments.[14]

Medigap policies and supplemental insurance

The need for additional coverage to help fill in for Medicare's cost sharing and deductibles became evident soon after enactment of the program in 1965. For the poor elderly population, Medicaid provided this coverage by paying the Medicare premium, deductibles, and cost sharing as well as providing supplementary benefits under Medicaid such as prescription drug coverage. However, for those able to afford coverage, a private health insurance market soon developed that offered "Medigap" plans to supplement Medicare coverage (Rowland, 1993). It is important to note that Medigap plans are designed to only reimburse the deductibles and coinsurance associated with Medicare covered services. Thus, the real focus of Medigap plans is on those uncovered risks associated with acute care services, not on long-term care strategies. As Medicare regulations changed to permit balance billing, the incentives to obtain Medigap coverage have increased.

Achieving health system goals through Medicare and Medicaid

After 1965, Congress and special interest groups used the incremental process of change to refine the systems of Medicare and Medicaid. Because the Medicare and Medicaid portions of the health care system were sufficiently large, these modifications had "spill-over" impact on the private sector and fee-for-service portions of the American system. Thus, health system goals of access, cost, efficiency and quality could now be achieved through regulations and legislation that modified the basic structure of Medicare and Medicaid.

During the 1970s, rising expenditures for health services prompted the federal government and the states to impose several "belt-tightening" measures. Their principal target was inpatient hospital expenditures, the most rapidly increasing cost component of medical care. Regulatory efforts during the 1970s also focused on changing institutional behaviors that were rooted in the structure of the American health care system. Regulations concentrated on reforming expenditures and health services controls, utilization review, and rate controls.[15] Cost control was again the principal issue of the health care debate in the 1980s. The primary focus of these reforms was on changing reimbursement strategies for hospitals and physicians. In 1982, Congress passed the Tax Equity and Fiscal Responsibility Act which introduced a capitated payment option under a prospective payment system (PPS). Then in 1984, Congress further curtailed Medicare costs by imposing a series of freezes on Medicare fees charged by doctors and by increasing the monthly premiums for Medicare Part B. The cost-control issue carried with it a concern for compromised quality of care, which special interest groups lobbied to retain.

Current policy issues: ensuring optimal quality at a threshold cost to elders and society

With the passage of Medicare and Medicaid, the volume and complexity of federal health legislation increased dramatically and medical expenditures exploded. General inflationary trends help explain only part of the growing medical costs faced by Americans. Because health-to-GDP expenditures have steadily increased, rising medical costs must be explained by factors directly related to the health care system itself, such as the growth in insurance coverage and third-party payers, demographic trends of the population, and increasing technology.

Third-party payments

The most important contributor to rising costs in the US healthcare system has been the growth in third-party payments for medical care. Third-party payers are not health care providers, but are those who pay the charges to providers on behalf of patients. The primary third-party payers are Medicare and Medicaid, and private health insurance companies – chief among them are the Blue Cross-Blue Shield plans.[16] As health care utilization among the elderly and the poor increases because of new Medicare and Medicaid legislation, greater demands are placed on existing resources. Because the medical market lacks effective competition, an expanded supply of providers simply generates higher medical expenditures. Third-party payments contribute to cost increases by hiding the real financial burden from both patient and provider. Under FFS medicine, providers share increased incentives to offer as many services as possible for each patient who lacks the knowledge or financial incentive to stop increasing services.[17] The evolution of managed care insurers such as Health Maintenance Organizations (HMOs), Preferred Provider Organizations (PPOs), and Point-of-Service (POS) plans that attract members with lower coinsurance and deductibles has slowed the growth of patient out-of-pocket spending (Levit *et al.*, 1994).

The aging of the population

Aging patterns of the population also contribute to the overall increasing costs of medical care. When the twentieth century began, the elderly did not make up a large proportion of the US population. Only one in 25 people was age 65 or older and the population's median age was 23. The elderly were not isolated from society; they commonly lived with their families. The concept of retirement did not exist. More than two-thirds of men 65 and over worked. By the late 1930s, when Social Security was established, the elderly's share of the population had risen: one in fifteen people was 65 or older. Today the elderly constitute a larger proportion of the total population – 12.7 percent of the total population, or over 34 million persons (US Department of Commerce, 1997, pp. 831–832). By 2030, when the baby boomers (those born between the years 1946 and 1964) reach retirement age, there will be almost 60 million (US Bureau of the Census, 1996). Government benefits to the aged now account for more than one-fourth of the federal budget (American Association of Retired Persons [AARP], 1997).[18]

Since the 1950s, life expectancies have steadily increased. Today, mean life expectancy for males and females is 76.0 years (US Department of Commerce, 1997, p. 832). By 2030 mean life expectancies for males and females will increase to 78.6 years. Life expectancy at age 65 today is 16.9 years. In 2030 life expectancy at age 65 will increase to 18.8 years (Preston, 1993). This rapid growth and increased life expectancy of the elderly, particularly the oldest old, represents in part a triumph of the efforts to extend human life, but these age groups also require a disproportionately large share of special services and public support. Most older persons have at least one chronic condition and many have multiple conditions. The aged also have more instances of disability and of inability to perform the ordinary activities of daily living (ADL), such as bathing, eating, getting in and out of bed, and using the toilet, and the instrumental activities of daily living (IADL), such as heavy housework, grocery shopping, or preparing meals. By 2030, there will be large increases in the numbers of seniors requiring special services in housing, transportation, health care and nutrition. At this same time there will also be large increases in some of the most vulnerable groups, such as the oldest old living alone, older women, elderly racial minorities living alone, and elderly unmarried persons living alone. Large increases in the numbers of elders requiring formal care (mainly nursing home and hospice care) and informal care (mainly care at home) will also occur. Undoubtedly, over the next three to four decades the elderly will place greater demands on not only the health system, but will absorb a greater percentage of federal dollars by participating in various programs of public assistance such as Social Security, Medicare, and to a lesser extent, Medicaid (Manton, 1989; Manton, Corder, and Stallard, 1993).

Technology

Modern medical technology and its distribution is also a major contributor to the spiraling inflation of medical expenditures in the US. Medical research spending, mainly by the federal government between the years 1960–1993, contributed to about one quarter of the growth in medical expenditures (Peden and Freeland, 1995). Clearly, new diagnostic and treatment procedures such as magnetic resonance imaging, renal dialysis, neonatal intensive care units, chemotherapy, and coronary artery bypass surgery are tremendously expensive because of both the equipment costs and the specialized personnel needed to operate them (Luce, 1988). Whether these innovations achieve improved outcomes is the subject of important research focused on quality, cost and value of health care (Guadagnoli and McNeil, 1994).

Futile care

Recent attention has been placed on expenses incurred during the last year of life as well as providing futile medical services (or "futile care") in the final weeks and months of life when reasonable evidence suggests no hope for recovery. Several studies suggest that once critically ill patients were admitted to intensive care units (ICUs) (Schapira *et al.*, 1993b; Schapira, Stucknicki, and Bradham, 1993) or medical instensive care units (MICUs) (Lee *et al.*, 1994) their prognosis was poor. The growth of hospice care in the US is directly related to these issues and the goal of patient-centered quality of care (see D. Bradham, Chapter 5 this volume). If a broad interpretation of futility is assumed, unilateral limitations on measures to prolong life where the prognosis for survival is poor may be appropriate because of limited societal resources (Halevy, Neal, and Brody, 1996). The current debate surrounding the concept of futility involves multiple ethical issues, such as rationing of medical care, limiting life-sustaining interventions, and physician assisted suicide, that are beyond the scope of this chapter.

Public perceptions of health care

The American public's exaggerated expectations of medical science coupled with its fear of illness, old age and death also contribute in subtle ways to the overall rising costs of medical care. Billions of dollars are spent every year on visits to the doctor for colds, flu and other self-limiting illnesses. Americans have a tendency to treat these as abnormal conditions rather than as part of the human experience. Thus, the sick, and especially the aged, are increasingly referred to medical specialists, hospitals and nursing homes (Cochran *et al.*,

1996). Greater insurance coverage of mental illness and greater utilization of medical services by persons with mental illness and drug addiction has meant that more persons are now using the health care system (Richardson, 1988).

A new paradigm: prospective payment

Since the early 1970s total health expenditures have continued to increase at an alarming rate, with 10–12 percent of GDP going into health care, rather than education and other societal needs. Congress sought an incentive structure that would increase cost-efficiency. To achieve efficiency, cost reductions and utilization controls that would allow the continuance of high quality and high access, a mechanism of prospective payment with specified limits per case. The 1982 Tax Equity and Fiscal Responsibility Act (TEFRA) created a managed care capitated payment option under a prospective payment system (PPS). This new paradigm[19] placed providers at fiscal risk, which caused them to be more conscious of limited resources. In response, many hospitals implemented new services (see Figure 3.3) including ambulatory programs, satellite clinics, substance abuse programs, rehabilitation services, skilled nursing services, laboratory, and other ancillary services (Koch, 1988).[20]

Medicare HMOs

Managed care options have been incorporated in Medicare since the early 1970's. However, managed care did not become a major component of Medicare coverage until 1985 when the HCFA implemented changes enacted by TEFRA. Under TEFRA, managed care plans are paid a predetermined, per-enrollee payment to provide *all* covered services to Medicare enrollees. Medicare-managed care plans[21] are attractive for the elderly since coverage for outpatient prescriptions and some preventative treatments, such as hearing and eye exams, are often available without the copayments and deductibles of Part B Medicare (US DHHS, 1996). Because managed care allows a team approach to health care, treatment of chronic disease may be better managed under managed care rather than fee-for-service medicine. However, anticipated cost savings from the HMO program are difficult to realize because of enrollment flexibility and greater use of services by Medicare beneficiaries who are not enrolled in HMOs (US General Accounting Office, 1997; Morgan et al., 1997).

Physician payment reform

In 1989 and 1990, Congress acted to reform the method by which Medicare reimburses physicians. Under new provisions, an annual cap is now placed on Medicare physician payments. These reforms also provide a new scale of reimbursement called the Resource-Based Relative Value Scale[22] (RBRVS).

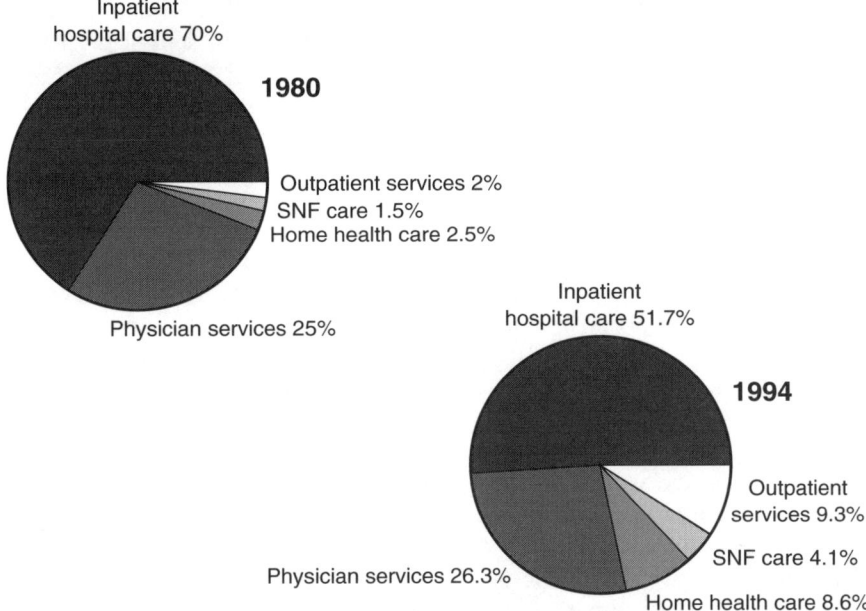

Figure 3.3 Distribution of Medicare spending comparisons between 1980 and 1994

Source: *Heatlh Care Financing Review, Statistical Supplement, 1996*, Fig. 11, p. 29. Baltimore: Health Care Financing Administration, Office of Research and Demonstrations.

The intended effect of RBRVS is not to save money on Medicare reimbursements directly, but to encourage broader use of lower-cost primary care and less use of high-cost specialty care, as well as to provide incentives for physicians to enter primary care medicine rather than medical specialties. Over time the RBRVS system should favor increased reimbursement rates for primary care physicians, while specialized physicians may see reimbursement rates rise more slowly or not at all (Hsiao *et al.*, 1992).

Access assessment: ensuring elder's access to medical care

Since the 1960s, public financing programs for health care have led to marked improvement in the availability and accessibility of medical care. Before Medicare and Medicaid legislation, only 50 percent of the elderly had any form of health insurance. Nearly all of the elderly are now covered for hospital and physician services under Medicare. In addition, Medicaid provides health insurance to over 38 million of the nation's low-income population, including insurance coverage to almost 5 million of the poorest elderly citizens (HCFA, 1998). Particularly for the elderly, the establishment of Medicare was successful in providing health insurance coverage and meeting its two main objectives:

remedying the failure of the private market to provide adequate health insurance for the elderly; and reducing the financial burden faced by older people (Rowland, 1993).

However, physical access remains a fundamental issue for those elderly dwelling in inner-city minority communities, the poor or near poor who do not qualify for public assistance programs, and the rural elderly. In America, medical care is maldistributed. Hospitals, nursing homes, clinics and health care professionals are disproportionately located in upper-middle class urban and suburban areas (Cochran *et al.*, 1996). Current population estimates indicate that 25 percent of the elderly reside in rural areas,[23] 45 percent in the suburbs, and 30 percent in urban[24] areas (AARP, 1997). Patterns of limited access contribute to the poor health and shorter life expectancy of those who live in rural areas, are poor, or live in inner-city minority communities (Pappas *et al.*, 1993).

Many problems still arise for the elderly that concern inadequate health insurance coverage and the high costs of health care that must be paid out-of-pocket despite public assistance programs. One reason for these problems stems from the fact that overall Medicare only covers 49 percent of the elderly's total health care costs. Medicare does not cover long-term care (chronic illnesses) in the community or in nursing homes, mental health care, or dental care costs, and nor does it pay for prescription drugs or durable medical products (eyeglasses, wheelchairs, or other medical sundries). These out-of-pocket expenses increase with age, and minorities and women carry the largest burden of these costs. Direct out-of-pocket medical expenditures for prescriptions and durable medical products comprise a large proportion of all personal health care expenditures.[25]

Another reason for disparity in the adequacy of health insurance among the elderly results from two major gaps in Medicaid coverage. First, only 36 percent of the non-institutionalized poor elderly receive Medicaid. Second, Medicaid's financing for the elderly, like Medicare, focuses on nursing home institutionalization, not on treatment of long-term chronic conditions (Estes and Binney, 1988). Nevertheless, several recent studies show that Medicaid has reduced income-related differences in access to care. These studies also suggest that poor persons enrolled in Medicaid are more likely than poor persons with no public or private coverage to have a usual source of care, higher rates of ambulatory visits, and more hospitalizations (Berk and Schur, 1998).

Health and aging policy at the crossroads

To meet the chronic health needs of an aging population, two major areas remain to be addressed: catastrophic coverage and the lack of public or private insurance coverage for long-term care (Rowland, 1993). Striking an effective balance between these policy priorities has led to failure to fill the remaining gaps in Medicare coverage.

The role of old-age interest groups: lessons from the 1988 Medicare Catastrophic Coverage Act

Since enactment of Medicare and Medicaid, the elderly have taken an increasingly significant role in the political process. They vote at much higher rates than younger age groups (US Bureau of the Census, 1997), and over the last three decades, there has been a tremendous increase in the number, membership, visibility and activity of old-age interest groups in the US. (The most powerful of these is the American Association of Retired Persons, or AARP, which boasts twenty-eight million members.) The inherent ability of old-age interest groups to develop a cohesive platform, coupled with high political efficacy, ultimately contribute to greater political access and responsiveness from elected officials (Binstock and Day, 1996). There is no better example of "interest-group politics" and its role in US health and aging policy making than events following the passage of the Medicare Catastrophic Coverage Act (MCCA) of 1988 and its subsequent repeal less than one year afterward.

In 1986, the federal government sponsored the development of proposals for public and private provision of catastrophic medical insurance, leading to the passage of the Medicare Catastrophic Coverage Act of 1988. However, Medicare beneficiaries had become aware that the real health-financing catastrophe lay not in acute care, but in long-term care. Under the new hospital financing system of prospective payment, patients were moved more quickly from Medicare-reimbursed acute-care hospital systems into informal care and sparsely reimbursed chronic-care systems. The AARP launched a national campaign to heighten public awareness of long-term care issues and pressure politicians to support long-term care coverage. Through candidate forums and intense media coverage, the campaign raised public consciousness, stimulated public discussion, and contributed to growing skepticism and dissatisfaction with the new catastrophic health insurance proposal because it did not address the issue of long-term care (Holstein and Minkler, 1991). Funding for Medicare catastrophic coverage was to be obtained from a special tax on Medicare recipients themselves, and this was seen as an infringement on their entitlement under the Social Security program (Aaronson, Zinn, and Rosko, 1994). The political pressure for repeal of the Medicare Catastrophic Coverage Act became so intense that AARP and other old-age interest groups reversed their initial support of MCCA and the Act was repealed in 1989, less than one year after enactment.

Long-term care

The second priority of aging and health policy since enactment of Medicare and Medicaid concerns the health care system's role in providing public assistance for long-term care. Several trends, most notably the increase in the elderly population, the rapidly increasing costs of nursing home care, and changes in family structure, have propelled the issue of long-term care to the forefront of the aging and health policy debate.

Under the US health care system, the costs of long-term care are not covered to any significant extent by private insurance or Medicare. For treatment involving long-term care, the elderly are left to rely on their own resources and, when those are exhausted, on Medicaid.[26] Major policy issues concerning long-term care involve questions of whether better financing methods can be found and in what segment of American society those responsibilities lie (Landers *et al.*, 1989). Sharply different views exist as to where the responsibility for financing long-term care belongs (Weiner and Illston, 1994). One view holds that the responsibility of financing long-term care should fall on individuals and their families and that the government should act only as a payer of last resort for those who are unable to provide for themselves. The opposing view is that the government should take the lead in ensuring comprehensive care for all older people, regardless of financial need (see D. Bradham in Chapter 5, this volume).

US aging and health policy: the next 40 years

As we have attempted to show throughout this chapter, aging and health care policies in America have evolved through a continual process of incremental changes that emerge from periods of compromise followed by implementation of new policy objectives to remedy current and potential problems. Implementation of public assistance programs such as supplemental security income, housing assistance and food stamps has resulted in substantial success in alleviating the worst affects of poverty, ill health, poor nutrition and inadequate housing. Remaining problems in housing for the elderly and low-income families still involve providing adequate, safe, and low-cost housing.

Social Security and federal-state programs such as OASDI and SSI have significantly reduced poverty among the aged and have alleviated many of the problems of retirement benefits. Retirement incomes of most elders have improved substantially in recent years, especially for those with adequate pensions and savings in addition to Social Security benefits, but those whose retirement depends entirely or largely on Social Security exist at or below the poverty line. Therefore, a two-class system among the elderly is an increasing reality. Pressing issues in Social Security policy remain, the most important of which is the relationship between the Social Security Trust Fund and the federal budget deficit. The immediate problem then with Social Security is that the surplus in Social Security payments counts against the deficit generated by current taxing and spending. In other words, the federal budget has borrowed from the trust funds, especially Social Security, to support recent trends in deficit spending. Those trust funds will have to be paid back however, when the baby boom generation starts to collect Social Security benefits. These payments would require an enormous tax hike or other borrowing from the general public – a solution that is less than palatable for almost all Americans.

Thus, current debate in Social Security reform focuses on how these programs should be financed, how long-term population trends will affect payroll taxes and benefits, appropriate retirement ages, and whether equity or adequacy of benefits should be more strongly emphasized.

Federal health care policy, particularly Medicare and Medicaid, has been successful in reducing the financial burden of health care for the elderly and poor and in addressing inequitable distribution by lowering financial barriers to medical care. Yet, serious burdens remain for much of the population and problems of access to care persist. The growing gap between financially secure and poor elderly persons exacerbates the equity-adequacy problem. Many of the remaining policy issues concerning public assistance programs for the aged involve the ability of current programs to balance acute and long-term care needs and to provide equitable access while practicing cost-containment strategies. As the new millennium approaches, the imbalance between available revenues and costs of public assistance programs is expected to grow rapidly. By 2010, overall GDP expenditures for Medicare alone will almost double (King, 1994). Current projections suggest that Medicare Part A, which is financed by payroll taxes, will be bankrupt by 2001. This imbalance is projected to grow rapidly as the baby boomers reach retirement age. While this imbalance is most acute and visible in the financing of Medicare and Medicaid, it applies equally to concerns in housing and income support.

From the standpoint of national policy in aging and health care, the challenge for the US well into the twenty-first century will continue to lie in meeting the demands of a rapidly growing cohort of elderly Americans placing greater demands on social insurance, public assistance, and health care programs.

Notes

1 In America, public assistance programs are generally thought of as "welfare." Programs are designed to help certain categories of persons whose circumstances place them in poverty: families who are temporarily unable to support themselves through no fault of their own or persons who are ineligible for social insurance but who deserve aid because their poverty is the result of age or disability. Thus, public assistance has traditionally only been available to children, or guardians of children, aged adults, and those who are disabled. Adults who do not fit this classification are assumed to be undeserving and are seldom eligible for assistance.

2 Although the Social Security Act did not include a health-insurance program, the President's Committee on Economic Security endorsed the principle of government-sponsored health insurance. However, President Roosevelt dropped the idea fearing its inclusion would endanger passage of the entire bill (Landers, Rovner, and McGuiness, 1989).

3 Government-sponsored health insurance first gained attention in 1798 when Congress established a government health insurance program for the merchant marines. In this program, sailors contributed a few cents a month to pay for hospital care provided in marine hospitals. This policy introduced the concept of a pre-paid health insurance plan. However, it was not until the early twentieth century that the idea of government-sponsored health insurance for the general public gained serious attention. That debate originated when the American Association for Labor Legislation (AALL), a group of lawyers, academics, and other professionals, lobbied in several states for enactment of health insurance legislation. In a parallel move, the American Medical Association (AMA) drafted health insurance bills that were later introduced in the New

York and Massachusetts legislatures. In 1917, the AMA's House of Delegates endorsed a health insurance plan comparable to an earlier AALL bill. Opposition to the idea of government sponsorship developed immediately. Opponents were in large part labor leaders who felt that a national health-insurance system would result in government control over the working class. In addition, labor leaders feared that government sponsorship would reduce new union memberships and provide management with a reason for withholding raises. Employers also opposed government sponsorship fearing their contribution would be excessive. In 1920, serious pressures from state medical societies prompted the AMA to reverse its position and oppose government-sponsored health insurance (Anderson, 1984; Landers *et al.*, 1989; Litman and Robins, 1984).

4 Under FFS, health services providers traditionally establish their own office, see only their own patients, and charge a separate fee for each individual service performed. If a patient sees more than one provider, the patient is billed separately for each service by each individual provider (Cochran *et al.*, 1996).

5 Under this financing system a fixed annual fee is paid per enrollee. Additionally, the provider is obligated to provide all necessary care, with no further fees. Nevertheless, a substantial component of the US health care system still practices under the traditional fee-for-service system.

6 Federal, state, and local governments provide a number of health-related services in the form of epidemic control, inoculations, health inspections, or veteran's care.

7 In 1994, annual expenditures from public and private sources for personal health care expenditures (PHCEs) amounted to 12.4 percent of the GDP. During that same year, total spending from all sources was $832.5 billion, a sum that amounted to an average of $3,074 spent for every man, woman, and child in the nation. Projections from the Health Care Financing Administration suggest that personal health care spending will continue to grow rapidly throughout the next decade. By the beginning of the new millennium, HCFA estimates that PHCE will exceed $1.3 trillion and will reach $2.0 trillion by 2005 (US Department of Health and Human Services, 1996).

8 Many of these proposals included provisions for government-sponsored health insurance available to all ages administered by the Federal government, and financed through payroll taxes. In 1945, President Harry S. Truman proposed a comprehensive medical insurance plan for all persons that would be financed through a 4 percent increase in the Social Security Act's OASI programs. Under this plan, Truman recommended coverage for hospitalization, doctor, nursing, laboratory, and dental services. Even though labor unions supported government-sponsored health insurance, opposition from the AMA, the private health insurance industry, and business groups was overwhelming. Truman's proposal met its demise when lobbying reached its peak in 1949-1950 with the AMA's dire warnings that national health insurance would mean "socialized medicine" and government interference in medical practice (Anderson, 1984; Lammers, 1983; Landers *et al.*, 1989; Lee and Benjamin, 1988).

9 Johnson's bill provided coverage for 60 days of hospital care, instead of 90 days, and also covered persons 65 and over. Almost on queue, the AMA mounted another campaign against government sponsorship. Arguing that the elderly needed more than just hospital benefits, the AMA introduced an alternative plan they called "eldercare." The eldercare plan called for voluntary comprehensive medical insurance for persons 65 and over, if their state government signed up for the program. The program would receive funding by matching federal-state funds and contributions from beneficiaries. A third plan emerged from the House Republican leadership introduced by the ranking member of the House Ways and Means committee, John W. Byrnes. The Byrnes bill provided a voluntary health insurance program for persons 65 and over to cover a proportion of most health care costs. This program would be administered by the federal government and financed by graduated premium contributions based on the individual's ability to pay, contributions from the states, and by annual appropriations from the federal government (Lammers, 1983; Landers *et al.*, 1989; Lee and Benjamin, 1988).

10 Nineteen million elderly persons gained eligibility for Medicare at its passing in 1965. Medicare beneficiaries now number more than 33.8 million persons who are 65 and over, 5.3 million who are permanently disabled, and over 257,000 persons suffering from end-stage renal disease (HCFA, 1998).

11 Medicare covers the following acute and extended care services: hospital care, physician services, post-hospital skilled nursing facility (SNF) care, home health care, laboratory and x-ray services, physical and speech therapy, rural health clinic services, and durable medical equipment and supplies.
12 During fiscal year 1998, coinsurance payments for hospitalization days 61–90 were set at $191 per day (HCFA, 1998).
13 During fiscal year 1998, coinsurance payments for lifetime reserve days were set at $382 a day (HCFA, 1998).
14 In 1993, nearly five million Medicare beneficiaries (13 percent) received some assistance from Medicaid buy-in agreements (Merrell et al., 1997).
15 With the countless proposals offered by the Nixon Administration, Congress, and interest groups, the 1970s also saw a resurgence of public debate over the issue of government-sponsored health insurance. These debates centered on the strengths and weaknesses of regulatory versus market-oriented reforms. Proponents of government-sponsored health insurance favored the implementation of strict controls over the health care industry as a precondition for expanding public financing of health care. Opponents of government-sponsored health insurance favored reforms that would encourage market forces to adopt more efficient methods of health care delivery and promote quality of care standards. By the close of the 1970s, however, the issue of national health insurance was replaced by a focus on domestic and economic issues (Bice, 1984; Koch, 1988; Landers et al., 1989).
16 A study conducted by Pedan and Freeland (1995) found that half of the 373 percent growth-per-capita medical spending from 1960 to 1993 was directly attributable to the growth of insurance coverage from third-party sources.
17 For example, between 1950 and 1980 the real, inflation-adjusted cost of a day in the hospital increased from $22 to $99 (a 450 percent increase). During this same period, direct patient out-of-pocket expenditures only increased from $7 to $9 (only a 29 percent increase) (US DHHS, 1982).
18 In 1987, even though older persons represented only 12 percent of the US population, personal health care spending by older persons accounted for 36 percent of all personal health care expenditures. These expenditures totaled $162 billion and averaged $5,360 per year for each older person.
19 Instead of reimbursing hospitals for their claimed reasonable costs, the new prospective payment system was based on a fixed amount, principally based on length of stay for treating each of 486 conditions called Diagnosis Related Groups (DRGs). The DRG system sorts patients into uniform, clinically compatible groups that have been categorized on the basis of traditional resources used by patients with similar diagnoses. TEFRA regulations gave bonuses to hospitals whose inpatient operating costs per discharge were less than the target rate. If a hospital's discharge costs fell below the target rate, the hospital was reimbursed 50 percent of the difference. Conversely, if a hospital's per-discharge costs were above the target, the hospital received a reimbursement at the target rate plus 25 percent. In this way, TEFRA provided the first incentive system for hospitals to lower their costs on Medicare discharges. An important effect that emerged under the new hospital-based incentive structure was that outpatient services yielded higher profits.
20 One of the criticisms of PPS holds that the DRG system may lead to "compression" in DRG prices. Under the compression model, the prices of the truly high-cost DRGs are set low relative to their actual costs; conversely, the prices of truly low-cost DRGs are set high relative to their costs. Proponents of the compression model claim that hospitals may discriminate against providing service to patients in the high-cost DRGs. Alternatively, compression may encourage some hospitals to specialize by efficiently treating high-cost services, such as services for stroke rehabilitation, chronic obstructive pulmonary disease (COPD), or coronary bypass, at more profitable rates (Koch, 1988). Increases in physician specialization also contribute to rising costs of health care.

Another criticism of the PPS system has been the tendency for hospitals to move some inpatient procedures to outpatient clinics. Under PPS, those procedures performed as part of an outpatient setting are not subject to the DRG-based system. Hospitals faced with declining revenues may place subtle pressures on health care practitioners to use outpatient services instead of inpatient services for specific high-cost procedures (Cochran et al., 1996). Thus, the real issue involves patient safety and quality of care.

There is also criticism of the current system of prospective payment involving the DRG system itself. Much of the debate concerns the fact that the current DRG system lacks a severity-of-illness scale for a patient within a specific DRG. Health services research analysts argue that the current DRG system is inherently biased, because patients with more severe illnesses are usually treated in urban tertiary-care hospitals. These hospitals are seen as a last resort for many patients who suffer from chronic long-term conditions (Altman and Ostby, 1993). Even though this problem appears to be real, no solution or alternative system for disease categorization has been offered.

21 Current enrollments show that about 3.7 million Medicare beneficiaries, or 10 percent of the Medicare population, are enrolled in Medicare HMOs (Butler et al., 1996). As of January 1997, more than 4.9 million Medicare beneficiaries were enrolled in 336 Medicare HMOs nationwide (HCFA, 1998).

22 Under RBRVS, Medicare reimbursement rates are set by evaluating the individual components required to produce physician services not by the prevailing rates of medical specialties. The actual cost components involved in setting reimbursement rates under RBRVS are the physician's work, practice expenses, and the cost of professional liability insurance.

23 For the rural elderly, access to health care has become an increasing problem. Incomes for rural elders are approximately 20 percent lower than metropolitan elders. Reasons for this disparity are low Social Security income, small savings, less widespread payment by private pensions, and few opportunities for part-time work. Lack of formal transportation systems coupled with lower income confounds both access to specialty services in rural communities as well as referral to specialty care services in more distant places. Hospitals in rural communities serve an economically constrained population that does not have widespread health insurance coverage. During 1994, rural community hospitals treated 16 percent of all Medicare inpatient admissions for chronic illnesses requiring multiple services. Yet, thousands of rural communities throughout America have no health care professionals at all. Over half of all hospital closures since 1983 have been in rural areas and one-quarter of all existing rural hospitals are in danger of closing (Alexy and Belcher, 1997). Fewer providers, limited health services, and lower allocation of funds may all contribute to the poorer health status found among the rural elderly (Haglund and Dowling, 1988).

24 Urban health problems arise from the complex interaction of socioeconomic factors, behavior, environment, and disease related to race and ethnicity. In inner-city minority communities, unemployment, lack of child care, violence, AIDS, teen pregnancy, drug abuse, homelessness, and environmental pollution all contribute to the decline in elder's access to care (McBride, 1993). Substantial racial gaps exist in incidences of stroke, heart attack and hypertension adding to the overall morbidity and mortality of minority groups within low-income areas (Frey, Jahnke, and Bullfinch, 1998). Differences in life expectancy and access to care are especially apparent within poor urban black and Hispanic inner-city communities. For example, in 1994, the average life expectancy for African Americans was 69.5, six years lower than that of whites (75.7 years) (Singh, Kochanek, and MacDorman, 1996). Most illnesses in the inner city, such as diabetes, hypertension and congestive heart failure, can be classified as ambulatory care-sensitive conditions, yet those from lower-income and minority groups frequently use emergency rooms as their primary source of care. Disparities between patients' access to care in low-income versus high-income areas are well documented in almost all US cities (Prewitt, 1997).

25 For example, in 1993 direct patient out-of-pocket expenditures were 20 percent (almost $150 billion) of all personal health care spending (US DHHS, 1996). In the same year consumer expenditures for prescription drugs totaled $48.8 billion, and durable medical products totaled $26.0 billion of all out-of-pocket patient spending (Levit et al., 1994).

26 Under the present health care system, the federal Medicare program is the dominant player in meeting the acute needs of the elderly, while long-term care organizations are primarily funded by state-run organizations financed under Medicaid programs (Weiner and Illston, 1994).

References

Aaronson, W.E., Zinn, J.S., and Rosko, M.D. (1994). The success and repeal of the Medicare Catastrophic Coverage Act: A paradoxical lesson for health care reform. *Journal of Health Politics, Policy and Law, 19*, 4, 753–771.

Achenbaum, W.A. (1978). *Old age in the new land: The American experience since 1790*. Baltimore, MD: The Johns Hopkins University Press.

Alexy, B., and Belcher, J. (1997). Rural elderly present need for nursing continuity. *Nursing Economics, 15*, 3, 146–150.

Altman, S.H., and Ostby, E.R. (1993). Paying for hospital care: The impact on federal policy. In E. Ginzberg (Ed.), *Health services research* (pp. 46–68). Cambridge, MA: Harvard University Press.

American Association of Retired Persons. (1997). *A profile of older Americans*. Washington, DC: AARP.

Anderson, G.F. (1997). In search of value: An international comparison of cost, access, and outcomes. *Health Affairs, 16*, 6, 163–171.

Anderson, O.W. (1984). Health services in the United States: A growth enterprise for a hundred years. In T.J. Litman and L.S. Robins (Eds.), *Health politics and policy* (pp. 67–80). New York: John Wiley & Sons.

Berk, M.L., and Schur, C.L. (1998). Access to care: How much difference does Medicaid make? *Health Affairs, 17*, 3, 169–179.

Bice, T.W. (1984). The politics of health care regulation. In T.J. Litman and L.S. Robins (Eds.), *Health politics and policy* (pp. 274–289). New York: John Wiley & Sons.

Binstock, R.H., and Day, C.L. (1996). Aging and politics. In R.H. Binstock and L.K. George (Eds.), *Handbook of aging and the social sciences* (pp. 309–330). San Diego, CA: Academic Press Inc.

Browne, W.P., and Katz, O. (1983). An introduction to public policy and sging. In W.P. Browne and O. Katz (Eds.). *Aging and public policy: The politics of growing old in America*, (pp. 3–18). Westport, CT: Greenwood Press.

Butler, R.N., Sherman, F.T., Rhinehart, E., Klein, S., and Rother, J.C. (1996). Managed care: What to expect as Medicare-HMO enrollment grows. *Geriatrics, 51*, 10, 35–42.

Cochran, C.E., Carr, T.R., Cayer, N.J., and Mayer, L.C. (1996). The double bind: income support or welfare dependence? (pp. 196-248), Health care: Unlimited needs, limited resources (pp. 249-294). In B.A. Gillett (Ed.), *American Public Policy*. New York: St. Martin's Press.

Estes, C.L., and Binney, E.A. (1988). Toward a transformation of health and aging policy. *International Journal of Health Services, 18*, 1, 69–82.

Frey, J.L., Jahnke, H.K., and Bulfinch, E.W. (1998). Differences in stroke between White, Hispanic, and Native American patients: The Barrow Neurological Institute Stroke Database. *Stroke, 29*, 29–33.

Glaser, W. (1984). Health politics: Lessons from abroad. In T.J. Litman and L.S. Robins (Eds.), *Health politics and policy* (pp. 305–339). New York: John Wiley & Sons.

Guadagnoli, E., and McNeil, B.J. (1994). Outcomes research: Hope for the future or the latest rage? *Inquiry, 31*, 1, 14–24.

Haglund, C.L., and Dowling, W.L. (1988). The hospital. In S.J. Williams and P.R. Torrens (Eds.), *Introduction to health services* (3rd ed., pp. 160–211). New York: Delmar Publishers.

Halevy, A., Neal, R.C., and Brody, B.A. (1996). The low frequency of futility in an adult intensive care unit setting. *Archives of Internal Medicine, 156*, 1, 100–104.

Health Care Financing Administration. (1998). Medicare deductible, coinsurance and premium amounts, 1998. Available online: http://www.hcfa.gov/stats/stats.htm.

Health Insurance Association of America. (1992). *Source book of health insurance data.* Table 2.1. Washington DC: Health Insurance Association of America.

Holstein, M., and Minkler, M. (1991). The short life and painful death of the Medicare Catastrophic Coverage Act. *International Journal of Health Services, 21,* 1, 1–16.

Hsiao, W.C., Braun, P., Becker, E.R., Dunn, D.L., Kelly, N., Causino, N., McCabe, M.D., and Rodriguez, E. (1992). Results and impacts of the Resource-Based Relative Value Scale. *Medical Care, 30,* 11 (suppl), NS61–NS79.

Keigher, S.M. (1991). Growing housing hardship among the elderly. In S.M. Keigher (Ed.), *Housing risks and homelessness among the urban elderly* (pp. 1–11). New York: The Hawthorn Press.

King, G. (1994). Health care reform and the Medicare program. *Health Affairs, 13,* 5, 39–43.

Koch, A.L. (1988). Financing health services. In S.J. Williams and P.R. Torrens (Eds.), *Introduction to health services* (3rd ed., pp. 335–370). New York: Delmar Publishers.

Kutza, E.A. (Ed.). (1981). *The benefits of old age.* Chicago: The University of Chicago Press.

Lammers, W.W. (1983). Public policy and the aging. In D.B. James (Ed.), *Issues in public policy: Public policy and the aging* (pp. 89–107, 145–170). Washington, DC: Congressional Quarterly.

Landers, R.K., Rovner, J., and McGuiness, C. (Eds.), (1989). *Aging in America: The federal government's role.* Washington, DC: Congressional Quarterly.

Lee, D.K., Swinburne, A.J., Fedullo, A.J., and Wahl, G.W. (1994). Withdrawing care: Experience in a medical intensive care unit. *Journal of the American Medical Association, 272,* 17, 1358–1361.

Lee, P.R., and Benjamin, A.E. (1988). Health policy and the politics of health care. In S.J. Williams and P.R. Torrens (Eds.), *Introduction to health services* (3rd ed., pp. 457–479). New York: Delmar Publishers.

Levit, K.R., Cowan, C.A., Lasenby, H.C., McDonnell, P.A., Sensenig, A.L., Stiller, J.M., and Won, D.K. (1994). National health spending trends, 1960–1993. *Health Affairs, 13,* 5, 14–31.

Litman, T.J., and Robins, L.S. (Eds.). (1984). *Health politics and policy* (Appendix 2, pp. 345–356). New York: John Wiley & Sons.

Luce, B.R. (1988). Medical technology and its assessment. In S.J. Williams and P.R. Torrens (Eds.), *Introduction to health services* (3rd ed.). (pp. 281–307). New York: Delmar Publishers.

Manton, K.G. (1989). National long-term care survey. University of Michigan. Internet, ICSPR number 09681.

Manton, K.G., Corder, L.S., and Stallard, E. (1993). Changes in the use of personal assistance and special equipment form 1982 to 1989: Results from the 1982 and 1989 NLTCS. *The Gerontologist, 33,* 2, 169–176.

McBride, D. (1993). Black America: From community health care to crisis medicine. *Journal of Health Politics, Policy and Law, 18,* 2, 320–336.

Merrell, K., Colby, D.C., and Hogan, C. (1997). Medicare beneficiaries covered by Medicaid buy-in agreements. *Health Affairs 16,* 1, 175–184.

Morgan, R.O., Virnig, B.A., DeVito, C.A., and Persily, N.A. (1997). The Medicare HMO revolving door: The healthy go in and the sick go out. *The New England Journal of Medicine, 337,* 169–175.

National Center for Health Statistics. (1997). *Health, United States, 1996–97 and injury chartbook* (Table 136). Hyattsville, Maryland.

Pappas, G., Queen, S., Hadden, W., and Fisher, G. (1993). The increasing disparity in mortality between socioeconomic groups in the United States, 1960 and 1986. *The New England Journal of Medicine, 329,* 2, 103–109.

Peden, E.A., and Freeland, M.S. (1995). A historical analysis of medical spending growth, 1960–1993. *Health Affairs, 14,* 2, 235–244.

Prewitt, E. (1997). Inner-city health care. *Annals of Internal Medicine, 126*, 6, 485–490.
Preston, S.H. (1993). Demographic change in the United States. In K.G. Manton, B.H. Singer and R.M. Suzman (Eds.), *Forcasting the health of elderly populations* (pp. 51–78). New York: Springer-Verlag.
Richardson, M. (1988). Mental health services: Growth and development of a system. In S.J. Williams and P.R. Torrens (Eds.), *Introduction to health services* (3rd ed., pp. 255–277). New York, Delmar Publishers.
Rowland, D. (1993). Financing health care for elderly Americans. In E. Ginzberg (Ed.), *Health services research* (pp. 126–160). Cambridge, MA: Harvard University Press.
Schapira, D.V., Studnicki, J ., and Bradham, D.D. (1993). Intensive care, survival, and expense of treating critically ill cancer patients. *Journal of the American Medical Association, 269*, 6, 783–786.
Schapira, D.V., Studnicki, J., Bradham, D.D., Wolf, P.A., Jarret, A.R., and Aziz, N.M. (1993). Heroic measures when treating patients with hematologic malignancies: The economic cost of survival. *International Journal of Oncology, 3*, 987–993.
Singh, G.K., Kochanek, K.D., and MacDorman, M.F. (1996). Advance report of final mortality statistics, 1994. *Monthly vital statistics report, 45*, (3 supp). Hyattsville, MD: National Center for Health Statistics.
Social Security Administration. (1999). *1999 SSI Annual Report*. Washington: US Government Printing Office.
Torrens, P. (1988). Historical evolution and overview of health services in the United States. In S.J. Williams and , P.R. Torrens (Eds.), *Introduction to health services* (3rd ed.). (pp. 3–31). New York, Delmar Publishers.
US Bureau of the Census. (1993). *Poverty in the United States: 1992* (Table 6). (Current population reports: Series P60–185). Washington, DC: US Government Printing Office.
US Bureau of the Census. (1996). *65+ in the United States* (Current population reports: Special studies, P23–190). Washington, DC: US Government Printing Office.
US Bureau of the Census. (1997). *Voting and registration in the election of November 1992* (Table 2). (Current population reports: Series P20–466). Washington, DC: US Government Printing Office.
US Department of Agriculture. (1998). Nutrition Program Facts. Food Stamp Program. Online, available HTTP: http://www.usda.gov/fcs/stamps/fspfor~1.htm.
US Department of Commerce, Bureau of the Census. (1997). *The statistical abstract of the United States* (117th ed.). Washington, DC: US Department of Commerce, Bureau of the Census.
US Department of Health and Human Services. (1982). *Final report: The 1981 White House Conference on Aging* (Vol. 1). Washington, DC: R.S. Schweiker.
US Department of Health and Human Services. (1996). *Health care financing review, Medicare and Medicaid statistical supplement*. (Figure 1, p. 10; Figure 11, p. 29; Figure 87, p. 179; and Figure 90, p. 185). Baltimore, MD: Health Care Financing Administration, Office of Research and Demonstrations.
US Department of Housing and Urban Development. (1998). Recommendations and Actions: HUD09: Consolidate Section 8 housing certificates and vouchers. Online, available HTTP: http://www.npr.gov/library/reports/hud09.html.
US General Accounting Office. (1997). Medicare HMOs: Potential effects of a limited enrollment period policy. Report to the Chairman, Committee on Finance, US Senate, GAO/HEHS-97–50. Washington, DC: US General Accounting Office.
Weiner, J.M., and Illston, L.H. (1994). Health care reform in the 1990s: Where does long-term care fit in? *The Gerontologist, 34*, 3, 402–408.

4 Changing meanings of frail old people and the Japanese welfare state

John Creighton Campbell

The passage of the *Kaigo Hoken* or Long-Term Care Insurance (LTCI) bill by the Japanese legislature in late 1997 signifies a major expansion, and indeed a qualitative change, in the development of social policy in Japan. Japan is only the second large country in the world to adopt a social insurance model for long-term care. The other such program was started by Germany in 1994, and was hailed by analysts as "virtually unparalleled in Western welfare states after 1975" (Goetting, Haug, and Hinrichs, 1994, p. 288) In fact Japan's program is much larger and in some ways more innovative than the prior German example.

The *Kaigo Hoken* program, when it starts in 2000, will collect premiums from all Japanese people with incomes aged 40 and above (including the elderly), and will provide institutional or community-based long-term care services to everyone 65 and over certified as having a physical or mental disability (and also to people over 40 with an "aging-type" disability such as Alzheimer's disease or stroke). The major differences with the German LTCI (*Pflegeversicherung*) program is that a lesser degree of disability is required for eligibility, the benefits are considerably higher at any level of disability, and benefits must be taken in services rather than as a cash allowance.

In this chapter I will try to place *Kaigo Hoken* into the context of the development of Japanese social policy by showing how it represents significant changes in basic assumptions.

Old-age policy in the Japanese welfare state

For several decades now, to a much greater extent than in any other advanced nation, social policy in Japan has been about the elderly. Since the late 1950s, most of the important policy changes in the social policy area, in terms of public attention, expense, or impact on society, have been explicitly aimed at the older people of the present or the future. These include:

- Universal public pensions in the late 1950s
- "Free" medical care for the elderly and the doubling of pension benefits in the "first year of the welfare era" in the early 1970s

- Major rationalization of the old-age health care and pension systems in the mid-1980s
- The "Gold Plan" to expand services for the frail elderly in 1990
- Long-Term Care Insurance in 1997

The only other social policy changes that are arguably of similar magnitude in this period would be universal health insurance (at the same time as universal pensions), reform in the unemployment compensation system in 1975, and imposition of effective cost-control in medical care in the early 1980s.

If we dropped one step down, to a medium level of magnitude or social significance, we would note such old-age policy changes as the development of service programs at the national and local levels from the mid-1960s, the raising of the permissible mandatory retirement age to 60 and a host of old-age employment-promotion programs from the mid-1970s, innovations in institutional care in the mid-1980s, and so forth. These would rank with relatively few developments in other social policy areas, including the children's allowance in the early 1970s, the Equal Employment for Women Act of 1985 and other gender-equality programs, or various changes in minority policy for *burakumin* and Koreans.[1] In short, Japanese social policy has largely been about the elderly.

There are two sets of reasons, negative and positive, for why old people have loomed so large in the recent development of the welfare state in Japan compared to other advanced nations. The negative reasons have to do with a lack of competition: first, problems like poverty, minority integration, unemployment, and so forth have not been absent in Japan but at least since the 1950s have not been as big as in many other countries; second, some problems such as discrimination against women or the disabled may be particularly bad in Japan in an objective sense, but for whatever reason have not been as politicized as elsewhere. The elderly have had a fairly clear field.[2]

On the positive side, it can be said that the elderly deserve particular attention in Japan. As everybody knows, their share in the population has been expanding at the most rapid rate in the history of the world, and before long Japan will have a higher proportion of old people than anyplace else – Japan as an "aging society" has been one of the most popular clichés for journalists, politicians and bureaucrats for many years. Moreover, it is widely believed, Japan's traditional ways of taking care of older people are breaking down or at any rate are clearly inadequate for their rapidly rising numbers. Therefore it is logical that something should be done.

It might also be argued that Japan's Confucian heritage of respect for elders makes this area of social policy much more attractive to everybody than programs aimed at other groups. When politicians have gotten behind major expansions of old-age policy, they saw the payoff much more as improving their image with voters in general than in gaining support from older people themselves.[3] In short, there are ample reasons why the story of the development of the Japanese welfare state for the last 40 years or so is mostly about policy for older people.

The evolution of old-age problems

Over that 40-year span, the nature of old-age policy has changed – or rather, after one set of perceived problems was addressed with a new program or some other policy change, attention moved on to another set of problems. I have characterized this evolution of "problem consciousness" through the 1980s as going through three stages (Campbell, 1992):

- *Rōgo mondai*, the "aging problem," or people worrying about what will happen to them when they get old. The response was expansion of public pensions in the 1950s and early 1960s.
- *Rōjin mondai*, the "old-people problem," or concerns about poverty, lack of medical care and other plights of current old people. These were addressed with a series of new programs or big expansions in the early 1970s.
- *Kōreika shakai mondai*, the "aging-society problem," or the impact of so many old people on Japan's overall economy and society (or more specifically fiscal system). These concerns led to rationalizations of the pension, old-age medical care and social welfare systems associated with "administrative reform" (*gyōsei kaikaku*) in the 1980s.

Of course, these problems never went away: each drew at least some attention continuously, among decision-makers and specialists if not necessarily the general public. All the various programs for the elderly were adjusted incrementally from time to time, and for that matter the understanding of the nature of each problem itself might change profoundly. In particular, the "old-people problem" came back to prominence in the late 1980s, but in a different enough form to constitute a new stage in the evolution of old-age policy and, perhaps, of the Japanese welfare state as a whole.

The old old-people problem

The initial large-scale public awareness of the *rōjin mondai* that emerged around 1970 had two direct sources and a key background condition. One source was active proselytizing on behalf of the plight of older people, mainly by Ministry of Health and Welfare (MHW) officials interested in expanding various service programs.[4] The second source was direct action by a political entrepreneur, Tokyo's progressive governor Minobe Ryōkichi, who initiated "free medical care" for the elderly partly to differentiate his own people-oriented platform from business-dominated Liberal Democratic Party (LDP) policies. The background condition was super-rapid economic growth, which was bringing a more and more obvious and deplorable gap in quality of life between younger participants in the boom (real wages roughly tripled from 1960 to 1970) and older retirees – the generation whose sacrifices in war and recovery had made prosperity possible.

With a lot of oversimplification, the old-people problem that emerged in that era, and the corresponding changes in public policy, can be characterized as having two dimensions. The distinction was between "normal" older people and those seen as needing special help – for the most part defined by whether or not the older person was living with his or her children.

Policy for "normal" old people

In 1970 a substantial majority of the elderly lived in the same household with a child, in what was conventionally seen as the traditional Japanese way. Under the surface, however, the older person's role within the household was changing. In what we could call the "pure" traditional pattern, based on a farming or shop-owning household, the father would stay in charge until he handed over the headship of household and farm or shop to his designated heir (ideally the oldest son). In exchange, he and his wife, or his widow, would be cared for by the heir's wife. On the one hand, the older people would be deeply respected; on the other, they would become dependent on the younger couple in all aspects of life, including financial support.

Actually even in the olden days there were many exceptions to this pattern, but the point here is that by the 1960s and 1970s this "pure" traditional form applied only to a small minority of cases. For most households, no longer was there a transfer of authority over its source of income from old to young – the house itself was now the main asset to be handed over in exchange for care. This decline of the older generation's economic bargaining power was matched by a deterioration in their legal authority (under the postwar reforms) and no doubt in their status based on social norms as well. Clearly even the older people who lived with children were in a much weaker position than in the "traditional" household, at least as it was seen in the national nostalgia.

Many Japanese saw this weakness and dependency as unfortunate. It was sad for the old people and it was bad for the young people as well since they were expected to take care of their parents (or worse still, parents-in-law) without much direct compensation. The resulting resentments and backbiting threatened to poison everyday life within the household. These perceptions, along with more the general sense of social and economic fairness to the older generation mentioned earlier, brought a series of policy changes that would lessen dependence among "normal" older people. Special loans so people could add an extra room to their house, senior centers that would get the mother-in-law out of the house (and hair) of the wife for a while, and various sorts of life-enrichment (*ikigai*) programs were expanded rapidly, and much discussed. However, by far the most important policies were pensions and medical care.

That is, from the 1960s into the 1980s, pension benefits were improved step by step. The first stage was seen as allowing the old people to give their grandchildren gifts or pocket money, but before long it was regarded as normal for the older couple to pull their own weight or a bit more in keeping the household going economically (by covering all their own costs, or by contributing to the overall budget). Similarly, "free" medical care (providing treatment without the individual copayment, which had been 50 percent until the early 1970s) meant that older people could now get medical care without having to ask their children for the money. In fact usage of care by older people shot up quickly, from being much lower than among the middle-aged to much higher, indicating that the financial constraint had been quite significant.

Although direct evidence is hard to come by, it may be safely assumed that these public programs did substantially change dependency relationships within the household. The interesting point compared with western nations is that even though the elderly were now much less dependent, the pattern of living together with children was still regarded as normal in Japan. In fact, although coresidence continued to decline, the rate of change was the same (about a one-percent drop a year) in the period when pensions and other benefits were rapidly improving as in the earlier period when they were on a much lower plateau.

Policy for "left-out" old people

Turning now to the other aspect of the *rōjin mondai*, the concern for the "non-normal" older people who did not live with their children, we might first observe that the continuous decline in the coresidency rate is a classic half-full or half-empty question. On the one hand, its moderate pace and the fact that even today more than half the 65+ population lives with children in Japan (compared to no more than 15 percent in other advanced nations) seem to indicate stability. On the other hand, particularly around 1970, the same trend was widely cited in Japan as indicating rapid social change.

That is, the reason why people thought that family care would no longer be enough was not that old people were getting poorer or sicker – the opposite was the case – but was that the Japanese family was changing or even disintegrating. The shift from a household-based to a company-based economy left older people with no economic role, urbanization left elders behind in the countryside, houses in overcrowded cities were too small for an extra bedroom, an emphasis on "my-home-ism" and even conjugal love made the small nuclear family the ideal middle-class lifestyle. The wistful hope of the time was for a lifestyle of *kaa tsuki baba nuki*, "with car without grandma."

All these factors were seen as causes of the decline in cohabitation, which would soon intensify so that more and more older people would not be able to live with their children. Those are the people perceived as having to rely on the government – indeed, the commonest term for elders needing special attention at the time was *hitorigurashi*, "living alone" (and in common parlance this category was blurred with elderly couples living independently). The second dimension of the policy response to the "old-people problem," starting in the 1960s and accelerating in the 1970s, was programs aimed at needy elderly in this sense, such as old-people's homes, nursing homes, home helpers, various sorts of checks or alarms in case of sudden illness, and so forth.

Of course, low income or a physical or mental disability also were part of neediness, but mainly in combination with a lack of family support – just being poor or sick was not as legitimate a subject for public responsibility as "living alone." That point is clear from the way eligibility was determined. Virtually all of these programs were administered by local governments (though most partially financed by the national government), so to obtain the service or admission to a home one would apply to the municipal government or the Welfare Office (*Fukushi Jimusho*). That is, these programs were managed similarly to public assistance, and there was usually either a means test for eligibility or (later in the period) a sliding scale for payments depending on income.

However, anecdotal evidence indicates that the means test often was not applied very rigorously, and even with sliding scales many people paid nothing or small amounts even if they had a decent income. That was true for "live-alones" (and elderly couples). Older people living with their children, even when their own incomes or the household income were low, found it very difficult to be approved. With regard to home helpers (the largest community-care program), provision to other than live-alones was never prohibited in the regulations, but it was approved very rarely.

An even more telling example is nursing homes. This program had been started back in 1963 in part as a response to the problems in old people's homes (*yōgo rōjin hōmu*) caused by residents with more medical needs than could be handled by their limited staff. However, they were still very much welfare (*fukushi*) institutions – due to pressure from the medical side of the Ministry of Health and Welfare, they had to be called "special care homes for the aged" (*tokubetsu yōgo rōjin hōmu*) rather than any term that had a medical or nursing connotation. And although in principle these institutions were supposed to be for people who needed medical care, admission decisions were made by local welfare bureaucrats, using no explicit medical criteria, and in fact many nursing home residents were not very disabled at all.

On the other hand, relatively few people admitted to nursing homes had any relatives who even conceivably were able to offer support. Probably the most-told anecdotes about Japanese old-age policy are tales of rejections for nursing-home admissions because a daughter-in-law or daughter was available. If she was employed she would be told just to quit. The conventional wisdom had it that the only way an ailing elder with children could get into a nursing home would be to convince the local bureaucrat in charge that the family members hated each other so much that living together would be impossible. This picture is exaggerated but was not without truth.

To recap, the underlying rationale for most Japanese social policy for older people divided them into two groups: those who lived with their children, for whom the main goal was to lessen dependency and achieve a measure of equality; and the "live-alones" who might require substantial support from the government to lead a decent life. I should emphasize that both of these goals were significant and worthwhile. They were quite progressive compared to the implicit government stance prior to the 1960s – that older people living with their families needed no government care, and those without families should get only minimal help (public assistance or an old-people's home). However, this approach was clearly becoming unrealistic in the late 1980s.

The new old-people problem

Since this is not a narrative account of Japanese old-age policy, I will not pause long for the policy changes of the early to mid 1980s, the era when the "aging-society problem" of the impact on overall economic and social conditions came to the fore. Many observers see this as a time of major cutbacks, a successful effort to "roll back the embryonic efforts at state support for social welfare," and a return to reliance on the traditional family system (Pempel, 1989). It is true that a lot of conservative rhetoric about a "Japanese-style welfare society" supports that view, but the impact on actual policy was much more moderate. In fact, my interpretation is that the pension and health-care systems for older people were rationalized and made practical by reforming some of the unworkable or unrealistically generous innovations of the enthusiastic early 1970s (Campbell, 1992, Chapters 9–10). Certainly both aspects of the response to the "old-people problem," dependency-reduction or equalization policies for "ordinary" older people, and the policy of expanding institutional or community-based care for those left out of the family system, continued without major change.

Toward the end of the decade, moreover, an impression grew that these responses were not enough and, in effect, that the "old-people problem" itself had to be rethought. Perhaps one source of this impression was actually the conservative rhetoric itself, which emphasized the "crisis" of rapid population aging on the one hand and the virtues of warm family care on the other. To many Japanese that seemed a contradiction – they saw the family as strained by the burdens of caring for older people even now, let alone when the numbers would be so much greater in the future. The point that care by families really meant care by women, and that more and more women were interested in outside employment, was also being expressed with increasing force.

Ideological contradictions aside, at the practical level it was becoming apparent that existing programs for the aged were inadequate or inappropriate. The most dramatic evidence was that enormous numbers of older people were living in hospitals, most with little or no need for intensive medical care. The big surge in admissions had come soon after "free medical care" started in 1973. The reforms of the early 1980s had added only a small daily copayment so that even with some extra charges it was often cheaper to live in a hospital than at home. It was easy to get in – a doctor at the hospital (if a small hospital, usually the owner) just had to give an appropriate diagnosis for admission; there was no procedure (and little incentive) for discharge if the patient improved. Such patients were profitable enough particularly in the early years to bring a boom in private hospital construction and no doubt some active recruiting of patients.

Nursing homes or for that matter some kind of "sheltered housing" would have been adequate for most of these people. However, the former had too few beds, and a major expansion would have required a lot of public capital investment. The latter had not really been developed in Japan except for old-style old-people's homes. Both were means-tested "welfare" programs and so stigmatized in most people's eyes. Similarly, home helpers and the other community-based services that could help keep frail people out of institutions altogether were too scarce and were usually means-tested and stigmatized.

Another important point is that many of these elderly long-term hospital residents did have families and got along with them fine. They could be living with their children – and should be, under the usual assumptions – but they or their children or both preferred not. If more community-based services or sheltered housing were available to people with families, at reasonable cost and without the welfare stigma, perhaps most of them would not want to go into a hospital (which was not in most cases a very attractive environment).

Having so many old people in hospitals severely undercut the assumptions underlying Japanese old-age policy. For example, it was long contended that the low percentage of the elderly in nursing homes (just over 1 percent of the 65+ population) was evidence of a distinctive Japanese preference for family over institutional care – in fact one often hears this claim even today, even though when one adds in long-term elderly inpatients in hospitals the institutionalized proportion goes up to around normal levels for advanced countries (a bit above 6 percent, slightly higher than in the United States).

To policy makers, embarrassment about the high rate of hospitalization was less a difficulty than various practical problems. Hospital care is intrinsically expensive, even in Japan, and even after a set of reforms in the 1980s that made hospitals with many elderly patients more like nursing homes, with fewer doctors and more aides, and with reimbursement on a capitated (per patient-day) rather than fee-for-service basis. These reforms did help constrain costs to an extent but did not decrease usage very much – after all, there were now all those beds to be filled.

A second problem about hospitalization is that it is paid for by health insurance, which was under increasing fiscal strain mainly due to rapidly growing expenditures on old-age health care, especially inpatient care. Most of this spending actually comes directly from the health-insurance premiums paid by younger people via a cross-subsidization scheme; they were complaining about the added burdens and the government was finding management of health insurance finance increasingly difficult.

Cutting down on hospitalization thus became an important policy goal, and the idea that the best way to prevent expensive institutionalization is to provide more community-based services became common among Japanese social-policy experts, as indeed it had among their colleagues in other advanced nations.[5] Combined with the heightened worries among citizens about the implications of population aging for themselves and for Japanese society – as perceived by a powerful entrepreneurial politician – this diagnosis led to a major policy change in 1990.

The Gold Plan

The Gold Plan, or Ten-Year Strategy to Promote Health Care and Welfare for the Elderly, was the invention of Hashimoto Ryūtarō. He drew on his varied experiences as Minister of Finance, Secretary-General and therefore chief election strategist of the Liberal Democratic Party, and long-time "boss" of the social-policy field (including service as Minister of Health and Welfare). His main purpose was to counter attacks from the Japan Socialist Party (JSP) on the new consumption tax, enacted in spring, 1989, that had already contributed to a crushing LDP defeat in the summer Upper House election. The Gold Plan was a campaign promise before the February 1990 general election to demonstrate that consumption tax revenues were in fact needed to meet the problems of the aging society, and would not (as the JSP had alleged) be frittered away on military spending and the like.

The plan itself called for an enormous increase over ten years in community-based services for frail older people, by expanding existing programs (e.g. tripling home helpers, and still bigger increases in day care and short stay) and creating some new ones (e.g. home care centers). Institutional care was initially not given special attention, but after a strong protest from provider groups and specialists, who were a bit more realistic about the potentials of community care for the very frail, it was decided also to more than double nursing-home beds (See Chapter 2 by D. Maeda, this volume.)

Campaign promises and grandiose government plans are as likely to fall by the wayside in Japan as elsewhere, but the Gold Plan turned out to be real. Most of its yearly targets were being met, and in 1994, realizing that even these numbers were quite inadequate to meet demand, officials devised a New Gold Plan with higher targets and had it approved with no difficulties by the cabinet. The great popularity of the community-based services, once available, effectively refuted another element of the old conventional wisdom, that Japanese would not want outside services coming into their homes unless in extremis.

Indeed, the underlying logic of the Gold Plan, old and new, was that these services were for "ordinary" old people, not just for those unfortunate enough to get left out of the traditional family. In practice as well as in rhetoric, older people living with children were welcomed, means-testing was abolished or sharply attenuated, and the application process was simplified (e.g. for many services the application went to the local home care center rather than the Welfare Office). The term "care" (*kaigo*) came into common parlance – it sounded new and unstigmatized, and did not exclude medical care the way "welfare" (*fukushi*) did.

It is fair to say, then, that the Gold Plan signified a major expansion of the Japanese welfare state by acknowledging that ordinary people, not some residual social category like people without families, are legitimate recipients of special governmental help. That is an important step beyond the government's earlier assumption of some responsibility for equalization, by redistributing money to make up for older people not having jobs and being likelier to get sick. But was the Gold Plan itself a real solution to the problem of care for the frail elderly?

The need to do more

For several reasons, the Gold Plan can be called *chūto hanpa*, a halfway remedy. It was too small to fulfill the implicit promise of government responsibility for the frail elderly. For a time it appeared that it could simply be expanded incrementally – the New Gold Plan – but in fact it lacked the financial and administrative infrastructure required for a larger program. Facing up to the question of what kind of infrastructure should be adopted led to a further important step in the development of the Japanese welfare state.

Although the Gold Plan was a great leap forward in provisions for frail older people, it was not big enough to be a comprehensive solution to the problem on the one hand, was too big to manage on the other. Even at the original Gold Plan levels, services for frail old people were getting unwieldy. On top of a set of intractable old problems – notably the irrational differences in burdens, services, management, and quality among the three main forms of institutional care (hospitals, nursing homes, and "old-age health facilities") – there were increasing difficulties in operating the proliferating community-based services. There was no real coordination, standards for eligibility were unclear, and the management of the various organizations providing services was far from systematic. All these problems would become much more serious with a big expansion, as would the overarching issue of how it would all be paid for.

In essence, there were three possibilities: standing pat, extending the logic of the Gold Plan by creating a comprehensive system of governments services financed by tax revenues, or changing course and taking a social insurance approach.[6] Standing pat would have been tough. First, there were two big pressures for change: active support from the general public, and government officials' worries about the serious difficulties they would face in health care and other policy areas if the problems of the frail elderly were not effectively handled. Second, it is hard to see what could have been done about eligibility, deciding who should get services on some consistent basis. Third, the managerial and financial problems noted above would have been a continued irritant. Doing nothing was not an attractive alternative.

Scandinavian style vs. social insurance

So, in my view, it was virtually necessary to invent a new system. The most obvious direction is what can be called the Scandinavian model: a comprehensive system of services provided by government employees, paid for by tax revenues passing through the regular budget, with decisions about eligibility and how much service is needed left up to a government official (often at the agency providing the service). Of course there are many variations within this framework, particularly in the interface with medical care and other social programs and the division of responsibility between municipal, regional and national government. Note also that the Scandinavian model is associated with high levels of service and cost, but structurally it can also operate with quite severe limitations on spending (as in the United Kingdom today).

This approach to care for the frail elderly grew out of welfare programs (poor houses, public assistance) for the poverty-stricken, but in Scandinavia it went far beyond such origins and became an explicit legislative right to such support for all citizens, along with something close to granting eligibility to anyone who asks for it. In recent years the quantity of services has to some extent been limited by budget restrictions on providers, but the level of benefits is certainly quite high by any standard.

There is no indication that Hashimoto Ryūtarō had the Scandinavian model in mind when he proposed the Gold Plan. However, the contents of that plan were picked up from Japan's existing programs, which were mainly within the social welfare tradition, and then from policy ideas espoused by specialists in and around the Ministry of Health and Welfare, particularly its welfare (*fukushi*) side centered on the Bureau of Social Affairs. These officials and their associated provider interest groups and experts were deeply influenced by British and Scandinavian social policy. Then and still today, they were convinced that having government directly provide services that would be paid for from tax revenues is the fairest and most efficient way to take care of frail older people.

The historical lineage of the Gold Plan, the beliefs of most providers and specialists in the field, and the fact that in the early 1990s the Scandinavian model was really the only systematic, comprehensive approach to care for the frail elderly that anyone knew much about would all seem to make this direction the logical one for Japan. However, it had two big political disadvantages: it required too much tax money, and it was too bureaucratic.

The alternative was a social insurance system. The fact that a program along those lines was enacted in Germany in 1994 provided legitimacy for that approach, although it is likely that Japan would have taken this course even without the prior example. Its financing was more feasible, since 50 percent of the costs would be covered by a new social insurance contribution, which was thought to be more palatable than a tax increase. The other 50 percent would come from taxes, though oddly enough this was a plus rather than a minus for the Ministry of Finance, which normally can be expected to oppose new spending. That is because the Ministry was desperate to hike the new consumption tax from 3 to 5 percent, and LTCI provided a popular pretext for doing so.

It is also odd that such a big new government program could be perceived as anti-bureaucratic. The key point is that the social insurance approach establishes a genuine right to receive services based on explicit eligibility standards, rather than having to ask some bureaucrat for help. The benefits are seen as coming from one's own past contributions rather than other people's taxes. And there is more room for consumer choice and the market.

The latter argument was quite attractive in Japan among conservative politicians and indeed for the general public. Anti-bureaucracy sentiments are nearly as widespread in Japan as in the United States. Given all the anecdotes about arbitrary denials of services at the Welfare Office and the like, the idea of giving the individual the right to choose was naturally popular. Frequently expressed notions were that old people themselves would be given the power to achieve an independent life and the system should be "user oriented."[7] Many also thought that market demand and competition would be the best way to stimulate the creation of new services on a large scale, and to ensure responsiveness and quality, as compared with relying on local government officials to be competent and energetic enough to do the job.

These points help explain why the more market-based social insurance model was popular once it was proposed, but perhaps more important at the early stages was support from an influential group in the social policy field – the bureaucrats and academics connected with health insurance, notably the leading promoter of a new program for long-term care, Okamitsu Nobuharu.[8] In a way the philosophical debate between social welfare and social insurance principles as most applicable to long-term care emerged as a factional struggle between two wings of MHW officialdom, in which the bureaucrats associated with the Social Affairs Bureau, and their allies among practitioners and experts, put up enough of a struggle to drag out the process but in the end decisively lost.

A Japan–Germany difference: services not cash

Although *Pflegeversicherung* provided the model for *Kaigo Hoken*, the two systems are not identical. In several important respects Japan looks much more generous than Germany:

- A lower threshold for eligibility
- Much higher allowances for a given level of disability
- A less rigorous assessment process that excludes a voice for the insurance carrier
- No caps on overall spending growth.

There are several reasons why Japan would opt for a larger and "softer" system than Germany, and I will just mention them briefly. On the Japan side, first, the fact that both nursing home and especially hospital care was already almost completely covered by government or health insurance for most older people, without a means test, meant that the top-level benefits had to be high enough to match. Second, not a few older people were getting more-or-less free community-based services even though they were not really very disabled; fears of knocking them out of the new system required the lowest category (which is called "needing aid" rather than "needing care," *yōshien* vs. *yōkaigo*) at about $500 a month, expected to cover about half the beneficiaries at enormous cost. Third, the eligibility process was made independent of local government (who are the insurers) largely in reaction to the arbitrary and highly bureaucratic system of old.

These considerations did not apply to Germany. I will not go more deeply into that system here, except to note that spending on LTCI in Germany is very carefully hedged, not only at the micro level of having eligibility decided by doctors that work for the insurers, but at the macro level by prohibiting any spending except from the specific social insurance premiums, and by specifying ceiling amounts in the legislation – not even cost-of-living adjustments can be made without passing a new law.

The reason for these tight strictures, I think, lies in the decision-making process. LTCI in Germany was the product of a debate between political parties who had been fighting over social insurance for decades. The aspects of LTCI that were seen as problematical and so became controversial were the same issues that these parties always fought about, mainly about how it should be financed, and (reflecting some bitter experiences of the past) how long-term spending could be kept from getting out of control. Incidentally, the German debate almost ignored several points that are actually quite fundamental to the problems of long-term care (especially in the community, the main focus), such as what services are appropriate, who should provide them, and how complex "care plans" should be drawn up and supervised. That was because they were new and did not fit comfortably into a discourse about social insurance.

Japan talked long and hard about those aspects because many participants in its debate, which mostly took place in and around the Ministry of Health and Welfare, were vitally concerned with service delivery in general and what would happen to existing clients in particular. On the other hand, lacking the institutional legacy of debates over social insurance along these lines, issues about financing received little attention. In fact, the single most surprising fact about the enactment of *Kaigo Hoken*, in my view, is that the opposition from *fiscal* conservatives was so weak. But then, *social* conservatives did not play the role one might expect either – a point raised by another comparison with the German program.

It was noted earlier that a key argument for the social insurance model in Japan was based on consumer sovereignty and market competition. Of course, consumer choice would be maximized and the strain on government capacity minimized if beneficiaries simply received a cash benefit, leaving them to obtain whatever long-term care services they wanted on their own. Presumably many would compensate a family member for providing care, or maybe just keep the money and somehow make do. German LTCI does offer such a cash allowance, although its value is lower than if the service option is selected, and in fact some 80 percent of beneficiaries made that choice (which incidentally meant that overall spending was much lower than had been estimated at the start).

The main rationale for the cash allowance in Germany was the desire to maintain support by family members; it was thought that a daughter could be tempted away from looking for a regular job if she were paid by her parent for delivering care. In fact, the system pays social security premiums for the caregiver to make this role even closer to regular employment. Some conservative politicians in Japan called for a cash allowance for similar reasons, to reward and maintain the role of the family in caregiving, but the idea did not draw much support from the public or among specialists and never got very close to being included in the law.

Remarkably enough, a key reason why the cash allowance did not succeed in Japan was the power of an essentially feminist idea – that current patterns of care for the elderly exploit women, and the only way that situation would be changed is by a massive increase in the use of formal services. A cash allowance might raise the family's standard of living a bit, but in most cases would not really liberate the caregiver. This argument was put forward forcefully during the process of preparing the draft legislation by women who were MHW advisory committee members, perhaps accounting for why the cash allowance alternative was excluded early on, but it is notable that this point of view continued to prevail even when the discussion became more public.[9]

So on the one hand, Japan had decided not to expand long-term care services provided directly by budgeted funds; on the other, by not offering a cash allowance, it precluded the possibility that many beneficiaries would choose to purchase services informally, from family members or acquaintances, or perhaps not at all. The alternative that was left is in effect a voucher system: the beneficiary would be allocated a certain amount of "money," but it could be used only to purchase designated services from an approved provider. The provider might be a government agency, but it could also be a nonprofit community organization, a hospital, or a commercial profit-making company.[10]

So far as I know, there is no precedent in the world for such a large-scale introduction of a voucher system, and the question of how all these services can be developed so quickly is hard to answer. Everyone is worried that a couple of million people will suddenly have all this purchasing power and they will have nothing to buy. Although at the early stages the most intense pressures will probably center on demand for institutional care, because many people now on waiting lists for nursing homes in urban areas will now have a "right" to be admitted, the fact that rates of institutionalization (including hospitals) is already at rates comparable to other advanced nations indicates that one way or another enough beds can probably be found.

The situation for community-based care is different. Current usage rates are relatively low in Japan; local surveys imply that the number of people eligible for LTCI will be two to four times the number currently receiving any sort of services (many at very low levels). In principle, it would seem that all the new money to come from LTCI would be enough to pay for the new services, and since most community-based services (unlike institutions) do not require much capital investment, enormous up-front spending should not be required. Still, is it realistic to expect that enough entrepreneurs and the necessary labor force will appear spontaneously? Municipal governments have been given a vague responsibility to see that enough services will be available, but it is not clear how they are to carry out this role.

It will be fascinating to see how this massive social experiment will play out. My guess is that the problem of inadequate supply will cause a lot of trouble for a couple of years, but in fact the market will work and community-based services will expand rapidly to meet demand (although to the discomfort of social welfare professionals, hospitals will probably dominate the market). I think the likelihood of overspending is a much more serious concern – in early small-scale tests of the assessment mechanism, both the numbers deemed eligible and the levels of service granted came out higher than the government had estimated. It is not uncommon around the world for new entitlement programs to be much more expensive than anticipated. Even the official estimates for *Kaigo Hoken*, which do not appear realistic, call for over $50 billion of spending per year by 2010 – if that is underestimated even just by 20 percent or so, the implications for fiscal policy and indeed for the overall social security system would be serious.

Conclusion

But this essay is not intended to be a comprehensive assessment of *Kaigo Hoken*. My aim has been to place this large new program into the context of the development of the welfare state. One point is that, in my view, this is the first time that Japanese social policy really deserved to "make the news" internationally. In this era of overall retrenchment, long-term care for the frail elderly is today the area where expansions of the welfare state in the advanced nations are most likely. Japan's program did take off from an earlier German example to an extent, but it is considerably bigger, and its reliance on vouchers is quite distinctive. If it works, this approach may become an important model for other nations.

Second, this program is of course a big and very important step for Japan. In terms of the quantity and (one hopes) quality of services available to frail elderly people, Japan could before long be near the Scandinavian level, albeit without as much bureaucracy. That is an enormous policy change. Frailty among the elderly even when they are ordinary people – not those left out of the system due to poverty or not having relatives available – is now seen as a risk that should be borne by society rather than the individual or family.

Third, what does this new program say about the role of families in the Japanese welfare state? When the Gold Plan was enacted, it was derided by many progressive feminists as just another gimmick to keep Japanese women in the house taking care of mothers-in-law. If *Kaigo Hoken* paid a cash allowance, as in Germany, criticism along those lines might be quite fair, but the massive increase in formal services that is planned now is intended to transform how care is really delivered.

It is true that policymakers in Japan as in Germany (and for that matter in Sweden and everywhere else) do hope to preserve the important role that family support now plays in the lives of frail older people, and that (more distinctively in Japan) this role should continue to be played within the same household in most cases. Nonetheless, *Kaigo Hoken* should bring a great improvement in the independence and quality of life of both the frail older person and the family caregiver, and should on those grounds be regarded as a great advance for the Japanese welfare state.

Notes

1 These are sweeping generalizations but I hope not foolhardy; in any case my general point about the relative weight of old-age policy in the Japanese welfare state does not rest on any particular judgment here. I have documented the old-age policy changes elsewhere (Campbell, 1992); some other cases were treated by Upham (1987).
2 Note I use a rather conventional definition of social policy here – if anti-pollution, regional development, protection of small business, mass education of a particular type, and other governmental policies with important social consequences were included in "the welfare state" old-age policy might not look quite so prominent.
3 Note there is no interest group in Japan remotely like the American Association of Retired People (Campbell, 1992, pp. 366–67).
4 Their tactics included the high-profile National Conference for a Rich Old Age in 1970, a direct imitation of the American White House Conference on Aging (which had exactly the same purpose) (Campbell, 1992, p. 120).
5 The proposition that more community-based services would save money by preventing institutionalization is commonplace among specialists, and was a rationale for significant policy developments in Scandinavia, Holland and elsewhere and experiments even in the United States.
6 Abstractly speaking, it was also possible to go backwards – cut back on public services and think instead about encouraging private long-term care insurance or other American-style solutions. As we will see, some market-based notions did become influential, but there were no serious calls for a full-scale retreat from Gold Plan commitments.
7 E.g. in the 1994 Cabinet-approved "Welfare Vision for the 21st Century" – see the English version of the MHW White Paper (Ministry of Health and Welfare, 1997, p. 108).
8 Before being disgraced when he was Vice-Minister for taking bribes, Okamitsu was known as the chief disciple of Yoshimura Hitoshi, who from the late 1970s had espoused American-style health economics ideas in a series of leadership posts at the ministry. (Campbell and Ikegami, 1998, Chap. 2).
9 In September, 1999, the Ministry of Health and Welfare responded to criticism that community-based care facilities were inadequate in many rural areas by authorizing the employment of a family member as a home helper, as long as no more than half of her work hours were devoted to care of her own relative.
10 Prefectural governments will have the power to approve and oversee providers.

References

Campbell, J.C. (1992). *How policies change: The Japanese government and the aging society*. Princeton: Princeton University Press.

Campbell, J.C., and Ikegami, N. (1998). *The art of balance in health policy: Maintaining Japan's low-cost, egalitarian system*. New York: Cambridge University Press.

Goetting, U., Haug, K., and Hinrichs, K. (1994). The long road to long-term care insurance in Germany: A case study in welfare state expansion. *Journal of Public Policy, 14*, 285–319.

Ministry of Health and Welfare. (1997). *Annual report of health and welfare 1995–1996*. Tokyo: Ministry of Health and Welfare.

Pempel, T. J. (1989). Japan's creative conservativism: Continuity under challenge. In F.G. Castles (Ed.), *The comparative history of public policy* (pp. 149–181). Cambridge: Polity Press.

Upham, F.K. (1987). *Law and social change in postwar Japan*. Cambridge MA: Harvard University Press.

5 Critical issues in health care for the US elderly

Beyond the millennium

Douglas D. Bradham

Identifying critical issues in a broad area such as aging is highly dependent on one's perspective. The premise for this chapter is that aging policy in the US is inextricably linked to health care policy for elders (see B. South and D. Bradham, Chapter 3 in this volume). The key assumption is that current trends influencing health care needs and the financing of requisite services affect tomorrow's events. It is also assumed that changes to such far-reaching policies will be minimal, which is characteristic of US health policy (Bradham, 1985). The perspective taken by this health economist in clinical geriatrics research focuses the analysis on four aspects of the future's long-term health care issue. These include:

- the changing needs of older adults
- the role that formal and informal health care play in meeting those needs and the costs of that care
- the public and private financing mechanisms that are required to meet these costs
- public policy options for provision of or financing of care.

This analysis is based on a period in the near future when another "demographic imperative" will face the American scene – the decades of baby boomer retirements, 2010–2030. Without a quantified estimate of the expected service requirements and the ability of individuals and family to pay for or provide these services, reasonable recommendations for public or private alternatives cannot be offered.

This analysis is dependent upon and strengthened by the context represented in the other chapters of this volume. It must be conducted with an appreciation of the types of services and needs for caring that are involved. These are found throughout this volume. The pressures on families, the elders themselves and national governments can not be ignored. Grasping the inter-relationships of the national and an individual's needs requires an immersion into many perspectives focused on the topic of "caring for elders in late life." Examining the policy-related aspects of long-term health care for US elders distills several issues that are critical for successful health care in the early decades of the new millennium for those over 65. The logic of the investigation flows along the lines of Figure 5.1.

Figure 5.1 suggests that demographic trends produce changes in factors that determine needs for long-term care (LTC). LTC needs are also influenced by changes in socioeconomic trends, which determine the purchasing capability of individuals and families. That is to say, socioeconomic trends affect the ability of the elderly to finance their health care services, as do general economic trends. There is often a gap between actual long-term care needs and the elder's personal financing capacity. That gap may require either family or public subsidy if these services are to be realized. Understanding this affordability gap of LTC services provides insight into viable public policy and private solutions that might be considered reasonable to elders, their families and society. Riley (1996) and then Ory, Cooper and Siu (1998) indicate that the elderly are no longer passive about their health care system. Although special interest political activists have long been active, in the most recent decade, voters' concern about the affordability gap has heightened their attention to health care policy and candidates' views. Elders' political impact on US health care policy is summarized by South and Bradham in Chapter 3 of this volume. Evidence of a responding political will from other age groups is growing. By weighing the private affordability against public sentiment to finance elders' services, several issues are crystallized where public policy may be helpful.

This analysis synthesizes published evidence regarding projected trends in the elderly's economic status and health care needs for three decades of the next century. A portion of these data is included in the attached figures to assist further inspection of the issues.

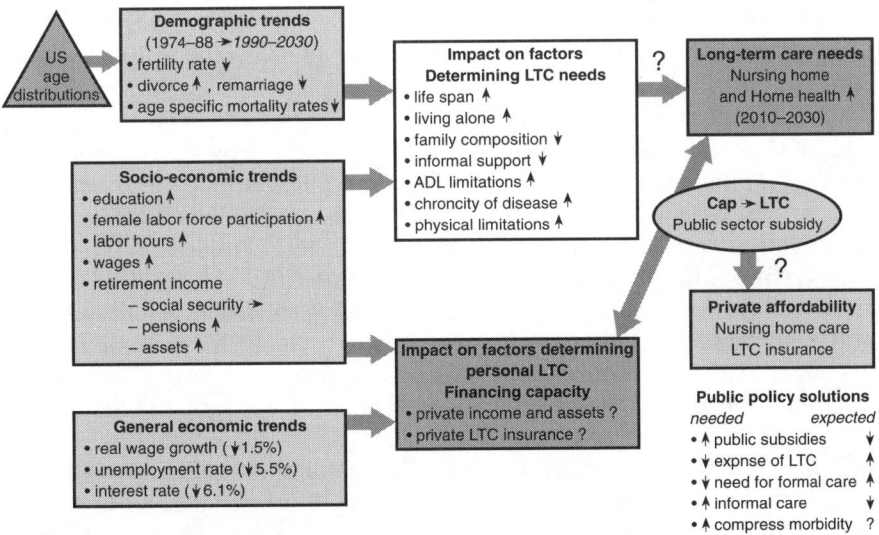

Figure 5.1 US elder's long-term care nexus and public policy options

Precursors to LTC need and financing

Two population-level factors are key precursors to LTC need determinants. There is of course a lagged effect. Demographic trends in one generation directly affect the types and prevalence of medical conditions found in the older age groups in future decades. Additionally, socioeconomic trends influence family size and composition, as well as the elder's and family's financial position at retirement. The availability of informal care through family members is dependent on family size, employment, income and wealth. At a population level, these trends modulate the level and types of needs seen in future elder cohorts. Using data from the 1974-to-1988 period, we can project the level of need and financial situation, to derive the US LTC affordability gap for 2010 and 2030.

Demographics trends

The 1990 US age distribution, with 32.2 million over 65, will be modified by falling fertility, increased divorce and declining remarriage rates to increase that number and proportion in 2010 and 2030. Declines in the age-specific death rates will accentuate these trends, resulting in estimated elderly populations of 44.6 and 72.5 million in 2010 and 2030. These are increases over 1990 of 38 percent (in 2010) and 125 percent (in 2030), using an optimistic view regarding declines in mortality rates, as shown in Figure 5.2 (Zedlewski and McBride, 1996).

Factors determining long-term care needs

Demographic trends like this will change the informal support and the quality of life of the elderly (Feasley, 1996). Life spans will be extended. The result is older age distributions with more than 72 million over 65, as shown in Figure 5.2. Increased chronic disease burdens will accompany these extended life spans (Hoffman *et al.*, 1996a; Liu *et al.*, 1990). Thus, the elderly will exhibit more physical limitations, less functional ability and multiple diseases throughout longer lives, as displayed in Figure 5.3. Nearly twice as many elders in the community will exhibit activities of daily living (ADL) limitations. That is an increase from 14.3 percent in 1990 to 15.8 percent in 2030. A legacy of smaller family sizes and increased international mobility of children will reduce family and informal support. Nearly 26.9 million elderly will be living alone in 2030 (see Figure 5.4). This is more than a twofold increase in solitary elders, which suggests an increased need for formal long-term care (e.g., home health and nursing home care, or group dwellings). Nursing homes will be home to 5.3 million in 2030, nearly a threefold increase from 1990 (1.8 to 5.3 million) (Figure 5.4). In 2030, 7.3 percent of the elderly will need to be in nursing homes, as compared to 5.6 percent in 1990. The increased demand for formal health care services is seemingly unavoidable (Blaum, Liang, and Liu, 1994). These

Critical issues in health care for the US elderly 101

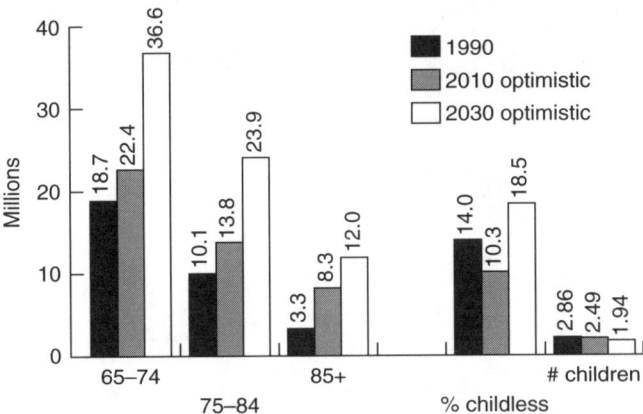

Figure 5.2 US Elderly age composition (in millions) and fertility history of women
Source: Zedlewski and McBride, 1992, Table 3, p. 257.

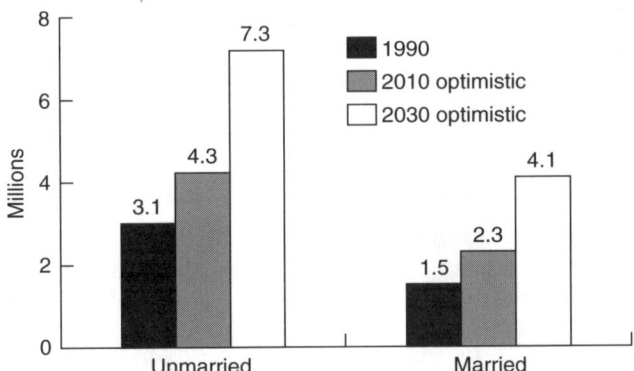

Figure 5.3 US elderly in the community with ADL limitations, by marital status 1990–2030
Source: Zedlewski and McBride, 1992, Table 3, p. 257.

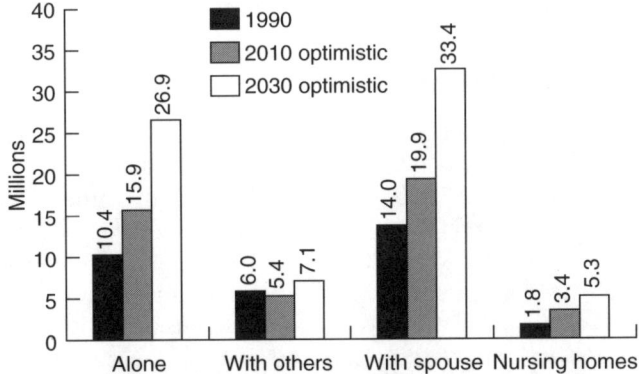

Figure 5.4 Living arrangements of US elderly 1990–2030
Source: Zedlewski and McBride, 1992, Table 3, p. 257.

102 *Assuring care: government policies and programs*

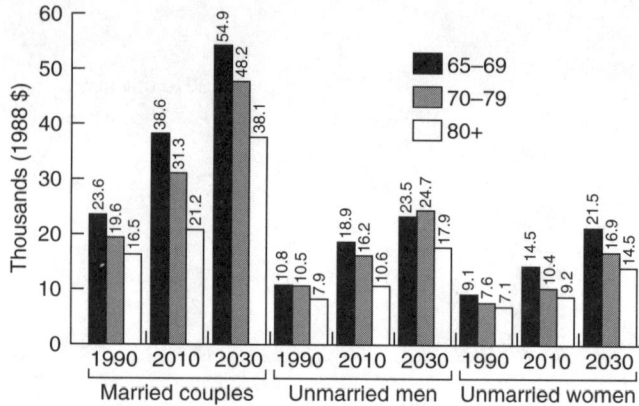

Figure 5.5 Income of US elderly by marital status 1990–2030 (in 1988 dollars)
Source: Zedlewski and McBride, 1992, Table 4, p. 259.

trends have not been ignored by the private sector. Several international hotel conglomerates have already initiated marketing campaigns for assisted-living facilities. Community groups are sponsoring group dwelling arrangements.

Socioeconomic trends

Socioeconomic trends will exacerbate these influences. With increased educational levels, more women will successfully manage careers with longer work hours and for longer durations. Retirement ages will be delayed to age 67 starting in 2000. The rewards will be increases in personal assets, pensions and retirement incomes. The cost will be fewer retired couples. Married couples will account for 2.3 of 44.5 million in 2010, or 5.1 percent. In 2030, 4.1 of 72.5 million elders will be married, or 5.6 percent. In 2010 and 2030, those elders (65 or older) who are married will have significantly larger personal incomes and associated wealth than will the unmarried (Figure 5.5). Unmarried women will remain in the most difficult position.

General economic trends

Although difficult to predict over the period of 1990 to 2030, current estimates indicate that real wages will decline slightly (1.6 percent to 1.5 percent) (Zedlewski and McBride, 1992). Thus, while declining unemployment (6.5 percent to 5.5 percent) and falling interest rates (6.2 percent to 6.1 percent) will generate positive impacts overall, for the elderly they spell reduced public and private capacity for retirement support. That is because falling unemployment leaves fewer children available to serve as adult caregivers and lower interest rates reduce the income streams from assets that could purchase caregiver support or nursing home care when required.

The declining relative proportion of employed Americans (versus retirees) will place an increased burden on fewer workers for public support of entitlement programs, which are public subsidies for the elderly (Medicare) and poor (Medicaid). This will occur at a time when increased taxes are politically and economically improbable with declining real wages.

Personal capacity long-term care financing

There are very few viable sources for financing the expected increase in long-term care demand. Current estimates indicate that 50 percent of long-term care expenses are paid privately, 38 percent by federal and state governments and the remaining 12 percent by other government sources (Lucas, 1996). Increased public subsidies are one source to meet the requisite financing, yet in the past public entitlements of Medicare and Medicaid have contributed significantly to the governmental deficit and increases in these programs are under severe constraint in the current political climate. In fact, 1997 saw considerable reduction in public welfare funds, including the accompanying health services of Medicaid.

Current political trends suggest that declining domestic program spending will be the norm as the country attempts to reduce deficits or to allocate debatable surpluses with declining tax revenues. A continued strong performance in the US economy may soften this trend. Global economic trends could exacerbate the issue. The impact and continuance of the deficits themselves are controversial. However, the institutional memory of the strong relationship between public sector health care subsidies and huge, unforgiving deficits will not fade during the next four decades.

Other sources for financing long-term care are private. The elderly and their families can use private incomes and assets directly to purchase required services when received. Additionally, private dollars can be used indirectly through prepayment of long-term care insurance, medical retirement accounts and other personal financing mechanisms, which are growing in popularity. Private sources become more important because of the expected decline of the public sector. The critical issue is whether the elderly can afford such private health care financing options. Published data addressing income distributions, nursing home use and expenses and other factors can assist our understanding of this critical alternative to public financing.

Long-term care affordability in 2010 and 2030

Projections of the needs for nursing home care and for long-term care insurance when compared to the elderly's personal financial conditions are quite revealing. (In these analyses long-term care insurance can serve as a surrogate for alternatives in pre-paid private financing like medical retirement accounts and home equity financing.) Nursing home care in the US can be expensive (Short et al., 1992). According to the Health Care Financing Administration (HCFA) statistical data, Medicare-financed skilled nursing home charges for the aged amounted to $353 per day in 1994 on average. With the 1994 average length of stay of 27.4 days, the expense per stay averages $9,754 (US Department of Health and Human Services, 1996). That expense in 2030 will be $28,271, assuming a 3-percent annual inflation rate. Yet, according to recent estimates, within their remaining lifetime, elders are expected (39 percent at age 65 to 49 percent at age 85) to use nursing home care for 1.0 to 1.1 years, respectively (Murtaugh *et al.*, 1997). Thus, the associated expense would be $128,845 to $154,614, in 1994 dollars. To place such an expense in proper perspective we must inflate them to our projection years, where the smaller amount becomes $206,758 in 2010 and $373,429 in 2030, assuming an average 3-percent annual inflation rate. Moreover, incomes of the elderly (in Figure 5.5) are estimated to be at levels such that only 7.9 percent and 10.1 percent of the elderly will be able to afford this care without a subsidy in 2010 and 2030 (in Figure 5.6). Again, unmarried women will be most disadvantaged. Recall from Figure 5.4 that an estimated 7.3 percent will be in nursing homes, yet those are usually the individuals with the lowest incomes and least likely to privately finance their care (Cornman and Kingson, 1996).

With private income marginally effective as a financing option, the alternative to public subsidy is private financing through long-term care insurance or another form of prepayment. Without pre-funding from middle age the affordability of these prepayment schemes for those over 65 is not promising when premiums are purchased as individuals (Lucas, 1996). Affordability improves when lower-priced group-purchased premiums are available. Still, to achieve coverage for more than 40 percent of the elderly, as shown in Figure 5.7, would require a willingness to spend 7.5 percent of their fixed retirement budgets for this *single* insurance premium (Zedlewski and McBride, 1992). This level of allocation to insurance would be over five times the proportion expended for *all* insurance by elderly retirees in 1987, as shown in Figure 5.8 (Nieswiadomy and Rubin, 1995). Thus, this mechanism also seems an unlikely alternative. An alternative, similar to Japan's, would be public financing (to pool the risks) with contributions beginning at mid-life (to lower the premiums). The mandated pre-funding option for middle-aged adults amounts to an extension of Medicare, and that is a tax that politicians are currently unwilling to discuss. Without tax incentives or mandates, pre-funding is not likely on a large scale, because the individual risks are perceived to be small.

Public policy issues and potential solutions

If current trends continue, we are left with difficult public policy issues regarding a growing need for formal health care in an increasingly chronically ill elder population, which is steadily increasing, both in numbers and as a proportion of the total US population. That population will have difficulty purchasing the required care privately. The situation described by our analysis above indicates that the status quo will not achieve successful aging and long-term care after

Critical issues in health care for the US elderly 105

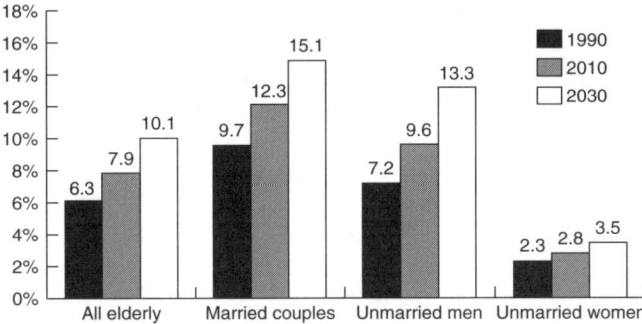

Figure 5.6 Who can afford nursing home care – percent of US elderly whose income is greater than 100 percent of nursing home costs

Source: Zedlewski and McBride, 1992, Fig 2, p. 263.

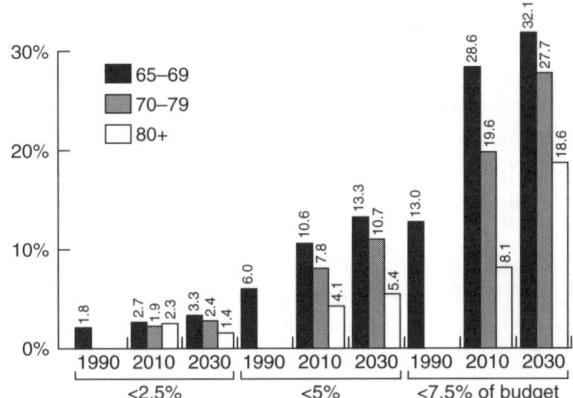

Figure 5.7 Who can afford LTC insurance – percent of US elderly whose income is greater than 100 percent of LTC insurance costs

Source: Zedlewski and McBride, 1992, Table 6, p. 269.

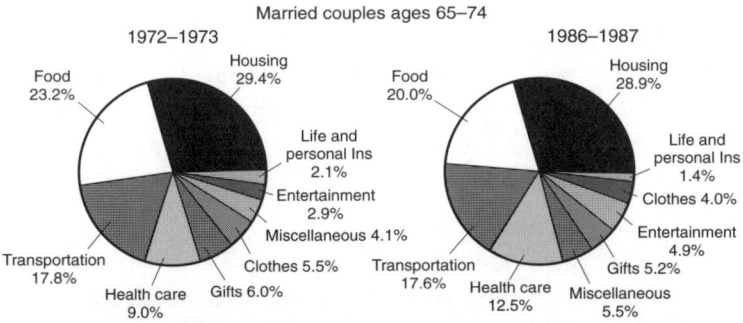

Figure 5.8 Annual expenditure shares of US elderly retirees

Source: Nieswiadomy and Rubin, 1995.

the millennium. Thus, the American public needs to find alternatives. Table 5.1 summarizes the critical issues, the traditional policy responses, some new alternatives and the likelihood of implementation, given past and current inclinations.

LTC will be unaffordable

The analysis examined above indicates that less than 10 percent of all elders will be able to afford the requisite long-term care in 2030, based on income and assets. For each individual, the perceived risk for needing LTC services is relatively small when compared to other issues of family, career and general welfare. There is confusion about what current health insurance plans will pay for. So, there are few who invest in prepaid LTC insurance plans to fund these services. In the past, when faced with the absence of individual capacity to finance health care, the federal and state governments enacted entitlement and subsidy programs of Medicare and Medicaid, which are funded by employee taxes. By pooling resources and risks in this manner, the cost to each individual is significantly reduced. These programs for elder's health care financing could be extended. By expanding home health and nursing home coverage, the needs described above could be accommodated. However, alternative national policy is necessary for several reasons. Such an extension of Medicare and Medicaid would require a considerable tax burden on a shrinking employed cohort. Experience with such intergenerational injustice implies difficulty for this option. Even in prosperous times, support for Social Security and related health care programs suffer from resentment of employee taxes for someone else's retirement. The political will seems insufficient to expand Medicare and Medicaid. This traditional policy alternative is unlikely.

Private financing through LTC Insurance will be insufficient

Private financing of expected LTC needs is possible by pooling risks and early investment in LTC insurance plans that are designed to pay for portions of the expected service needs (Meiners, 1983, 1984; Rubin and Meiners, 1989). These plans, while growing in number, have not reached sufficient acceptance to enable their playing a large role in offsetting the future national expenses described above. Although some segments of the elder populations will be economically better off, the estimates above suggest little increase in such investment for private financing of LTC. This "preventive" investment alternative suffers from the same lack of perceived risk and lack of knowledge among middle-aged individuals.

With incentives from federal and state governments and large corporations, enrollments in LTC insurance plans would increase, which would lower premiums and increase the future cost-sharing potential between public and private sources. These incentives could be similar to Individual Retirement

Table 5.1 Critical issues in health care for the US elderly

Critical issues for US LTC after the millennium	Traditional and new policy alternatives	Likelihood of implementation
LTC will be affordable to no more than 10 percent of elders with sufficient personal financial capacity (e.g., income and assets).	Increased public subsidies required for remaining 90 percent. • Perhaps a means-tested arrangement for Medicare and Medicaid extensions.	**Unlikely**, given current political and tax trends, as well as history of federal and state entitlement programs.
Private financing of LTC through insurance plans will not be sufficient to close the gap.	Increased public incentive for private investments in LTC insurance will be required. • Perhaps an income tax credit. • Perhaps an income tax deduction.	**Unlikely**, given current political and tax trends.
Informal caregiving will be insufficient to fill the service needs.	Increased incentives for informal care support are required. • Perhaps an income tax credit for trained, certified employees in a role below Home Health Aide. • Perhaps a welfare-to-workforce incentive for trainees and trainers.	**Both options are possible**, since more elders will live alone and fewer informal family caregivers will be available; thus, caregiver market will exist.
Overall, (formal) health care expenditures will be too large for individuals and society.	Increased public financing for outpatient, home-based and/or evidence-based physician care may shift more resources to most cost-effective care. • Perhaps HCFA rules will specify reimbursement for specified outcomes in providers' populations. • Perhaps a tax credit or HCFA contractual requirement to provide health promotion incentives to individuals at mid-life and beyond.	**First option is unlikely**, since market-driven health care and society has potentially reached the margin of its impact and there remain many unsubstantiated health care procedures and interventions; however, further invasion of medical practice by policy-makers will not be accepted. **Second option is possible**; however, evidence of outcomes and effective mechanisms must be documented.

Accounts (IRAs) and Medical Trust Account (MTA) incentives of the 1980s, where investments were partially deductible from income taxes and the proceeds non-taxable. A more engaging alternative would be to provide income tax credits for the investments in any of these plans. Since funds in IRAs, MTAs or LTC insurance plans can be used to offset the expected LTC expenses, society's fiscal outlay in the future would be reduced. From the public policy maker's perspective, a credible incentive today would provide a larger cost-sharing opportunity for future national and state expenses. Again, the past suggests that this approach is unlikely to be enacted. Actually, IRA and MTA tax incentives have been reduced in the past decade and almost eliminated over recent years. The result has been a reduction in the number of citizens participating in these retirement options. New tax credits would be unlikely, given the current mood of national and state policy-makers.

Informal care support will be insufficient

Fewer informal family-member caregivers will be available. Couples will reach retirement with fewer children than past generations. Furthermore, fewer couples will reach retirement age still married. More elders will live alone in 2010 and 2030 due to fewer marriages and increased divorce rates. Thus, the need for informal caregivers will be heightened. As shown in the secondary analysis above, delaying or avoiding the formal long-term care expenditures gains considerable value to society, whether supported publicly or privately. This can be accomplished through informal caregiving to various degrees. Informal caregiving is valuable to society. From an economic perspective, voluntary informal caregiving shifts LTC expenses from society to the volunteering individual and/or family member.

Sparse research is available to document the long-suspected economic value of caregiving (Sevick and Bradham, 1997). However, as the demographic trends described continue to evolve, the reality in economic terms of these "labors of love" will be obvious. A society that recognizes this contribution and places value on it will see the economic logic of reimbursement or tax-incentives for family-centered care of its elders. Japan's policies have placed high regard on encouraging traditional family-centered caregiving for elders, with payment possible. US policy in the past has relied on a medical paradigm to deny family members reimbursement for their voluntary contributions.

There are truly personal benefits for caregiving to elders in later life. Moving Japanese and American caregiving experiences are revealed in this volume. They take place in various settings (e.g., home, hospice and others) and underscore the personal value to be gained for the elder and the caregiver. However, to be successful at a national level in the US, larger numbers of caregivers must be found than voluntary motives will provide. The opportunity costs not being gainfully employed, but rather providing such caregiving, will increase as fewer informal caregivers are available. Encouraging family or non-family to engage in this supportive activity is critical.

A US policy that explicitly recognizes the economic value of the caregiving role, even when provided by a family member, would benefit everyone involved. Such a policy, whether by reimbursement (income) or through tax incentives (income tax credit or deduction) would encourage the informal care of the elderly. A caregiver policy would explicitly recognize the economic value of this role. This policy could accomplish other recent national goals by encouraging caregiving as a bridge from subsidized welfare to a productive role in the workforce. For the same reasons, society and individuals can benefit from formal policies that incorporate subsidies to health care providers for developing the low-skilled labor force that is required to meet the expected demand for caregiving early in the next millennium. This labor pool is difficult to maintain, in reality. These are high-turnover positions, based on home health and nursing home manpower research. This is in part due to low wages and low respect among the health professionals. Furthermore, the turnover rate deserves an explicit economic offset to the personnel and the firms willing to pursue this training and entry-level development. Demonstration projects in this area are underway to examine implementation issues (e.g., Maryland Department of Human Resources, Family Investment Program, Welfare-to-Work Demonstration Projects; James A. Haley Veterans Medical Center in Tampa, Florida).

These options could generate a significant improvement in meeting the needs of the elderly in a relative short period, as policy changes go. Within a decade, more services could be available at the community level and within a generation, a more family-centered caregiving basis for informal long-term care might be institutionalized. Mechanisms of gaining respect for this role must be established well in advance of the looming crisis. Carefully evaluated demonstrations are necessary today to improve our judgement of the potential impact of such policies. It is also important in crafting these policies to remember that the caregiver's needs must be considered in estimating service demands, not just those of the care receiver, which is the norm (Anderson et al., 1998).

Overall (formal) health care and associated expenditures must be reduced

The data examined above clearly describe increases in overall use of health services by the elderly. Increased numbers of elders with longer lifespans will exhibit more conditions that are chronic, requiring more medical management. Policies to directly reduce services are unpopular and unlikely given increased chronicity of disease in a growing elderly population, who characteristically vote to protect these services.

However, an alternative for policy that would impact on this future must capitalize on the movement among members of the affected cohort to increase self-responsibility for health and health care, which is a promising trend for the elderly of the future. This change, if supported by policy, would represent a cost sharing with the patients themselves while they are younger. It could be in the form of investments in prepaid insurance policies, described above, or by encouraging health promotion in mid-life and beyond. Like other policy options with long-term benefits, this incentive must be both credible and significant or the perceived small risk will reduce their relative importance to each individual. The rationale for this policy option requires brief elaboration.

Recently, Medicare Health Maintenance Organizations (HMOs) have been found to be reducing preventive services and raising premiums to the elderly. Now that managed care markets are near capacity, competitive forces are focused on service scope and content. Long-term preventive and health promotion activities are prime targets for cost-cutting management practices. This is especially true when elders can transfer to other providers in periods as short as six months, lowering the provider's incentive for preventing future health care consumption. Thus, those preventive services that are not likely to reduce short-run health consumption are discontinued. While this may be financially logical for the managed care firm, it makes no sense for society. Since Medicare HMO contracting by the Health Care Financing Administration (HCFA) represents society's perspective rather than the firm's, these contracts could more strongly secure these long-term benefits for the beneficiaries. Thus, preventive *and* health promotion interventions should be an equal priority to that of acute pain relief (Harris et al, 1989). Reimbursement regulations could specifically support documented health promotion behavior (e.g., smoking cessation; weight loss; and/or increased organized physical activity). Such a policy may be most effective as an individual tax credit; however, a corporate-level incentive for major employers (e.g., multinational corporations) and major providers of care (e.g., managed care and HMOs) would be more manageable.

Such a policy would be based on the concepts of the "compression of morbidity and mortality" theory, which was first described by James Fries in 1980. Fundamentally, the concept is that through health promotion for middle-aged and the elderly, both self-responsibility and health are improved (both mental and physical), which in turn reduces medical needs, increases independence and reduces health care use and expense. At a population level (e.g., major employers, insurance plans, managed care and HMOs), this could be quite powerful (Fries *et al.*, 1993). There is sparse documentation of the potential savings to society from compressing morbidity through health promotion, although the literature is growing. However, like the case for seatbelt use, straightforward logic does not equate to changed behavior. Effective incentives must be found. A review of the morbidity compression framework and description of some research underway may lend more credibility to this important and practical policy option.

Health promotion in older adults: motivation and theoretical framework

The importance of chronic diseases among older Americans, the related high cost of secondary and tertiary health care, and their combined increases in the future motivates a need to bring health promotion interventions from clinical trials into actual clinical practice for both the middle-aged and the elderly who are at risk for cardiovascular disease and its sequelae. There is an increase in cardiovascular disease (CVD) among older Americans and one can logically expect an associated increase in treating the complications of CVD in long-term care services (Elward and Larson, 1992; Schneider and Guralnik, 1990). These services will mean expenses for health care consumed over an expanding life span of these older adults (Christersen, Long, and Rodgers, 1987; Manton and Vaupel, 1995). Secondary and tertiary care in the form of major surgery and extended care compose the majority of these potentially avoidable expenses (Bindman et al., 1995; Ellencweig and Pagliccia, 1994; Weissman et al., 1991).

"Preventive gerontology" is not a new concept (Bierman and Hazzard, 1985; Hadley, 1995). Actually implementing it in a long-term managed care environment is a challenge that must be undertaken in order to efficiently meet the future needs of these older Americans (Nelson et al., 1997; Omenn, 1994). Anne Somers clearly stated the challenge in her foreword to *Practicing prevention for the elderly* (Lavizzo-Mourey et al., 1989).

The challenge now facing those of us who share this conviction is threefold:

- to strengthen the science base linking specific risk factors to specific disease outcomes and linking specific modification in these risk factors to modified outcomes
- to translate these basic scientific findings into practical guidelines that can be used by the public, physicians and other caregivers to prevent or postpone individual disease and disability
- to devise organizational, financial and other socioeconomic modalities and policies to permit the incorporation of the new science base and prevention technologies into routine health care for the American people.

Clinical researchers have developed primary, secondary and tertiary interventions to reduce CVD risks and improve independence, functional ability, survival and quality of life for older adults (Boult et al., 1996; Ettinger et al., 1997; Harris et al., 1989; Katzel et al., 1995; Tinetti et al., 1995). Among suitable interventions for exportation to ambulatory practice are several behavioral modifications (i.e., smoking cessation, exercise, weight loss, etc.) through aggressive risk factor management (ARFM) of CVD risk factors (e.g., hypertension, diabetes, obesity and sedentary lifestyle).

In order for managed care decision-makers to confidently embark on system-wide implementation of health promotion interventions, evidence of value and cost-effectiveness in actual practice must be obtained (Docteur, Colby, and Gold, 1996; Fries et al., 1993). This applied investigation of outcomes management has been called "the basic science of health care reform" (Bradham, 1994; Ginzberg, 1991). To link aging and health promotion to health care expenditure reduction is embodied in the "compression of morbidity" into the expanding years of older adults. Such evidence is growing (Fries, 1997; Vita et al., 1998). Under the conditions described above, there is an obligation for a public policy of health promotion (Pellegrino, 1981).

112 *Assuring care: government policies and programs*

The "compression of morbidity" paradigm

The conceptual framework supporting this position of mandating health promotion services was first described by James Fries, MD, in 1980 and further clarified in his 1990, 1996, and 1997 publications. Fries estimates that a *nearly 25 percent reduction in health care expenditure was achieved* through an exercise program alone in a runner's club as compared to community-based controls over an eight-year period (Fries, 1997), and another study found a reduction in health care expenditure over an even longer period in university alumni with low-risk profiles (Vita *et al*, 1998). The paradigm provides a potent strategy for reducing the health care burden of older adults.

The "morbidity compression" paradigm, shown in Figure 5.9 (Fries, 1996), recognizes that:

- most health conditions are chronic rather than acute
- these conditions may be asymptomatic in late middle age
- many are behavior-related
- the burden of such illnesses occurs in the later years of life (i.e., among older adults).

The strategic intervention is to provide middle-aged and older adults with *secondary* prevention through health promotion and preventive services to delay or prevent morbidity (line II in Figure 5.9) and *tertiary* prevention following CVD to improve the quality of the expected longer life span (line III in Figure 5.9). Secondary prevention improves function and survival by early interventions at the preclinical or asymptomatic phase of disease, while tertiary prevention mollifies the symptoms in order to maximize survival and function of the diseased older adult (Lavizzo *et al.*, 1989). Among secondary preventive interventions are:

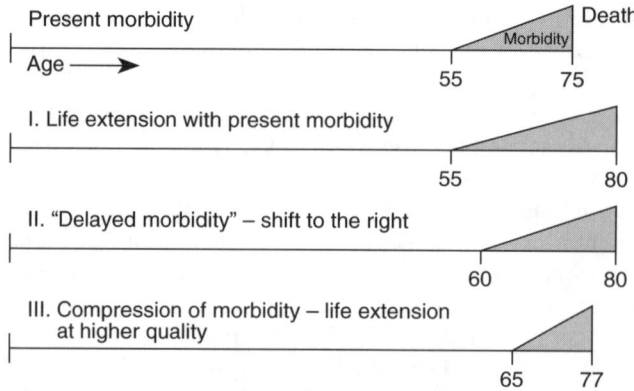

Figure 5.9 Compression of morbidity

Source: Fries, 1996

- behavioral modifications (e.g., smoking cessation, exercise, weight loss, etc.) for the ARFM (e.g., exercise, nutrition, weight loss, etc.) of CVD risk factors (e.g., hypertension, diabetes, hyperlipidemia and obesity) and
- preventive care (e.g., general physicals, lab screening for CVD risk factors, flu vaccines, cancer screening, etc.).

An example of tertiary prevention is rehabilitation of older patients with peripheral arterial disease (PAD), heart failure and stroke.

In a period of health care reform where health services' benefits and costs are being brought into balance, this overarching clinical strategy to obtain health care value is compatible with an increased role for preventive and primary care. This strategy facilitates and depends on an enhanced patient-centered responsibility for one's own health status.

Significance of older adult health promotion

The importance of middle-aged and older adult health promotion research that focuses on integrating health promotion into clinical practice and assessment of the short- and long-term impact of chronic disease prevention is evidenced in the burden of chronic conditions among the elderly and the associated secondary and tertiary health care resources consumed by these patients. The estimated total population with chronic diseases is expected to increase by 21.2 percent from 1995 to 2010 to reach a level of 120 million and by another 23.3 percent from 2010 to 2030 to a level of 148 million (see Figure 5.10). *The*

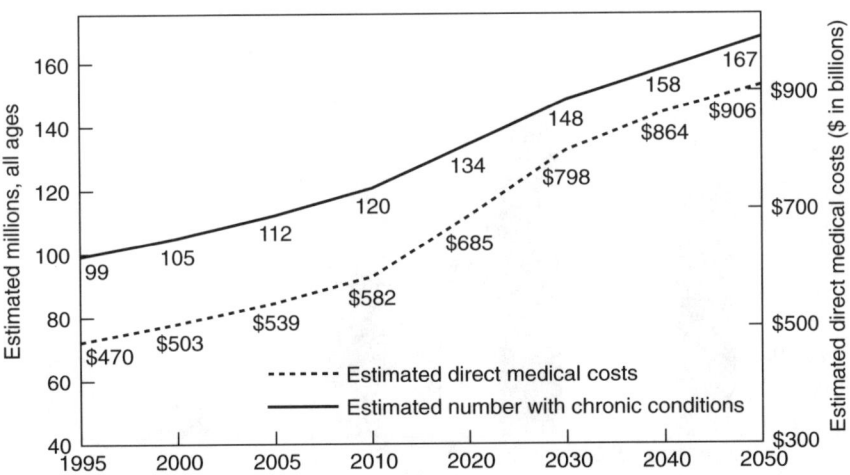

Figure 5.10 Estimated number of persons and direct medical costs for persons with chronic conditions in the US., 1995–2050

Source: Hoffman, Rice, and Sung, 1996

elderly compose 30 to 50 *percent of this chronic diseased population*. Managed care market pressures, reduced services, public support and incomes will exacerbate the pressure for long-term care, as described above (Chisholm and Hahn, 1995; Cowper *et al.*, 1993; Iglehart, 1996; Welch, 1996). *Morbidity compression could reduce the cost and need for services by 15 to 25 percent.*

Forty-five percent of non-institutionalized Americans are estimated to have at least one chronic condition with their direct health expenses accounting for nearly 75 percent of all US health care expenditures or approximately $425 of $650 billion in 1990 (Hoffman, Rice, and Sung, 1996). The remaining $234 billion in direct expenses came from the patients, their employers and their families. *Forty-one percent of the direct expenses for chronic care were from public payers of Medicare, Medicaid, the Department of Veterans Affairs and other state and local assistance programs* (see Figure 5.11). In contrast, public funds paid for only 19 percent of acute treatment. Thus, directly reducing the impact of chronic diseases in older adults will directly affect public financing of health care. Given this resource allocation, health promotion for older adults is a public policy option (Kane, 1994).

Thus, if a 15 to 25-percent reduction in these annual health care expenses (similar to Fries, 1996) can be obtained for older adults, then a considerable expense in private and public funds will be saved and be available for others at a time of immense pressure for these funds, all other factors held constant (Fonseca *et al.*, 1996). This is a controversial issue, but long-term evidence is beginning to emerge. Vita *et al.* (1998) found in a three-decade follow-up study of 1,741 university alumni, that health behaviors (e.g., smoking, diet and weight, and exercise) in midlife are predictors of subsequent disability, and their

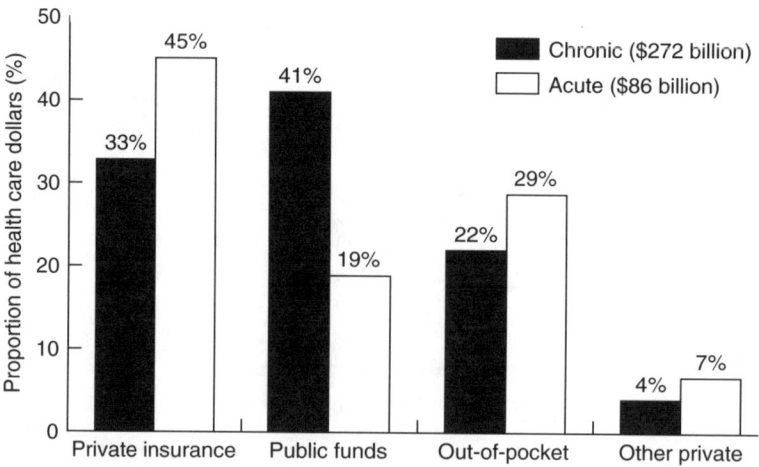

Figure 5.11 Percent of US health care dollars by payer for acute versus chronic conditions, 1987

Source: Hoffman, Rice, and Sung, 1996

disability is delayed to later life. Morbidity was compressed into fewer years at the end of life.

Although this transition from prevention theory to actual practice has received some attention, the health care reform environment from 1996 to 1999 generated more incentives for adoption of such successful interventions (Chisholm and Hahn, 1995; Lewis and Rose, 1991). Because of telecommunications technology for remote electronic linkages, the approach need not rely on maintaining the hospital- or clinic-based sites as were used in the mid-1980s, but can capitalize on the managed-care philosophy of gate-keeping and distributed ambulatory care clinics (Bradham, Morgan, and Dailey, 1995). The initial design of optimal delivery mechanisms must explore options of community-based exercise and weight-loss programs, as well as home-based programs, with telemedicine linkages. Finally, the crush of practice demands on today's clinicians has improved their receptivity to computer-assisted reminders for various guidelines for care, preparing the way for computer-aided feedback systems to inform patients and clinicians of achievement in lowering CVD risk factors (Haynes, Hayward, and Lomas, 1995). Off-site health promotion activity can potentially be conducted, monitored and integrated into chronic disease management – for example, diabetes care.

Conclusions

Several critical issues for health care of the US elderly that will arise early in the new millennium have been examined. The potential role of national and state policy makers in proactively countering the projected trends have been described. Suggested options for policy in the US have been delineated. Many of these have counterparts in Japan's relatively more comprehensive aging policies described elsewhere. It is necessary for US policy makers and citizens, who are concerned by the issues of caring for elders, whether through formal health service or informal caregiving, to embrace the discussion and motivate changes for improving the quality of elders' collective lives. Many contributors find reasons to be positive about the health status gains to be achieved among the elderly, while raising concerns about the uncertainty of society's ability to finance this care (Lee and Skinner, 1999; Cutler et al., 1996).

In the probable absence of private initiatives to accomplish the prescribed changes of increased caregiving and health promotion, society must act. Because these "issues" will not become "crises" for another decade or two, they require considerable motivation to be proactive. In the case of such preventive measures, it is often "for the protection of the general welfare" that governmental intervention is undertaken. In other arenas, for instance, the environment, global warming, seatbelt use and the threat of terrorism, national governments have initiated action prior to the crisis point, because to wait would be irresponsible. Japan has undertaken aging initiatives to forestall the impact of their aging society. Will the US? Can we afford to do nothing? Examples and experiments in many countries can be studied. Potential demonstration projects in the US can be initiated. However, in the case of informal caregiving and health promotion a fundamental change is required now.

References

Anderson, R.A., Bradham, D.D., Hueser, M.D., Wofford, J.L., and Colombo, K.A. (2000). Caregivers' access to assistance caring for functionally impaired elderly persons and their unmet needs for supportive services. *Journal of Health Care for the Poor and Undeserved*.

Bierman, E.L. and Hazzard, W.R. (1985). Middle age: Strategies for the prevention or attenuation of chronic diseases of aging. In R. Andres, E.L. Bierman, and W.R. Hazzard (Eds.), *Principles of geriatric medicine* (pp. 862–866). New York: McGraw Hill.

Bindman, A.B., Grumbach, K., Osmond, D., Komaromy, M., Vranizan, K., Lurie, N., Billings, J., and Stewart, A. (1995). Preventable hospitalizations and access to health care. *Journal of the American Medical Association, 274*, 305–311.

Blaum, C.S., Liang, J., and Liu, X. (1994). The relationship of chronic diseases and health status to health service utilization of older Americans. *Journal of the American Geriatrics Society, 42*, 1087–1093.

Boult, C., Altmann, M., Gilbertson, D., Yu, C., and Kane, R.L. (1996). Decreasing disability in the 21st century: The future effects of controlling six fatal and nonfatal conditions. *American Journal of Public Health, 86*, 1388–1393.

Bradham, D.D. (1985). Health policy formulation and analysis. *Nursing Economics, 3*, 167–172.

Bradham, D.D. (1994). Outcomes research in orthopedics: History, perspectives, concepts and future. *Athroscopy, 10*, 493–501.

Bradham, D.D., Morgan, S., and Dailey, M.E. (1995). The information superhighway and telemedicine: Applications, status and issues. *The Wake Forest Law Review, 30*, 145–167.

Chisholm, S.W. and Hahn, M.A. (1995). Emerging veterans health administration geriatric and extended care initiatives. *Geriatric Nursing, 16*, 42–47.

Christersen, S., Long, S.H., and Rodgers, J. (1987). Acute health care costs for the aged Medicare population: Overview and policy options. *The Milbank Quarterly, 65*, 397–425.

Cornman, J.M. and Kingson, E.R. (1996). Trends, issues, perspectives, and values for the aging of the baby boom cohorts. *Gerontologist, 36*, 15–26.

Cowper, D.C., Manheim, L.M., Weaver, F.M., and Pawlow, A.J. (1993). Mix and match: VA and non-VA care for elderly veterans. *VA Practitioner*, 41–44.

Cutler, D.M., McClellan, M. Newhouse, J.P., and Remler, D. (1996). Are medical prices declining? *National Bureau of Economic Research*. Working paper no. 5750.

Docteur, E.R., Colby, D.C., and Gold, M. (1996). Shifting the paradigm: Monitoring access in Medicare managed care. *Health Care Financing Review, 17*, 5–21.

Ellencweig, A.Y. and Pagliccia, N. (1994). Utilization patterns of cohorts of elderly clients: A structural equation model. *Health Services Research, 29*, 225–45.

Elward, K. and Larson, E.B. (1992). Benefits of exercise for older adults: A review of existing evidence and current recommendations for the general population. *Clinical Geriatric Medicine, 8*, 35–50.

Ettinger, W.H. Jr., Burns, R., Messier, S.P., Applegate, W., Rejeski, W.J., Morgan, T., Shumaker, S., Berry, M.J., O'Toole, M., Monu, J., and Craven, T. (1997). A randomized trial comparing aerobic exercise and resistance exercise with a health education program in older adults with knee osteoarthritis: The Fitness Arthritis and Seniors Trial (FAST). *Journal of the American Medical Association, 277*, 25–31.

Feasley, J.C. (Ed.). (1996). *Health outcomes for older people: Questions for the coming decade.* Washington DC: National Academy Press.

Fonseca, M.L., Smith, M.E., Klein, R.E., and Sheldon, G. (1996). The Department of Veterans Affairs medical care system and the people it serves. *Medical Care, 34,* MS9–MS20.

Fries, J.F. (1980). Aging, natural death, and the compression of morbidity. *New England Journal of Medicine, 303,* 130–135.

Fries, J.F. (1990). The compression of morbidity: Near or far? *Milbank Quarterly, 67,* 208–232.

Fries, J.F., Koop, C.E., Beadle, C.E., Cooper, P.P., England, M.J., Greaves, R.F., Sokolov, J.J., Wright, D., and the Health Project Consortium. (1993). Reducing health care costs by reducing the need and demand for medical services. *New England Journal of Medicine, 329,* 321–325.

Fries, J.F. (1996). Physical activity, the compression of morbidity, and the health of the elderly. *Journal of the Royal Society of Medicine, 89,* 64–68.

Fries, J.F. (1997). Exercise and the health of the elderly, *American Journal of Geriatric Cardiology, 6,* 24–32.

Ginzberg, E. (Ed.) (1991). *Health services research: Key to health policy.* Cambridge, MA: Harvard University Press.

Hadley, E.C. (1995). The science of the art of geriatric medicine. *Journal of American Medical Association, 273,* 1381–1383.

Harris, S.S., Caspersen, C.J., DeFriese, G.H., and Estes, E.H., Jr. (1989). Physical activity counseling for healthy adults as a primary preventive intervention in the clinical setting. *Journal of American Medical Association, 261,* 3590–3598.

Haynes, R.B., Hayward, R.S.A., and Lomas, J. (1995). Bridges between health care research evidence and clinical practice. *Journal of American Medical Association, 2,* 342–350.

Hoffman, C., Rice, D., and Sung, H-Y. (1996). Persons with chronic conditions: Their prevalence and costs. *Journal of American Medical Association, 276,* 1473–1479.

Iglehart, J.K. (1996). Reform of the Veterans Affairs health care system. *New England Journal of Medicine, 335,* 1407–1411.

Institute for Health and Aging. (1996). *Chronic care in America: A 21st century challenge.* San Francisco: University of California.

Kane, R. (1994). Making aging a public health priority. *American Journal of Public Health, 84,* 1213–1214.

Katzel, L.I., Bleecker, E.R., Colman, E.G., Rogus, E.M., Sorkin, J.D., and Goldberg, A.P. (1995). Effects of weight loss versus aerobic exercise training on risk factors for coronary disease in healthy, obese, middle-aged and older men: A randomized controlled trial. *Journal of American Medical Association, 274,* 1915–1921.

Lavizzo-Mourey, R., Day, S.C., Diserens, D., and Grisso, J.A. (Eds.). (1989). *Practicing prevention for the elderly.* Philadelphia: Hanley and Belfus.

Lee, R., and Skinner, J. (1999). Will aging baby boomers bust the federal budget? *Journal of Economic Perspectives, 13,* 117–141.

Lewis, B., and Rose, G. (1991). Prevention of coronary heart disease: Putting theory into practice. *Journal of the Royal College of Physicians of London, 25,* 21–26.

Liu, K., Manton, K.G., and Marzetta, B.L. (1990). Morbidity, disability and long-term care of the elderly: Implications for insurance financing. *Milbank Quarterly, 68,* 445–492.

Lucas, D. (1996). Managed competition with prefunding: The solution for long-term care. *Milbank Quarterly, 74,* 571–597.

Manton, K.G., and Vaupel, J.W. (1995). Survival after the age of 80 in the United States, Sweden, France, England, and Japan. *New England Journal of Medicine, 333,* 1232–1235.

Meiners, M.R. (1983). The case for long-term care insurance. *Health Affairs*, *2*, 55–79.

Meiners, M.R. (1984). Long-term care insurance: Premium estimates for prototype policies. *Medical Care*, *22*, 901–911.

Murtaugh, C.M., Kemper, P., Spillman, B.C., and Carlson, B.L. (1997). The amount, distribution and timing of lifetime nursing home use. *Medical Care*, *35*, 204–218.

Nelson, L., Brown, R., Gold, M., Ciemnecki, A., and Docteur, E. (1997). Trends: Access to care in Medicare HMOs. *Health Affairs*, *16*, 148–156.

Nieswiadomy, M. and Rubin, R.A. (1995). Changes in expenditure patterns of retirees: 1972–73 and 1986–87. *Journal of Gerontology: Social Sciences*, *50B*, S274–S290.

Omenn, G.S. (1994). Prevention policy: Perspectives on the critical interaction between research and policy. *Preventive Medicine*, *23*, 612–617.

Ory, M.G., Cooper, J., and Siu, A.L. (1998). Toward the development of a research agenda on organizational issues in the delivery of healthcare to older Americans. *Health Services Research*, *33*, 287–297.

Pellegrino, E.D. (1981). Health promotion as public policy: The need for moral grounding. *Preventive Medicine*, *10*, 371–378.

Riley, M.W. (1996). Scientific basis for re-inventing health care. Prepared for panel on Identifying Research Priorities: Perspectives from Policy and Practice, by National Institute on Aging, Program on Age and Structural Change. Washington, DC.

Rubin R.M., and Meiners, M.R. (1989). Private long-term care insurance: Simulations of a potential market. *Medical Care*, *27*, 182–193.

Schneider, E.L., and Guralnik, J.M. (1990). The aging of America: Impact on health care costs. *Journal of American Medical Association*, *263*, 2335–40.

Sevick, M.A., and Bradham, D.D. (1997). Economic value of caregiver effort in maintaining long-term ventilator-assisted individuals at home. *Heart and Lung*, *26*, 148–157.

Short, P.F., Kemper, P., Cornelius, L.J., and Walden, D.C. (1992). Public and private responsibility for financing nursing home care: The effect of Medicaid asset spenddown. *Milbank Quarterly*, *70*, 277–298.

Tinetti, M.E., Inouye, S.K., Gill, T.M., and Doucette, J.T. (1995). Shared risk factors for falls, incontinence and functional dependence: Unifying the approach to geriatric syndromes. *Journal of American Medical Association*, *273*, 1348–1353.

US Department of Health and Human Services. (1996). *Health Care Financing Review, Statistical Supplement*. (Table 37 pp. 274–5 and Table 41 pp. 284–9). Baltimore, MD: Health Care Financing Administration, Office of Research and Demonstrations.

Vita, A.J., Terry, R.B., Hubert, H.B., and Fries, J.F. (1998). Aging, health risks, and cumulative disability. *The New England Journal of Medicine*, *338*, 1035–1041.

Weissman, J.S., Stern, R., Fielding, S.L., and Epstein, A.M. (1991). Delayed access to health care: Risk factors, reasons, and consequences. *Annals of Internal Medicine*, *114*, 325–331.

Welch, W.P. (1996). Growth in HMO share of Medicare market, 1989–1994. *Health Affairs*, *15*, 201–214.

Zedlewski, S.R., and McBride, T.D. (1992). The changing profile of the elderly: Effects on future long-term care needs and financing. *Milbank Quarterly*, *70*, 247–275.

Part II
Providing Care
Professional caregivers

6 We live too short, and die too long

On Japanese and US physicians' caregiving practices and approaches to withholding life-sustaining treatments

Michael D. Fetters and Marion Danis

Comparative research on Japan and the United States

The work in this book examines the intersection between culture, policy makers, and those who provide and receive care "on the ground." The clinical arena is a pivotal interface between health care policy and culture, with physicians having a great deal of power in clinical decision-making, and organized medicine exercising a great deal of political power in health care policy decisions. Because both health care policy and culture-specific ideas about death and aging inform clinical decision-making, physicians' perspectives are crucial in the examination of care and meaning in late life. In this chapter, we begin by presenting four reasons for studying approaches to life-sustaining treatments in Japan and the United States. Based on empirical research, we examine physicians' approaches to withholding life-sustaining treatments in Japan and the United States and draw conclusions about the implications of these for health care policy makers.

Cross-cultural inquiry is invaluable for understanding the values and beliefs that form the moral fabric of our society, a fact well illustrated by recent work on Japanese and Western bioethics (Hoshino, 1997a). Four compelling reasons to compare approaches to the use of life-sustaining technology in Japan and the United States are:

- both countries are experiencing rapid growth in their elderly populations with concomitant questions about appropriate use of life-sustaining treatment for this group
- both countries are concerned about spending increasing proportions of their gross domestic products (GDPs) on health care
- both countries have ready access to costly medical technology
- the values and belief systems of Japan and the United States are very

different. As we struggle with end-of-life issues, we may learn from each other's approaches.

Aging populations

As in many developed countries, the populations of Japan and the United States are aging at an unprecedented pace, with an expected growth peak in the next 25 to 30 years. The Japanese population of 65 years and older is projected to nearly double from about 12 percent in 1990 to about 23 percent by the year 2015 (Ministry of Health and Welfare, 1991). The US Bureau of the Census estimates that the United States population over 80 years old will grow from about 3 million to over 6 million in the same time frame, and will increase to over 15 million people by the year 2050 (Randall, 1993). Given the prevalence of chronic and terminal illnesses in elderly populations, the economic burden of providing health care for the elderly is a major concern for policy makers in Japan and the United States. These demographic changes have important implications for health professionals and caregivers on the ground as well, as there will be increasing demands to provide both the medical and everyday physical care of the elderly. Since chronic and terminal illnesses common in the elderly demand more intensive outpatient, inpatient, and chronic institutional care, future health care expenditures in Japan and the United States are expected to increase further.

Increasing health care expenditures

Health care expenditures in Japan and the United States are increasing to enormous proportions. In 1996, the United States spent about 14.2 percent of its gross domestic product on health care, compared to approximately 7.2 percent in Japan (Anderson, 1997). Clearly, the greater the proportion of the GDP allocated to health care, the smaller the proportion available for other national needs. In the United States, ethicists and policy experts like Daniel Callahan, former director of The Hastings Center, an independent bioethics research institute, have advocated limiting health care expenditures (Callahan, 1987). Callahan, for example, argues that medical expenditures have outpaced and will continue to outpace our ability to pay for them, and that rationing of medical care is inevitable. Using the metaphor of "the ragged edge of technology," he illustrates how many high-tech clinical innovations drive up medical costs while having only a marginal impact on patient care (Callahan, 1990). Expenditures on technology are drawing attention in Japan as well. Makoto Kikuchi has been a leading proponent for medical technology assessment in Japan. His research has revealed that medical expenditures increased from about $50 billion in 1975, when the production of medical engineering equipment first became widespread, to about $110 billion in 1985

(Kikuchi, 1991). Since increasing health care costs are related to high utilization of medical technology in both countries, there is a need to understand in greater detail physicians' caregiving practices and clinical decision-making processes.

Medical technology use in Japan and the United States

Medical technology is available and extensively used in both Japan and the United States. Although the United States, unlike all other major industrial countries, lacks some form of universal health insurance and places a lower emphasis on public health than many other countries, it is a world leader in the discovery and application of medical technology. As a consequence, the technology is not only available, but also widely used – indeed one of the defining features of US medicine is its aggressive nature (Payer, 1996). Possibly contrary to our own good, the widespread availability of medical technology has resulted in a "technological imperative" to use medical technology because it is available rather than because it leads to improved outcomes (Koenig, 1988). This overly aggressive use of medical technology, at times contrary to the patient's own wishes, was partly behind the passage of the Patient Self-Determination Act, which took effect in 1991. This legislation was designed to inform patients of their right to prepare advance directives for treatment and to empower them to refuse life-sustaining treatment (Omnibus Budget Reconciliation Act of 1990). The passage of this act is both a clear indication of Congressional concern about the aggressive use of end-of-life treatment and an indication that patient preferences are expected to dictate use of life-sustaining treatment. The high percentage of US hospital beds allocated to intensive care relative to other counties is yet another indication of aggressive end-of-life care in the United States (Chalfin and Fein, 1994).

As in the United States, medical technology is widely available and utilized in Japan. The installation rates of computed tomography (CT) scanners, dialysis equipment, and various other medical engineering equipment in Japan are the highest in the world (Kikuchi, 1991). There is a penchant to use this medical technology, especially for screening and diagnostic purposes. One example of the aggressive use of medical technology is the yearly Japanese physical (*kenkō shindan*), which is widely encouraged and practiced in Japan. The *kenkō shindan* is very technology-centered, as even in the most basic form it typically includes extensive blood work, chest X-ray, urinalysis, electrocardiogram, and upper gastrointestinal series – all items that are no longer recommended in the periodic health examination in the United States and Canada (Canadian Task Force, 1979; US Department of Health and Human Services Public Health Service, 1994; US Preventive Services Task Force, 1996). More expanded testing in the so-called "human dry dock" exam (*ningen dokku*) frequently includes ultrasound of the abdomen, spirometry, and upper and lower endoscopy, and in the most aggressive form *ningen dokku* may include computed tomography or magnetic resonance imaging of the brain (Hinohara, Touma, and Tajima, 1991).

Ultrasound and computed tomography are frequently used as diagnostic and surveillance tools in outpatient practice as well. While therapeutic use of medical technology appears to be more limited in Japan than the United States, there is clearly an aggressive nature to Japanese medicine.

The rapid increase in new types of medical technology and their rapid diffusion into the clinical setting, combined with the rapidly growing elderly population, have led to the common use of advanced life-prolonging treatments in Japan and the United States. Concerns have been raised about the costs to society relative to the meager benefit derived, though we hasten to acknowledge that there has been much debate about the extent to which the use of high-tech care at the end of life contributes to the high cost of care, or the extent to which high costs could be prevented (Scitovski, 1984; Emanuel and Emanuel, 1994; Lubitz, Beebe, and Baker, 1995; Emanuel, 1996). All told, these trends have focused attention on the difficult ethical problems related to withholding and withdrawing technology-intensive treatments. Resolution of such ethical conflict requires a better understanding of the values and belief systems in the US and Japan.

Differing values and belief systems

There is increasing interest in the United States in understanding how medicine reflects its culture (Freund and McGuire, 1995; Stein, 1990), how cultural and social differences influence health outcomes and quality of care (Helman, 1994; Kleinman, 1980; Kleinman, 1995; Kleinman, Eisenberg, and Good, 1978; Steiner, 1992; Orr *et al.*, 1995), and how US medical culture differs from the medical cultures of other countries (Hafferty and McKinlay, 1993; Payer, 1996). Clearly, decision-making about such issues as euthanasia, surrogate parenting, brain death, and organ transplantation creates ethical dilemmas not limited by national boundaries. Clinical approaches to resolving issues vary from country to country due to differences in values and belief systems in the respective cultures. There are many classic and more recent works on the relevance of culture to medicine in Japan in relation to East Asian medicine (Lock, 1980), medicine generally (Ohnuki-Tierney, 1984), menopause (Lock, 1993), brain death and organ transplantation (Lock and Honde, 1990; Feldman, 1994; Ohnuki-Tierney, 1994; Lock 1996a; Lock, 1996b; Lock, 1997; Ohnuki-Tierney, 1997), cancer disclosure (Long and Long, 1982; Elwyn *et al.*, 1998), mental health (McDonald-Scott, Machizawa, and Satoh, 1992), and the role of the family in medical decision-making (Tamura and Lau, 1992; McDonald-Scott, Machizawa, and Satoh, 1992; Fan, 1997; Hoshino, 1997b; Fetters, 1998; Long, 1999; Long, 1997a).

There is also a developing literature on physicians' approaches to life-sustaining treatments in both the United States (Society of Critical Care Medicine Ethics Task Force, 1992; Asch, Hansen-Flaschen, and Lanken, 1995; Hanson *et al.*, 1996) and Japan (Fukaura *et al.*, 1995; Asai at al., 1997). Still, there has been very little research designed to compare Japanese and US physicians' approaches to end-of-life decision-making (Sirio et al., 1992; Asai, Fukuhara, and Lo, 1995). An analytical study comparing intensive care unit (ICU) utilization in Japan and the United States suggests that better outcomes of intensive care could be achieved in the United States with fewer ICU beds, as in Japan (Sirio et al., 1992). Survey research by Asai et al.(1997) revealed Japanese physicians to be more aggressive with end-of-life treatments in response to case scenarios than Japanese-American physicians. Moreover, the Japanese physicians were more likely than their Japanese-American respondents to ignore the patient's request to withdraw life-sustaining interventions. To our knowledge there have been no previous investigations designed to compare the nature of end-of-life decision-making for elderly patients in Japan and the United States. The ongoing work of Susan Long (Long, 1999; Long, 1997a; Long, 1997b) and many contributors to this book is illuminating these morally compelling issues from an "on-the-ground" perspective.

Hence, the conflicts created by changing demographics, pressures to use the latest technological treatments, and economic pressures to limit their use have forced patients, their families, and physicians in Japan and the US to make difficult treatment decisions that in aggregate have profound health care expenditure implications. On the ground, in the hospitals, decisions to withhold life-sustaining treatments are literally life-or-death decisions. For patients and family members, these decisions affect not only the timing but also the manner of death. A decision to withhold treatment from a patient may deprive the patient and the family of enormously meaningful time together. Decisions to continue treatment may also result in suffering for the patient, family, staff, and friends. Clearly, the personal stakes for caregivers and patients are very high. Yet the stakes for society are high as well. Given society's competing demands for public health services, as well as other societal priorities, health care policy makers in both Japan and the US cannot ignore the complex, heart-wrenching decisions that must take place. In the following discussion, we present US and Japanese physicians' reports of their approaches to withholding life-sustaining treatments for elderly patients.

Methods

This project began in the United States as descriptive research to understand patients' and physicians' preferences for decision-making about end-of-life treatments (Danis et al., 1996; Hanson et al., 1996). Data collection for the US arm of this research began on October 1, 1990 and continued until July 31, 1993 at a university hospital in North Carolina. A Japanese arm was added in 1992 to compare Japanese physicians' approaches to end-of-life decision-making with US physicians' approaches. Data collection occurred from June until August 1992 at a university hospital in rural Japan.

The US arm used a sequential enrollment protocol which first prospectively enrolled patients with a diagnosis associated with an approximately 50 percent six-month mortality and then enrolled the attending and resident physicians providing care for these patients. Patient enrollment criteria included:

- 50 years of age or older
- either severe chronic lung disease, severe heart disease, or metastatic cancer
- admission to the medicine, gynecological oncology, or the family practice service.

These data have been reported in detail in previously (Danis et al., 1996). All participating US physicians were involved in the treatment of at least one patient with short life expectancy at the time of the interview; further details on recruitment and the primary findings of the US arm of this research have been reported previously (Hanson et al., 1996). Because the Japanese arm of the study was conducted to obtain parallel data on physicians' approaches to end-of-life care, a sequential patient-physician enrollment protocol was not utilized. Rather, Japanese physicians were randomly selected from the hospital roster of clinical internal medicine-related departments. Physicians from these departments were excluded if they were not actively providing medical care to adults or if they were from a department that did not routinely provide terminal care.

Instrument

First developed in English for the US arm of the study, the data-collection instrument contained both structured and semi-structured questions and was administered in person by an interviewer. The same questions were asked of all participants. The initial questions were based on two clinical vignettes (65-year-old with severe congestive heart failure and 65-year-old with metastatic cancer), and subsequent questions addressed variables such as permanent unconsciousness, futile treatments, resource allocation, and participant demographics (Hanson et al., 1996). To make the instrument culturally relevant for Japan, several items required deletion or changes in wording. Furthermore, two questions were added to inquire about physicians' experiences with cancer disclosure. After translation of the instrument into Japanese, it was translated back into English and reviewed for accuracy by two bilingual speakers.

In the US, the instrument was administered by trained interviewers who then transcribed each interview. The first author (MDF) was trained by the primary interviewer of the US arm and conducted the interviews in Japan. Tapes of each 30–60 minute interview were then transcribed by native Japanese speakers. In order to make the Japanese transcripts accessible to monolingual English-speaking research assistants, each transcript was independently translated into English by both a bilingual Japanese native and a bilingual American native.

This chapter reports the results from the open-ended question, "Under what circumstances are you inclined to withhold life-sustaining treatments?"

Analysis

Content analysis of the transcribed text involved:

- multiple readings of the transcripts
- coding scheme development
- coding and recoding of the interviews
- quality control measures.

The analysis team included a physician (MDF) and two graduate students. This group reviewed each transcript at least three times and developed a coding scheme from identified themes. This iterative process required serial coding and recoding of transcripts until the coders agreed that the coding scheme was capturing the major concepts of the text. Each coder also kept a coding diary as a reference on the use of codes and to note data falling outside the coding scheme. At least two people coded each transcript, with discrepancies negotiated at a review session. A third coder adjudicated irreconcilable differences between the first two coders. Coding disagreements were more common in the early phases of the analysis. Most differences arose from omissions or from using different codes with similar meaning. After reconciliation, the codes were inserted by a word processor into the transcripts for use in the content analysis. We sought to maximize trustworthiness of this research by working independently during both development and implementation of the coding scheme.

Results

Demographics

The demographics of the participating physicians are summarized in Table 6.1. Most participants were male physicians trained in internal medicine. While most US participants reported their religion as either Protestant (46 percent), Catholic (17 percent), Jewish (14 percent), or other (15 percent), most Japanese participants reported their religion as Buddhist (63 percent) or none (33 percent). The Japanese physicians were slightly older and had a narrower range of years in practice.

Decision-making about withholding life-sustaining treatments

Content analysis of the transcribed interviews revealed factors Japanese and American physicians consider when making decisions about withdrawal of

Table 6.1 Demographics of participating physicians

	US n=158 No.	(%)	Japan n=30 No.	(%)
Gender				
Female	27	(17)	2	(7)
Male	131	(83)	28	(93)
Specialty				
Internal medicine	142	(90)	26	(87)
Gynecology	6	(4)	–	(0)
Family medicine	–	(0)	2	(7)
Anesthesia	–	(0)	1	(3)
Critical care	–	(0)	1	(3)
Other	10	(6)	–	(0)
Religion				
Protestant	72	(46)	1	(3)
Catholic	26	(17)	–	(0)
Jewish	22	(14)	–	(0)
Buddhist	–	(0)	19	(63)*
Shinto	–	(0)	2	(7)*
None	15	(10)	10	(33)
Other	23	(15)	–	(0)
	Median (range)		Median (range)	
Age (years)	39.9	27–69	41.8	30–59
Years in practice	8.2	0–39	13	4–32

* One individual reported practicing both Buddhism and Shintoism

life-sustaining treatment. These are listed in Table 6.2. In the following discussion, we present the spectrum of factors considered by these physicians in decreasing order of frequency and illustrate how emphasis on these factors differed between Japanese and US physicians. For some factors, we provide the percentage of physicians in both groups who articulated a given point. The limitation of this data is that some physicians may simply not have remembered the factor. In contrast, this more spontaneous approach may provide a more honest indication of the factors relevant to their decision-making and may also give some indication of the relative importance of the major factors in Japan and the US. These factors are presented cumulatively; that is, no one physician could be identified as considering all these factors when interviewed since all statements were offered spontaneously.

Across the board, both groups indicated the importance of treatment attributes, and in a related vein, the nature of the illness. A large number of physicians in both groups also emphasized patient attitudes and attributes. While many physicians in both groups indicated a need to know family preferences, the Japanese physicians clearly afforded greater weight to family preferences than the US physicians. To round out the discussion, we end with examples of how physician attitudes influence care and note the relative

Table 6.2 Factors influencing decision-making

A	*Treatment and illness factors*	
	1	Treatment effectiveness
	2	Treatment harm
	3	Alleviating pain and suffering
	4	Nature of illness
	5	Co-morbidity and prognosis
B	*Patient factors*	
	1	Patient preferences
	2	Patient communication
	3	Quality of life
	4	Patient age
	5	Patient competence
	6	Patient understanding
C	*Family factors*	
	1	Family preferences
	2	Family suffering
	3	Family understanding
D	*Economic and legal factors*	
	1	Costs
	2	Legal issues

unimportance of social factors such as costs and legal issues in these physicians' approaches to withholding life-prolonging treatments.

Treatment and illness factors

Treatment attributes were among the most important factors discussed, as illustrated by the number of times these factors were raised by the participating physicians during their interviews. Sixty-seven percent (n = 20) of the Japanese respondents and 55 percent (n = 87) of the US physicians deemed treatment attributes relevant for decisions to withhold life-sustaining treatment. The overwhelmingly dominant topic of discussion about treatment attributes related to questions about the effectiveness of available life-sustaining treatment.

Treatment effectiveness

In relation to treatment attributes, the most common rationale for withdrawing life-sustaining treatment was that the treatment was ineffective and would not significantly change the patient's course of illness. Some physicians referred to this as futility, while others simply regarded the treatment as ineffective. Forty-three percent (n = 13) of the Japanese physicians and 45 percent (n = 71) of the US physicians reported considering treatment ineffectiveness when deciding to withdraw life-sustaining treatment, or treatment effectiveness when deciding to continue such treatment. While there was broad agreement about the importance of treatment effectiveness, there was little consensus about what constitutes effectiveness or ineffectiveness. These doctors used a variety of descriptors for lack of effectiveness, such as "nil," "remote," "poor," "probability of effectiveness of less than 1 percent," "less than 10 percent," "less than 25 percent," and "less than 30 percent." Some were willing to withhold treatments based solely on estimations of futility and lack of effectiveness. This group is exemplified by one physician who said, "If the treatment is not going to work, you don't do it. That seems pretty obvious, but you wouldn't believe how often that is not followed." Most physicians, US and Japanese alike, conceded that defining "effective," "ineffective," and "futile" in the clinical theater is quite difficult. Given that fact, an even greater number indicated that notions of futility really had to be considered together with other factors such as patient consciousness, presence of dementia, and/or risk of suffering.

Treatment harm

Both US and Japanese physicians also indicated a need to know about potential harms from treatment. Side effects of the intervention itself or toxicity that could be expected to result as a consequence of the treatment were factors raised specifically by 30 percent (n = 9) of the Japanese physicians and 9 percent (n = 14) of the US physicians. Harmful consequences of treatment could include functional sequelae such as neurologic compromise from stroke as a complication of resuscitation, or aesthetic harm such as edema from progressive renal impairment. The possibility of prolonging death rather than prolonging life was recognized as a real danger in caregiving for terminally-ill patients.

Alleviating pain and suffering

Physicians in both groups were averse to causing pain or suffering as a consequence of life-sustaining treatments but cognizant of the difficulty in predicting circumstances that would clearly lead to suffering as a result of treatment. Among all who addressed the issue, there was virtually unanimous agreement that measures should be taken to prevent or alleviate pain whenever possible. For many participants, the threat of a life-sustaining treatment perpetuating suffering was among the most powerful of reasons for withholding treatment.

Nature of illness

Illness severity inevitably has an influence on the effectiveness of the treatment. Generally speaking, the more advanced the illness, the lower the probability of treatment being effective. Both groups of physicians emphasized factors such as the nature of the illness and the presence of co-morbidities for making decisions about whether to withdraw treatment. These physicians sought information about whether the illness was acute or chronic and wanted to know the etiology of the exacerbating illness. They also found it helpful to determine the degree to which the patient's illness responded to treatment over time. For example, one explained:

> If I can't make a significant dent in the improvement of their clinical status in three or four days, I consider backing off depending on the other medical problems present. I am less inclined to be pushed by age; I am more inclined to be pushed by the severity of the underlying medical problems.

Thus, the natural history of the disease is relevant for making a decision on whether to withdraw life-sustaining treatment. Is the illness reversible, and can the patient return to a baseline level of functioning as a result of treatment? These physicians reported the need to know about the general health of the patient – information with relevance for the overall prognosis. For some, the nature of the illness was sufficient information to determine whether to withdraw life-sustaining treatment. Others reported a need to know whether the illness was a technology-dependent illness, such as a patient in a comatose state intubated and ventilated on the respirator, or if, for example, in the United States, the patient was a candidate for organ transplantation.

Co-morbidity and prognosis

Yet another issue reported as relevant by these physicians was co-morbidity. They inquired about the nature of pre-existing or co-existing disease. They were interested in specific co-morbidities such as dementia, depression or other psychiatric illness, alcohol or substance abuse, or cancer. Some felt the latter was an important issue, while others did not. A second consideration related specifically to the patient's prognosis. Some physicians mentioned the importance of prognosis only in general terms, while others sought to clarify the meaning of "terminal." Was the patient's death imminent within minutes to a week? Did "terminal" indicate an intermediate time frame of weeks or months? Or did "terminal" mean the patient's inevitable death from the disease might be a year or more away? While many physicians sought this information, some were forthcoming in their assessment that accurate prediction of length of survival is difficult. Although a terminal stage of disease was frequently cited as the basis for withholding life-sustaining treatments, a minority of physicians were quick to point out the difficulty inherent in defining the word "terminal."

Thus, the nature of treatments and patients' underlying illnesses in terms of the severity of their primary problem as well as co-morbid problems have an impact on the long-term prognosis and thus on physicians' willingness to pursue or withhold treatments. However, this is strongly tempered by patient factors, especially patient preferences for treatment.

Patient factors

Like treatment attributes, the patient's wishes and the patient's ability to communicate preferences for treatment emerged as highly important factors in these physicians' decisions about withholding life-sustaining treatments. Indeed, patient preferences were identified as relevant by a majority of physicians in both countries. Other patient factors such as quality of life, age, competence, and patient understanding also figured prominently for some physicians in both countries.

Patient preferences

Many US and Japanese physicians indicated that they considered the patient's preference for treatment. Fifty-two percent (n = 16) of the Japanese physicians and 59 percent (n = 94) of the US physicians responded by asking for the patient's preference. The Japanese physicians typically asked, "What is the patient's will?" (*kanja no ishi*) or "What is the patient's preference?" (*kanja no kibō*). For many of them, this was their first response to questioning, and qualitatively the most important information. For others, patient preferences were lumped together with family preferences almost as if they were inseparable. The role of family preferences will be addressed in greater detail below. Others indicated patient preferences as one of several factors that they would consider when making decisions about whether to offer or withhold treatments.

There were also various degrees of importance attributed to patient preferences by the US physicians. Among the physicians who discussed patient preferences, a majority weighed patient preferences as the most important factor in their decision-making. Other factors were relevant not for the physician to make a decision, but to assist the patient in making an informed decision. A minority indicated that they would weigh patient preferences among other considerations such as treatment effectiveness, prognosis, age, etc. Some physicians in both countries felt strongly that if a patient wanted to have a treatment, it would be unethical to withhold it. Likewise, some indicated that they would only withhold treatment if that was the express wish of the patient. However, a handful of US physicians indicated that if the treatment was not expected to work, the patient would not get the treatment. Many others indicated that while patient preferences were of prime importance, some circumstances would make them reluctant to adhere strictly to a patient's preferences. They might act, for example, by providing a requested treatment, but not as aggressively.

Intra-group variations aside, there was an overall qualitative difference between the US and Japanese physicians. The US physicians who asked about patient preference essentially wished to delegate the decision to the patient. That is, "the patient's preference" was equated with "the patient makes the decision." Eliciting the patient's preference was tantamount to eliciting their informed consent to a procedure or intervention without which treatment would not proceed. In Japan, there were certainly some doctors who followed this approach. However, the more common pattern among Japanese participants was the presumption that "patient's preferences" should be used to inform the doctor's decision about what treatments to use. Thus, while patient preferences were reported as important factors by both the Japanese and US physicians, preferences were frequently synonymous with the patient making the decision in the US, whereas patient preferences in Japan tended to be valued as information to be used in the physician's decision-making process.

Patient communication

For US physicians, especially those who follow a "patient decides" model, communication is central for determining the patient's preferences. Direct communication with patients is the means for presenting the different treatment options, their benefits and risks, and for ascertaining the patient's understanding of these factors. Not surprisingly, these physicians inquired as to whether the patient was able to communicate his or her wishes or needs. Many of the US physicians presented an image of sitting down with the patient to have a detailed discussion about the current situation, risks, and benefits of treatment. In contrast, the Japanese physicians more typically used a longer course of time to get to know the patient and to determine the patient's preferences. Several reported using family reports of their past discussions with the patient to learn what the patient's opinion might be. Reports of discussions between family members and the patient were asked for by many more Japanese than US physicians. Some Japanese physicians pointed out the difficulty of having such serious discussions with someone whom they had just met. Such frank discussions might be construed as disrespectful, especially if the patient was older and of higher social status than the physician.

One area illustrating differences in communication patterns is the use of advance directives for treatment preferences. Some US physicians advocated having a discussion with patients about their preferences for life-sustaining treatments prior to occurrence of illness. This proactive approach was seldom mentioned by the Japanese physicians. While the Japanese physicians commonly asked whether the patient had previously indicated treatment preferences in the event of life-threatening circumstances, the possibility of direct, advance discussions with the patient about his or her preferences initiated by the physician was apparently not an option these physicians routinely exercised. Some US physicians emphasized that they actively withheld information about treatment possibilities when they deemed that the treatment was not a plausible option. In other words, these physicians operated on a belief that only "realistic treatment options" should be communicated to the patient. Discussing non-options was not an issue raised by the Japanese physicians.

Quality of life

Either direct references to the term "quality of life" or allusions to quality of life were very common among both the Japanese and US physicians. Some simply referred to quality of life. Other doctors suggested that they would be inclined to withhold life-sustaining treatments when they were reasonably confident that the patient would not have a good quality of life regardless of what treatment was employed. Physical and mental suffering were both articulated by the physicians as reasons for withholding life-sustaining treatment. Physical suffering usually implied pain. Twenty-three percent (n = 7) of the Japanese physicians and 10 percent (n = 16) of the US physicians indicated that the patient's suffering from pain was a factor that would support withholding life-sustaining treatment. Both groups were generally opposed to using life-sustaining treatments if the net effect would be to prolong physical or mental pain or suffering, even if the treatment might prolong the patient's life for an extended period of time. An indicator deemed important by both groups of physicians concerned the patient's ability to ambulate. A patient being bedridden, especially after a long course of treatment, was cited by both Japanese and US physicians as a reason to withhold life-sustaining treatment.

Patient age

Some physicians indicated that age was an important factor. Twenty percent (n = 6) of the Japanese physicians and 8 percent (n = 13) of the US physicians mentioned age as relevant when determining whether to withhold life-sustaining treatment. Both Japanese and US physicians made similar comments about the relationship between age and life-sustaining treatment. Some specified the years beyond which consideration of longevity becomes a particularly important factor, though there was disagreement as to what specific age should be the cutoff, with the two commonly mentioned limits being 80 years and 90 years. Others stressed the importance of physiological age rather than chronological age. Others indicated age as relevant when considered in combination with other non-medical factors and co-morbidities. No one cited advanced age as sufficient reason in itself to withhold life-sustaining treatment. Only if the very old patient was deemed incompetent or unable to make a decision would some physicians be willing to withhold life-sustaining treatment. Others were adamantly opposed to the use of age as a criterion for determining whether to withhold life-sustaining treatment and sought instead to understand the patient's preferences or to evaluate the severity of the underlying illness.

Patient competence

Some Japanese and US physicians alike described the patient's mental function as important for making a decision to withhold life-sustaining treatment. For this variable, only 7 percent (n = 2) of the Japanese physicians and eight percent (n = 12) of the US physicians inquired about patient competency when asked about the circumstances in which they would withhold life-sustaining treatment. A small number of physicians inquired about the patient's consciousness. While some US physicians inquired about the patient's level of consciousness and cognitive abilities or impairment, such as patient senility, many also inquired about the patient's competence to make decisions. Japanese physicians were primarily concerned with whether the patient was conscious or comatose, rather than if the patient was competent.

Patient understanding

The data indicate that physicians believe a patient's understanding is relevant for making medical decisions in at least two ways. First, a patient's lack of knowledge about the implications of the use of life-sustaining treatment was cited as relevant. Physicians citing this commented on the difficulty of providing patients with an accurate picture of what a given treatment will involve. They stated that physicians' experiences with other similar cases may allow the physicians to foresee impending complications. Still, they think it may be very difficult both for the physician to convey the plausible outcomes and for the patient to understand the implications of pursuing life-sustaining treatments. This was reported by some to be especially true for end-of-life treatments which offered not a simple choice between life and death, but rather a more complicated array of possible outcomes, including living with return to baseline, living with some degree of impairment ranging from minor to severe, or death. Second, the patient's understanding was also reported by the physicians as relevant for a decision to withhold life-sustaining treatment based on the patient's understanding of that decision. For example, some of these physicians wanted to know if the patient could articulate the implications for a variety of treatment options and the plausible outcomes of those treatment options. If such a patient chose to terminate treatment, the physicians reported that it is easier to withhold treatment.

Family factors

The frequency of mentioning family or significant others proved to be quite divergent between the Japanese and US physicians. Family factors were raised by 57 percent (n = 17) of the Japanese physicians, whereas only 27 percent (n = 43) of the US physicians raised any issues related to the family or significant others in decision-making. Japanese physicians overwhelmingly referred to family involvement in decision-making in neutral terms. Only one somewhat negative reference was made – a physician indicated he would be less likely to provide aggressive treatment if the family had "abandoned" the patient in a long-term care hospital. In contrast, 19 percent (n = 8) of the US physicians' comments about family involvement made negative reference to the role of the family in terms of the family being obstructionist (n = 4) through demands or poor understanding of the disease process, the family as a source of legal problems (n = 2), or the family being dysfunctional or not supportive of the patient (n = 2).

Family preferences

The role of family preferences for withholding life-sustaining treatment was very different for these Japanese physicians and US physicians. Forty percent (n=12) of the Japanese physicians reported family preferences as important in decisions about whether to withhold life-sustaining treatment. Ten of them asked for the patient and family preferences, and two physicians never even mentioned seeking the patient's preferences but did ask about the family's preferences. In contrast, only about 10 percent (n = 15) of the US physicians acknowledged the family as relevant to decision-making while the patient was competent. Nine percent (n = 14) of the US physicians' references to family members or significant others related to surrogate decision-making by the family for incompetent patients. Patient incompetence did not play a central role for the Japanese physicians. One US physician stated he would seek family preferences only for a patient over the age of 90. As alluded to in the discussion of patient preferences, many Japanese physicians accorded family preferences an importance at least equal to that of the patient preferences. Yet as with patient preferences, it is unclear the extent to which family preferences determine the decision or serve merely as additional data to inform the physician's decision.

Family suffering

Japanese and US physicians were similarly concerned about the possibility of life-sustaining treatment causing a burden of emotional pain to the family. Situations in which treatments were perceived to cause family suffering fell into two categories: circumstances in which the physician saw suffering by the family, and those in which the physician anticipated family suffering based on the patient's prognosis. For example, a physician mentioned that if a patient experienced a cardiac arrest for which resuscitation was delayed for 10 minutes, a circumstance with a high probability of catastrophic brain damage, he would be reluctant to resuscitate due to the impact on the family. A few Japanese physicians commented that life-sustaining treatment could become an excessive burden, or that withholding would be appropriate for "situations when it seems the patient's family can't mentally bear ongoing treatment." Similarly, a small number of US physicians were concerned about how life-sustaining treatment could cause suffering for the family.

Family understanding

Some US physicians reported considering the various levels of family understanding about the disease process and the use of high technology treatments. These comments reflect physicians' need to make sure that the family understands the implication of decisions. As in the case of patients with faulty understanding of treatment options, when managing situations in which the family does not adequately understand the implications of the treatment, or has unrealistic expectations for the treatment, some doctors indicated a reluctance to comply with family preferences.

Economic and legal factors

In any research, that which is absent from the findings may be as informative as that which is found. In this study, few Japanese or US physicians volunteered cost as relevant to their decision to withhold life-sustaining treatment. When participants in either group did mention cost, their discussions were largely similar. In the small number of cases when cost issues were raised by either US or Japanese participants, they broached the idea that costs might be or possibly should be considered, if the treatment was very expensive and the expected benefit was very minimal. An even smaller number raised questions about who actually bears the weight of the costs – society or patients and their families. Japanese physicians had relatively little commentary about overall health care costs for society, and the US physicians also seemed reluctant to discuss the issue of cost. Their references to cost were typically vague mentions about the costs of treatment in general or that life-sustaining treatments can cost a "ton of money" or "break the bank." Others were more candid about their aversion to using cost as a factor in decision-making, but reported the reality that cost does become a consideration in circumstances when the proposed intervention is highly expensive and there are questions about the effectiveness of the treatment. Some tried to assess whether there were outrageous costs for the expected result, that is, would the incurred costs have a tangible effect on health care outcomes. One Japanese physician indicated his sense that the publicity about brain death simply resulted in redirecting attention away from the more important common problem of caregiving for patients in vegetative states, whose health care costs are extremely high. Another expressed the opinion that withdrawal of life-sustaining treatments is appropriate if there is a risk of creating financial problems for the patient and the family. US physicians similarly indicated a concern about wasting family or patient resources.

It was no surprise that Japanese physicians rarely voiced legal concerns. There are fewer lawyers in Japan per capita than in the United States, and there seems to be a much smaller penchant for bringing suit in Japan. But it was surprising that only two of all the US participants raised legal issues as a relevant consideration for withholding life-sustaining treatment. Even in these two cases, the issue was raised more as though it were a peripheral, unusual issue. We expected there would be more medicolegal concerns raised, since the recent past has demanded physicians' conscious attention to legal aspects of clinical medicine (Richards and Rathbun, 1993; Leaman and Saxton, 1993).

Discussion

The main message that we derive from these interviews with Japanese and US physicians is that they think about similar concerns when deciding whether or not to utilize highly technological life-sustaining treatments at the end of life. The medical literature suggests that US physicians are accustomed to withdrawing treatments (Asch, Hansen-Flaschen, and Lanken, 1995) and use criteria such as age and severity of disease to make decisions about who receives cardiopulmonary resuscitation and intensive care (Hanson and Danis, 1991). In contrast, literature from Japan suggests that Japanese physicians are reluctant to withhold and withdraw life-sustaining treatment (Fukaura *et al.*, 1995; Asai, Fukuhara, and Lo, 1995; Asai *et al.*, 1997) although we were not able to make this assertion from our data. In making their decisions, the most frequently emphasized factors by both Japanese and US physicians were treatment effectiveness, patient preferences, and patient quality of life. We find three notable trends in these physician groups.

First, many Japanese physicians perceived the patient and the family as almost inseparable in decision-making. While many Japanese physicians indicated family preferences as highly compelling, only a minority of the US physicians mentioned this as significant. Among the Japanese physicians, family preferences were mentioned as relevant by 40 percent of the physicians compared to only 10 percent of the US physicians. In a small minority of cases, Japanese physicians cited family preferences as a factor without citing patient preferences. The tone of Japanese physicians' discussions about involving family members was much more neutral than many of the US physicians. These results are consistent with the growing body of literature about the central role of the family in medical decision-making in Japan (Hattori *et al.*, 1991; Tamura and Lau, 1992; McDonald-Scott, Machizawa, and Satoh, 1992; Fan, 1997; Hoshino, 1997b; Fetters, 1998; Long, 1999; Long, 1997a), and specifically its role in end-of-life treatment decisions (Fukaura *et al.*, 1995; Asai, Fukuhara, and Lo, 1995). In a prospective cohort study of do-not-resuscitate (DNR) orders at a teaching hospital in Japan, Fukaura *et al.* (1995) found that family members and physicians participated in all the DNR orders, but only 5 percent of the patients participated. For a subgroup of the US physicians in our study, family preferences were deemed relevant only when the patient was incompetent. Furthermore, a small number of the US physicians reported the family's role in a negative way, as if the family were obstructive to good decision-making, or a legal threat. These observations highlight a growing interest in examining the role of the family in decision-making. Indeed we should note that the conception of the family's role may be changing in the US (Hardwig, 1990; Nelson, 1992; Nelson and Nelson, 1993; Nelson and Nelson, 1995; Reust and Mattingly, 1996; Kuczewski, 1996; Nicholson, 1997). There is more recognition that the preeminence of the patient's perspective to the exclusion of the family's concerns may not necessarily be the most advisable approach.

Second, we find that when US physicians discuss these issues they refer to bioethical principles and policy that Japanese physicians do not typically refer to, including an emphasis on patient competence, informed consent in decision-making, the application of bioethical principles when thinking about the issues, and on a limited basis, the use of advance directives to plan end-of-life care. It is quite likely that these differences are a reflection of the bioethics movement in the US. This influence can be seen in a variety of publications over the last decade in the US from respected clinicians, ethicists, medical groups, and governmental commissions (President's Commission for the Study of Ethical Problems in Medicine and Biomedical and Behavioral Research, 1983; Wanzer *et al.*, 1984; Hastings Center, 1987; Wanzer *et al.*, 1989; Council on Ethical and Judicial Affairs, 1991; American Board of Internal Medicine, 1996; Council on Scientific Affairs, 1996; Institute of Medicine Committee on Care of the Dying, 1997). At the same time, previously published work examining the relationship between patient preferences and actual treatment use found in the US arm of this research indicated little systematic evidence that patient preferences determine life-sustaining treatment (Danis *et al.*, 1996).

Third, variation between the two groups in their approaches to patient involvement in decision-making were noted. While both US and Japanese physicians report the substantive importance of patient preferences, the difference in how patient preferences are reported to influence decision-making was striking. To many US physicians, the patient's preference is the decision, whereas for the Japanese, the patient's preference tended to be just one of the factors. This difference is reflected in the most common decision-making patterns found in the two groups. Japanese physicians were more likely to report considering multiple factors in their decision-making. This is consistent with previous work on decision-making about disclosure of a cancer diagnosis in Japan and the United States (Elwyn *et al.*, 1998). Japanese physicians seem to be concerned with many factors, and prefer to make decisions on a case-by-case basis rather than base decisions on a single factor such as treatment effectiveness, bioethical principles, or patient preferences.

There were four primary limitations of this research. First, the recruitment procedures for the US and Japanese arms of the study were not the same. Given that this research focused on physicians' approaches to end-of-life care, and that physicians in the US were actively providing care for at least one patient with a poor prognosis at the time of the study, and that the Japanese physicians were all recruited from internal medicine-related departments in which caregiving for terminally ill patients is common, we believe that the impact of the differences in recruiting on the results are likely to be minimal. Second, it is possible that a larger sample size in the Japanese arm would have resulted a broader range of responses. Similarly, both arms were conducted in university hospitals that service rural areas. Investigations from other settings might provide further variations in approaches to end-of-life caregiving. Third, these data were collected at the dawn of managed care's penetration into US medicine. Given the managed care emphasis on cost reduction, we cannot be sure whether these data reflect current practices in the varied managed care settings. We suspect that the range of behaviors is probably similar if not the same, but the most common behaviors, and US physicians' willingness to act in accordance with the decision-making patterns they described may have changed. Fourth, these data represent both Japanese and US physicians' self-reports of their behaviors, and there can be differences between self-reports and actual behaviors. Whether there is 100 percent correlation is probably not of great significance since our focus has been on describing the range of approaches and general trends. Furthermore, the range of findings identified here is consistent with our own observations as clinicians about caregiving at the end of life.

As a final note, we are compelled to call attention to intracultural and intercultural diversity as there are compelling data to refute the stereotypes of monolithic end-of-life decision making in Japan and the United States (Long, 1997a). In this chapter, we have made many comparisons and observed trends. We wish to acknowledge the salient diversity of these cultures and hope that our generalizations will be accepted as such, and not as stereotypes.

Health care policy implications

What then are the policy implications of these physicians' perspectives on caregiving in late life and use of life-sustaining treatment? These data suggest at least four relevant considerations.

We live too short and die too long

These physicians' experiences in providing care for terminally ill patients have given them an appreciation for the precious nature of life and the hazards of a prolonged dying process focused on keeping people alive rather than on the quality of their living. One Japanese physician shared his thoughts about his experience caring for an amyotrophic lateral sclerosis patient. He stated, "We had a patient with amyotrophic lateral sclerosis, the patient was conscious and had a 'mind' (*kokoro*). At home we connected the ventilator. I think we must think more about the problems of the aging of society." This respondent went on to discuss how the book *We live too short and die too long* by Walter Bortz (1991) influenced him to think about the quality of life that one lives and the fact that the dying process itself takes too long. His comments suggest that there may be a universal sense that on one hand, life is precious and worth living as long as possible. On the other hand, efforts to keep a patient alive with aggressive use of life-sustaining treatment can inadvertently result in the patient having a prolonged and agonizing existence up until the time of death. This message emphasizes the need to maintain and implement policies nurturing the positive aspects of living, while overturning existing and rejecting new policies that tragically prolong dying.

Decision-making processes vary enormously

There is much variation in the weight different doctors give to diverse factors in their decision-making about life-sustaining treatment. Likewise the literature indicates that there is variation among patients and families in their values and preferences for life-sustaining treatment (Gross, 1998). If there is a good match and physician actions are in concordance with patient and family desires, the variation in nature and duration of care that patients and families experience at the end of the patient's life may simply reflect the fact that each case has unique goals, needs, and manifestations of disease. But there is no mechanism to guarantee a good match between patient preferences and physician behavior and approaches. Under these circumstances the care that patients receive at the end of life may be a matter of chance. Such a situation is a concern for doctors, caregivers, and patients. Moreover, it may result in variable and unjust distribution of finite resources, thereby becoming a concern for policy makers as well. This struggle to use modern technology in facing the age-old problem of finding a graceful way to die supersedes cultural boundaries.

Balancing patient and family preferences with realities of physiology and economics of treatment

Advocates for patient autonomy might argue that patients should have the freedom to make decisions themselves or through a designated surrogate without considering costs or any other factors. On the other hand, unrestrained demand for end-of-life treatments may inevitably result in unjust distribution of the limited health care and societal resources. Nevertheless, costs were infrequently raised by these physicians as relevant for decisions about whether to withhold life-sustaining treatment. There are at least two plausible interpretations of this phenomenon. First, physicians believe cost considerations are largely irrelevant to clinical decision-making. Second, direct discussion of costs is socially taboo; allusions to costs can only be found tucked away and camouflaged in physicians' behaviors and discussions about futility. Physicians may simply mask health care rationing decisions as treatment effectiveness decisions. From the perspective of patients and families, physicians' reported neglect of cost considerations may be reassuring. In contrast, this may be an important area of concern for policy makers. Given the expanding elderly population, the anticipated greater need for care in late life, and the expanding availability and variety of high technology treatments, health care policy makers need to scrutinize the best means of balancing patient and family preferences with the economics of treatment.

Physician reports versus physician behaviors

A subject of considerable concern, particularly raised in the United States literature, is the degree to which physicians adhere to patient preferences. When physicians respond to surveys or interview questions about their approaches to patient care and decision-making, they may be reporting what they believe they ought to practice rather than what they actually do practice. The discrepancy between their reported behaviors and attitudes and how they actually practice may reflect their aspirations for their relationships with patients and family members. While this discrepancy may be disheartening, as has been the interpretation of the SUPPORT study (SUPPORT Principal Investigators, 1995), behavioral change is notoriously difficult to bring about, and it will likely take many years for practice patterns to change noticeably. Thus, the effectiveness of health care policies designed to provide a framework for ethical decision making should not be measured over the short term. Indeed, in the ancient practice of medicine, the passage of many years may be required before there are truly tangible behavior changes.

Acknowledgments

This research was made possible in part by the generous support of Dr Fetters, by the Japan-United States Educational Council (the Fulbright Japan Today Program) and the Robert Wood Johnson Clinical Scholars Program. Dr Danis and the project "Making choices and allocating resources near life's end" was funded by grant HS 06655 from the Agency of Health Care Policy and Research. Dr Fetters' participation and presentation of this paper at the Workshop, "Care and meaning in late life: Culture, policy, and practice in Japan and the United States" at Zushi, Japan was supported by the Abe Program.

References

American Board of Internal Medicine. (1996). *Caring for the dying: Identification and promotion of physician competency*. Philadelphia, PA: American Board of Internal Medicine.

Anderson, G.F. (1997). In search of value: An international comparison of cost, access, and outcomes. *Health Affairs, November/December*, 163–171.

Asai, A., Fukuhara, S., and Lo, B. (1995). Attitudes of Japanese and Japanese-American physicians towards life-sustaining treatment. *Lancet, 346*, 356–359.

Asai, A., Fukuhara, S., Inoshita, O., Miura, Y., Tanabe, N., and Kurokawa, K. (1997). Medical decisions concerning the end of life: A discussion with Japanese physicians. *Journal of Medical Ethics, 23*, 323–327.

Asch, D.A., Hansen-Flaschen, J., and Lanken, P.N. (1995). Decisions to limit or continue life-sustaining treatments by critical care physicians in the United States: Conflicts between physicians' practices and patients' wishes. *American Journal of Respiratory and Critical Care Medicine, 151*, 279–92.

Bortz, W. (1991). *We live too short and die too long*. New York: Bantam Books.

Callahan, D. (1987). *Setting limits: Medical goals in an aging society*. New York: Simon & Schuster.

Callahan, D. (1990). *What kind of life: The limits of medical progress*. New York: Simon & Schuster.

Canadian Task Force. (1979). The periodic health examination. *Canadian Medical Association Journal, 121*, 1193–1254.

Chalfin, D.B., and Fein, A.M. (1994). Critical care medicine in managed competition and a managed care environment. *New Horizons, 2*, 275–282.

Council on Ethical and Judicial Affairs, American Medical Association. (1991). Guides for the appropriate use of do-not-resuscitate orders. *Journal of the American Medical Association, 265*, 1868–1871.

Council on Scientific Affairs, American Medical Association. (1996). Good care of the dying patient. *Journal of the American Medical Association, 275*, 474–478.

Danis, M., Mutran, E., Garrett, J.M., Stearns, S., Hanson, L. C., Slifkin, R., and Churchill, L. (1996). A prospective study of patient preferences, life-sustaining treatment and hospital cost. *Critical Care Medicine, 24*, 1811–1817.

Elwyn, T.S., Fetters, M.D., Gorenflo, D.W., and Tsuda, T. (1998). Cancer disclosure in Japan: Historical comparisons, current practices. *Social Science and Medicine, 46*, 1151–1163.

Emanuel, E.J., and Emanuel L.L. (1994). The economics of dying: The illusion of cost-savings at the end of life. *New England Journal of Medicine, 330*, 540–544.

Emanuel, E.J. (1996). Cost savings at the end of life. What do the data show? *Journal of the American Medical Association, 275*, 1907–1914.

Fan, R. (1997). Self-determination vs. family-determination: Two incommensurable principles of autonomy. *Bioethics, 11*, 309–322.

Feldman, E. (1994). Culture, conflict, and cost: Perspectives on brain death in Japan. *International Journal of Technology Assessment in Health Care, 10*, 447–463.

Fetters, M.D. (1998). The family in medical decision-making: Japanese perspectives. *Journal of Clinical Ethics, 9*, 143–157.

Freund, P.E., and McGuire, M.B. (1995). *Health, illness and the social body*. Englewood Cliffs: Prentice Hall.

Fukaura, A., Tazawa, H., Nakajima, H., and Adachi, M. (1995). Do-not-resuscitate orders at a teaching hospital in Japan. *New England Journal of Medicine, 333*, 805–808.

Gross, M.D. (1998). What do patients express as their preferences in advance directives? *Archives of Internal Medicine, 158*, 321–324.

Hafferty, F.W., and McKinlay, J.B. (Eds.). (1993). *The changing medical profession: An international perspective*. New York: Oxford University Press.

Hanson, L.C., and Danis, M. (1991). Use of life-sustaining care for the elderly. *Journal of the American Geriatrics Society, 39*, 772–777.

Hanson, L.C., Danis, M., Garrett, J.M., and Mutran, E. (1996). Who decides? Physicians' willingness to use life-sustaining treatments. *Archives of Internal Medicine, 156*, 785–789.

Hardwig, J. (1990). What about the family? *Hastings Center Report 10*, 5–10.

Hastings Center, The. (1987). *Guidelines on the termination of life-sustaining treatment and the care of the dying*. Bloomington, IN: Indiana University Press.

Hattori, H., Salzberg, S.M., Kiang, W.P., Fujimiya, T., Tejima, Y., and Furuno, J. (1991). The patient's right to information in Japan: Legal rules and doctor's opinions. *Social Science and Medicine, 32*, 9, 1007–1016.

Helman, C.G. (1994). *Culture, health, and illness* (3rd ed.). Oxford: Butterworth-Heinemann.

Hinohara, S., Touma, H., and Tajima, M. (1991). *Ningen dokku manyuaru: Kenkō hyōka to shidō no pointo*. (Human dry dock manual: Points on health evaluation and guidance). Tokyo: Igakushoin.

Hoshino, K. (Ed.). (1997a). *Japanese and western bioethics: Studies in moral diversity*. In H.T. Engelhardt and S.F. Spicker (Series Eds.). *Philosophy and medicine: Vol. 54*. Dordrecht: Kluwer Academic Publishers.

Hoshino, K. (1997b). Bioethics in the light of Japanese sentiments. In K. Hoshino (Ed.), *Japanese and western bioethics: Studies in moral diversity* (pp. 13–23). In H.T. Engelhardt and S.F. Spicker (Series Eds.) *Philosophy and medicine: Vol. 54*. Dordrecht: Kluwer Academic Publishers.

Institute of Medicine Committee on Care of the Dying. (1997). *Approaching death: Care at the end of life*. Washington, DC: National Academy Press.

Kikuchi, M. (1991). Status of medical engineering technology assessment in Japan. *Frontiers of Medical and Biological Engineering, 3*, 3–15.

Kleinman, A., Eisenberg, L., and Good, B. (1978). Culture, illness, and care: Clinical lessons from anthropological and cross cultural research. *Annals of Internal Medicine, 88*, 251–258.

Kleinman, A. (1980). *Patients and healers in the context of culture: An exploration of the borderland between anthropology, medicine, and psychiatry*. Berkeley: University of California Press.

Kleinman, A. (1995). *Writing at the margin: Discourse between anthropology and medicine*. Berkeley: University of California Press.

Koenig, B. (1988). The technological imperative in medical practice: The social creation of a 'routine' treatment. In M. Lock and D. Gordon (Eds.), *Biomedicine examined* (pp. 464–496). Dordrecht: Kluwer Academic Publishers..

Kuczewski, M. (1996). Reconvening the family: The process of consent in medical decision-making. *Hastings Center Report, 26*, 30–37.

Leaman, T.L., and Saxton, J.W. (1993). *Preventing malpractice: The active solution*. New York: Plenum Medical Book Company.

Lock, M.M. (1980). *East Asian medicine in urban Japan*. Berkeley: University of California Press.

Lock, M.M. (1993). *Encounters with aging: Mythologies of menopause in Japan and North America*. Berkeley: University of California Press.

Lock, M.M. (1996a). Deadly Disputes: Ideologies and brain death in Japan. In S.J. Youngner and R.C. Fox (Eds.), *Organ transplantation: Meanings and realities* (pp. 142–167). Madison: University of Wisconsin Press.

Lock, M.M. (1996b). Death in technological time: Locating the end of meaningful life. *Medical Anthropological Quarterly, 10*, 575–600.

Lock, M.M. (1997). The unnatural as ideology: Contesting brain death in Japan. In P.J. Asquith and A. Kalland (Eds.), *Japanese images of nature: Cultural perspectives* (pp. 121–144). Nordic Institute of Asian Studies. Richmond, UK: Curzon Press.

Lock, M.M., and Honde, C. (1990). Reaching consensus about death: Heart transplants and cultural identity in Japan. In G. Weisz (Ed.), *Social science perspectives on medical ethics* (pp. 99–120). Philadelphia: University of Pennsylvania Press.

Long, S.O. (1997a). Living poorly or dying well: Culture and decisions about life supporting treatments for American and Japanese patients. Manuscript submitted for publication.

Long, S.O. (1997b). Reflections on becoming a cucumber: Images of the good death in Japan and the US. Paper presented at the Center for Japanese Studies, University of Michigan, September 11.

Long, S.O. (1999). Family surrogacy and cancer disclosure in Japan. *Journal of Palliative Care, 15*, 3, 31-42..

Long, S.O., and Long, B.D. (1982). Curable cancers and fatal ulcers: Attitudes toward cancer in Japan. *Social Science and Medicine, 16*, 2101–2108.

Lubitz, J., Beebe, J., and Baker, C. (1995). Longevity and Medicare expenditures. *New England Journal of Medicine, 332*, 999–1003.

McDonald-Scott, P., Machizawa, S., and Satoh, H. (1992). Diagnostic disclosure: A tale in two cultures. *Psychological Medicine, 22*, 147–157.

Ministry of Health and Welfare. (1991). *Health and welfare statistics*. Tokyo: Health and Welfare Statistics Association.

Nelson, J. (1992). Taking families seriously. *Hastings Center Report, 22*, 6–12.

Nelson, J.L., and Nelson, H.L. (1993). Guided by intimates. *Hastings Center Report, 23*, 14–15.

Nelson, H.L., and Nelson, J.L. (1995). *The patient in the family: An ethics of medicine and families*. New York: Routledge.

Nicholson, R.H. (1997). In the family's best interest. *Hastings Center Report, 27*, 4.

Ohnuki-Tierney, E. (1984). *Illness and culture in contemporary Japan: An anthropological view*. New York: Cambridge University Press.

Ohnuki-Tierney, E. (1997). The reduction of personhood to brain and rationality? Japanese contestation of medical high technology. In A. Cunningham and B. Andrews (Eds.), *Western medicine as contested knowledge* (pp. 212–240). Manchester, UK: Manchester University Press.

Omnibus Budget Reconciliation Act of 1990 (1990). Vol. Pub. L. No. 101–0508, pp. 4206, 4751.

Orr, R.D., Marshall, P.A., and Osborn, J. (1995). Cross-cultural considerations in clinical ethics consultations. *Archives of Family Medicine, 4*, 159–164.

Payer, L. (1996). *Medicine and culture.* New York: Henry Holt and Company.

President's Commission for the Study of Ethical Problems in Medicine and Biomedical and Behavioral Research. (1983). *Deciding to forgo life-sustaining treatment.* Washington DC: Government Printing Office.

Randall, T. (1993). Demographers ponder the aging of the aged and await unprecedented looming elder boom. *Journal of the American Medical Association, 269*, 2331–2332.

Reust, C.E., and Mattingly, S. (1996). Family involvement in medical decision-making. *Family Medicine, 28*, 39–45.

Richards, E.P., and Rathbun, K.C. (1993). *Law and the physician: A practical guide.* Boston: Little, Brown and Company.

Scitovski, A.A. (1984). The high cost of dying: What do the data show? *Milbank Quarterly, 62*, 591–608.

Sirio, C.A., Tajimi, K., Tase, C., Knaus, W.A., Wagner, D.P., Hirasawa, H., Sakanishi, N., Katsuya, H., and Taenaka, N. (1992). An initial comparison of intensive care in Japan and the United States. *Critical Care Medicine, 20*, 1207–1215.

Society of Critical Care Medicine Ethics Task Force. (1992). Attitudes of critical care professionals concerning forgoing life-sustaining treatments. *Critical Care Medicine, 20*, 320–326.

Stein, H.F. (1990). *American medicine as culture.* Boulder: Westview Press.

Steiner, R.P. (1992). Culture, family medicine and society. *American Family Physician, 46*, 1398–1400.

SUPPORT Principal Investigators. (1995). A controlled trial to improve care for seriously ill hospitalized patients. The Study to Understand Prognoses and Preferences for Outcomes and Risks of Treatments (SUPPORT). *Journal of the American Medical Association, 274*, 1591–1598.

Tamura, T., and Lau, A. (1992). Connectedness versus separateness: Applicability of family therapy to Japanese families. *Family Proceedings, 31*, 319–340.

US Department of Health and Human Services Public Health Service. (1994). *Clinician's handbook of preventive services.* Washington, DC: US Government Printing Office.

US Preventive Services Task Force. (1996). Cost-effectiveness and clinical preventive services. In *Guide to clinical preventive services* (2nd ed.) (pp. lxxxv-xcii). Baltimore: Williams & Wilkins.

Wanzer, S.H., Adelstein, S.J, Cranford, R.E., Federman, D.D., Hook, E.D., Moertel, C.G., Safar, P., Stone, A., Taussig, H.B., and van Eys, J. (1984). The physician's responsibility toward hopelessly ill patients. *New England Journal of Medicine, 310*, 955–959.

Wanzer, S.H., Federman, D.D., Adelstein, S.J., Cassel, C.K., Cassem, E.H., Cranford, R.E., Hook, E.W., Lo, B., Moertel, C.G., Safar, P., Stone A., and Vaneys J. (1989). The physician's responsibility toward hopelessly ill patients: A second look. *New England Journal of Medicine, 320*, 844–849.

7 Difficult choices

Policy and meaning in Japanese hospice practice

Susan Orpett Long and Satoshi Chihara

This chapter deals with a specialized type of care service, that of hospice. Hospice has a more limited variety of care recipients than that of general community or institutional care for the elderly because of its emphasis on end-of-life care for terminally ill patients. Its professional and volunteer workers provide services for adults of all ages, but its focus on care for the dying makes it relevant to concerns of elderly members of society, who are more likely to face serious illnesses, and more likely to be caregivers for family members nearing the end of life.

In Japan, the hospice concept has been imported from abroad, particularly from Great Britain where it originated. While hospice is administratively placed within Japan's medical system, it is offered by its advocates as a service whose philosophy of "care for the whole person" is intended to bridge the divide between medical and social welfare approaches. As an alternative model of care, hospice has been of great interest to the media and the public in recent years and there has been tremendous growth in the numbers of hospices and patients since the first Japanese hospice was opened in 1981. Yet in putting the hospice ideal into practice, its advocates have had to deal with a number of incongruities between hospice philosophy and its new cultural, social, and administrative home. The gap between ideal and practice is not, however, due to cultural lag, but rather to the complexities and uncertainties of the difficult choices to be made in end-of-life care.

This chapter explores incongruities and ambivalence surrounding hospice at both the level of policy and the level of personal meaning. After introducing the development of hospice in Japan, we investigate the place of hospice-type care in the ambivalent ideas expressed by ordinary Japanese people about the process of dying, the role of organized religion in Japan, and concepts of family which challenge the notion of individual autonomous decision-making upon which hospice is predicated.

These ideas about family are part of a wider conceptualization of interpersonal relations which also frame physician-patient relations. The idealized relationship of trust between physician and patient has been challenged by technological and organizational change in medicine itself and in the way its practitioners are viewed in the media. The local family practitioner making house calls has gradually come to be replaced, in image and in reality, by a medical team of specialists, located in a hospital and armed with the latest in medical technology. A longstanding relationship based on knowledge of each other's families and personal histories can no longer be assumed and thus the basis for physician benevolence has been undermined. While hospice philosophy anticipates team work and patient-centered decision-making, hospice practice in Japan continues to rely on physician leadership due to its institutional character and to government regulations of health care workers.

Lastly, we examine the ways in which national government policy has supported the development of this alternative model of end-of-life care, and yet has instituted regulations which are sometimes inconsistent with it. The Japanese Association of Hospice and Palliative Care Units has responded with its own guidelines, and increasing interest in home hospice may lead to resolution of some of the inconsistencies. Other areas of ambivalence will remain due to the very nature of end-of-life care, but the role of hospice seems firmly established in contemporary Japan. We consider the health care policy implications of this change.

Methodologies

The authors bring two distinct approaches to this work. Dr Chihara is trained in medical oncology and has devoted his career to caring for cancer patients. Since 1982 he has been associated with Seirei Hospice, Japan's first hospice, and currently serves as its director. He brings a wealth of clinical, administrative, and professional association experience to the question of the place of hospice in Japan and is a strong advocate of this model of care.

In contrast, Dr Long is trained in cultural anthropology, specializing in medical care, family, and caregiving issues in Japan. In 1996, she spent six months conducting a participant-observation and interview study of end-of-life decision-making in a hospice and other institutions in the Kansai area. These included a Christian hospital, a national hospital, and a private university medical school hospital, as well as interviews and observations during house calls of private physicians and visiting nurses. Her approach is focused on the daily interactions of patients, family, and staff; she takes a more analytical than advocacy approach to hospice practice.

Development of hospice in Japan

The modern hospice movement developed from the establishment of St Christopher's Hospice in London in 1967. Its founder, Dr Cicely Saunders, advocated a program for terminally ill cancer patients that would relieve the pain these patients experienced toward the end of their lives. This pain was recognized as a complex phenomenon that included not only physical, but also mental/emotional, social, and spiritual elements. This work could best be accomplished by the cooperative efforts of an interdisciplinary team of medical and social service professionals (Tsuneto, 1996a and 1996b), while the significance of the family in providing primary care was recognized. Volunteers provided assistance and support to the patients, families, and staff. (See Field and Cassel, 1997; Smith, 1985. Regarding volunteers in Japan, see Kitagawa, 1995.)

It did not take long for the hospice concept to reach Japan, for by the early 1970s, a number of medical professionals had already begun to explore the possibility of establishing hospice practice in Japan. There were a number of historical reasons for this interest. First, Japanese medicine in the 1960s and 1970s was becoming increasingly oriented toward high-technology diagnosis and treatment. Medical education and practice had long been specialized in Japan, but combined with the newer techniques and a growing national economy, medical care was increasingly hospital-centered. Birth and death moved from being a family-centered event in the home to a professionally synchronized occasion in the hospital in a process of medicalization of the human life course (Kashiwagi, 1995, 1997).[1]

Second, rapidly changing patterns of disease helped to create an interest in hospice care. Statistics from 1935 list tuberculosis as the leading cause of death; cancer was not among the top five causes of death until 1951 when it represented 7.9 percent of all deaths.[2] By the mid-1970s when plans began for the earliest hospices, cancer accounted for over 20 percent of all deaths in Japan. There is no sign of any deceleration in this trend. In 1995, the death rate from cancer was 211.6 per 10,000 population, or 28.5 percent of all deaths (Kōseishō, 1997, pp. 408 and 424). The attention of public health officials, the public, and the media has consequently come to focus on cancer.

A third factor in the development of hospice was a growing skepticism about doctors, and about "progress" in general. Reports of environmental disasters and iatrogenic problems filled the media in the late 1960s and the 1970s (Sonoda, 1988). News stories of students buying their way into medical schools and physicians making money by prescribing large amounts of medication increased skepticism about whether doctors were worthy of the public's trust.[3] Moreover, the notion of informed consent has a recent history in Japan. Physicians are frequently accused of prescribing excessive examinations and medications without sufficient explanation to or consent from patients. In fact, there is evidence from the 1970s that many patients disposed of a significant proportion of the medications they received from their physicians (*Yomiuri Shimbun*, 1977b). All of these things led to increasing distrust of physicians and caused them to become increasingly defensive about their practices. Physician-patient relations thus deteriorated (See Long, 1980, Chapters 2 and 3).

Thus, when hospice ideas were being introduced in the 1970s, people were beginning to note the discrepancy between the public's high expectations of modern, high-tech medicine and the reality that it had little to offer patients with advanced cancer that could not be treated surgically. Lengthy admissions to hospitals did not relieve the suffering experienced by patients in physical and mental pain. Hospice seemed to be an attractive alternative.

The earliest plans to establish hospices in Japan came from two sources. First, in the 1970s two Christian hospitals began planning for hospice wards which would be affiliated with yet distinct from the rest of the hospital. The first such unit was opened in 1981 at Seirei Mikatagahara Hospital in Hamamatsu, a hospital founded to care for terminally ill tuberculosis patients in 1931 by several young Christians with a strong commitment to the poor and sick. The establishment of the hospice ward was not unopposed even at Seirei, where some physicians argued that their duty was to prolong lives, not attend to the dying. A statistical portrait of Seirei's development is presented in Appendix 1 (see also Seirei Fukushi Jigyōdan, 1990).

Seirei Hospice was followed shortly by Yodogawa Christian Hospital in Osaka, whose hospice ward opened in 1984. These two programs have served as models for most subsequent development of hospice and palliative care institutions in the country, including the only Buddhist hospital-based palliative care program which opened in Nagaoka, Niigata Prefecture in 1993.[4] As of April, 1999, there were fifty-two licensed hospice and palliative care wards associated with hospitals in Japan, and an additional twenty to twenty-five institutions which offer palliative-type care outside of the government licensure system.

The second source of interest in hospice came from a few physicians in private practice. Most notable was Dr Sōichi Suzuki of Tokyo who began home hospice services in the early 1970s. He asserted that both patients and family members would benefit from home hospice care if they had available systematic support twenty-four hours a day, seven days a week which could respond to their needs. However, this type of hospice care, in contrast to American hospice which is primarily home-based, was slow to develop in Japan. Not only was the general trend still toward hospital-based medical care for the availability of high-tech equipment and staff convenience, but the Japanese universal insurance system provided such good coverage that some people claimed that it was less expensive (to the patient and family) to stay in the hospital than to live at home. In particular, with the introduction in 1973 of both the Health Care for the Elderly program (*Rōjin Hoken*, see Chapter 2 by D. Maeda and Chapter 4 by J. Campbell, this volume) and catastrophic medical care coverage, hospital care was available to all without regard to economic status, age, or employment history. As long as hospice care took place within a hospital, medical insurance would pay. Moreover, few physicians had the interest and specialized knowledge to provide hospice care at home, and there was insufficient support in home services from nurses and aides.

By the late 1980s the Ministry of Health and Welfare had decided to encourage the development of programs for the treatment of terminally ill patients. To promote palliative care and to establish standards for such programs, in 1990 the Ministry issued regulations for hospice and palliative care units connected with hospitals. Whereas the insurance system reimburses hospitals and clinics on a fee-for-service basis, the fees for the often low-tech, time-consuming activities of hospice care were low, making it difficult to recover costs, particularly of labor. Hospices argued that a reasonable per diem charge was necessary to maintain quality of care. The Ministry of Health and Welfare agreed that institutions which met the Ministry standards would be licensed by the government, making them eligible to receive per diem reimbursements.[5]

The Ministry regulations covered only three aspects of hospice practice: admission, staffing, and space. First, the regulations established that government-licensed programs are for the treatment of patients who are terminally ill due to a malignant neoplasm (cancer) or acquired immunodeficiency syndrome (AIDS). Admission or discharge must be decided by committee, and not by an individual physician.

Secondly, the regulations required that nursing and physician services meet all regular standards for hospitals in Japan. Beyond that, the nurse-patient ratio must minimally be two registered nurses per every three patients, compared with a one-to-three ratio on other wards. (Note that this total number of staff must cover patient care twenty-four hours per day, seven days per week.) The ward must also have at least one full-time physician who practices palliative care.

In addition, the regulations set standards for minimal space requirements (30 square meters per patient for the ward as a whole, and 8 square meters per patient in his or her room). More than half of the rooms must be single rooms; the extra fee for a single can be charged on no more than 50 percent of the rooms. A hospice or palliative care ward must also contain a family room, a kitchen for patient use, a small meeting room for family consultations, and a lounge.

Ideals, practices, and ambivalence

Some authors who have written about hospice practice in Japan have explained differences from Britain or the US as due to "obstacles" of Japanese culture (see Paton and Wicks, 1996). In our view, such an approach is problematical. First, it presumes that in countries other than Japan, hospice ideal and practice are the same, an assumption clearly challenged for the United States in David Barnard's chapter in this volume. In Japan, as in the US, people hold a variety of opinions and values. For example, they may simultaneously wish to enjoy autonomous decision-making about their medical care and yet want family closely involved in those decisions. These values are not always consistent, nor are they arranged in a fixed hierarchy, but rather are variously drawn upon as circumstances suggest their relevance. Thus, for dealing with a cold, a Japanese adult may decide on his or her own to seek medical advice and treatment, but the same individual might want a spouse or adult child along when consulting a physician for a problem that seems more serious. The "right" answers, even about *how* to make decisions, are not always clear, either to individuals faced with choices or to those involved with decisions about allocating societal resources. Claiming that culture is an "obstacle" overlooks the complexity of belief systems and social interaction and the significance of policy in shaping behavior. Neither culture nor policy *determine* behavior, but they do create parameters and allocate meaning to particular practices. In this section we look at how the reality of not always having one "right" answer leads to ambiguity and inconsistencies in individual and policy decisions, which in turn shape the reality of hospice practice.

Ideas about the "good death"

To the extent that hospice addresses the quality of death, Japanese notions about the "good death" influence perceptions about what constitutes good hospice care. Although images of Buddhist monks peacefully accepting fate as they face death (e.g. Blackman, 1997; for Buddhist influence on lay people, see Char *et al.*, 1996) might suggest one image of a good death in Japan, interviews provide evidence that there are many and conflicting notions about the best way to die (Long, 1997). *Pokkuri*, a sudden death without experiencing illness, is the ideal for the many people, including those elderly who regularly visit *pokkuri dera*, Buddhist temples which specialize in prayers for a quick dying (Woss, 1993; Young and Ikeuchi, 1997). Such a death is ideal because it avoids pain and suffering for the dying, as expressed by a physician specializing in internal medicine:

> What kind of death would be ideal? Hmmm. Maybe *pokkuri shinu*. Suddenly, like when you get up and you're brushing your teeth and you have a cerebral hemorrhage and die ... Because you wouldn't have to worry about things ...You wouldn't have to suffer with the complications of the disease and the inconvenience of being in the hospital for a long time. Yes, *pokkuri* death would be best.

Pokkuri death also prevents a person from becoming a burden (*meiwaku*) on the family.

Yet in interviews and discussions, other people pointed out that *pokkuri* death may be too quick, not allowing death to be a process of coming to terms, of giving life closure. Many people, both healthy and ill, said in the interviews that they wished to have time "to prepare." Preparation sometimes referred to arranging financial matters or handing over business clients. Often it meant the possibility of doing things the person wanted to do during his or her lifetime. For some people, it also seemed to mean a spiritual readying, a chance to convey final messages to loved ones, or to spend time together. One man in his seventies explained:

> I told [the doctor] from the beginning that I wanted to know whatever I had. [Why?] So I could prepare. [What kind of preparation?] Mentally, and financially, too. For three days after I was told I just felt stunned. I realized I couldn't do all the things I wanted to. I had just bought a computer and was going to learn how to use it. But then I started to pull myself together.

Such a readjustment of life goals and orientations takes time, and thus a gradual process of dying also is an ideal, as long as it is without pain. Many people believe that an ideal death is one that is *yasuraka*, peaceful. Others spoke of *rosui*, a gradual decline due to old age, as the ideal death.

These varying ideas about what constitutes a "good death" influence the way people view hospice care. There is a strong consensus that pain and suffering should be minimized if the death is to be a good one, and this leads many families and patients to an interest in hospice. Hospice workers define their central role as that of pain control, and present it as such to potential patients and families.

Beyond the elimination of pain, people sometimes associated hospice with an atmosphere in which a peaceful death could be achieved. A divorced woman in her late thirties who suffers from chronic gastrointestinal illness talked about what an ideal death meant for herself:

> In one sense it would be to have it quick so I wouldn't have pain – I'm not afraid of death, but I am of pain. On the other hand, I would want time to prepare. Maybe an ideal would be to go to a sanatorium, a place by the ocean or a lake where I could get ready and take walks by the sea and they would give me morphine for pain ... someplace quiet.

Hospice care was associated with this kind of image by a man in his late forties who was hospitalized in an intensive care unit after a first heart attack. He asked if hospice wasn't the place "where they let you die *yasuraka ni* (peacefully)." He continued, "That's what I'd want. If I had terminal cancer, I wouldn't want all that life-prolonging treatment." Hospice patients seemed convinced that hospice was in fact the best place for them to experience such a death, given their terminal cancer. Many expressed a sense of relief when they were admitted, believing that their pain would be controlled and that they would have time to "prepare." They also wished to avoid burdening family while maintaining their presence and support.

In the context of multiple interpretations of what a good death means, hospice plays a significant role. All of these goals may not be achievable simultaneously, presenting challenges to hospice staff. Hospice cannot offer a death that is *pokkuri*, but it provides pain control and care that relieves the family from assuming full responsibility for the patient. It offers a quiet and calm atmosphere in which to "prepare" for death over an extended period of time. Pain relief takes priority, while life-prolonging treatments are rejected. If these data suggest that hospice is consistent with many diverse ideas about the good death, it also suggests that to be successful, hospice practice must respond to these expectations with appropriate practices. Pain control must take priority; secondarily, patients should be given the opportunity to prepare for a peaceful death while minimizing the burden on family members.

Ambivalence about religion

The notion that mental "preparation" is part of a good death suggests that for at least some Japanese, there exists a spiritual element to the transition from the known life in this world to the unknown future (see also Ohnuki-Tierney, 1984). Yet if asked directly to name their religious preference, most contemporary Japanese respond that although their family maintains a relationship with a particular temple or shrine, they personally profess belief in no particular religion. More likely, they practice rituals from several traditions eclectically (and from an American religious perspective) with much skepticism and little commitment, as portrayed in Itami's well-know film, *Sōshiki* (*The Funeral*). In recent years, the activities of groups which claim to be religious organizations such as Aum Shinri Kyō have increased the public's distrust of the sincerity of religious motivation and action.

From its founding at St Christopher's as well as its beginnings in Japan, the hospice movement has been a Christian movement. Only about one percent of the population in Japan is Christian (*Japan Statistical Yearbook*, 1998), but Christianity has been a respected influence in Japan, particularly in the areas of education, medicine, and social services. But if few Japanese are Christian and many are skeptical about organized religion in general, how might hospice be relevant to their needs?

First, hospice workers emphasize that one does not need to be of any particular faith to be a hospice patient, only to understand the goals of hospice. Nonetheless, some patients, and even a hospice volunteer interviewed in Long's study, had initially believed that they were not eligible because they were not Christian. A number of patients commented (without being asked) that they believed that Christianity offered answers to the "problem" of death and a few indicated that they admired the stoicism of Christians in the face of death who could celebrate death as a rebirth with God. From the staff perspective, pain control was the primary goal, but chaplains were considered a critical part of the staff. Conversions to Christianity were not the principal goal of hospice, but were welcomed by the chaplains and Christian hospice staff. While patients seemed grateful for the care they received, most of those interviewed in Long's study remained skeptical or saw Christianity as too removed from their own lives to consider conversion.

Christianity also influences the practice of hospice more subtly in Christian hospitals as well through the goals and expectations of the staff. As part of the patient's psychosocial and spiritual care, the staff works to promote reconciliation, forgiveness, service to others, acceptance of death, and perhaps an understanding of one's relationship with God, all from a Christian perspective.[6] At a physician-nurse conference for the discussion of patients who had died recently, his nurse spoke admiringly of the way Mr Matsumoto, an elderly Christian man, had spent his last days:

> He was supported by his Christianity; he knew his diagnosis and prognosis and understood what hospice is. Having a positive attitude [*maemuki*] and

pain control were his goals for the hospitalization. He was cheerful [*akaraku*] and calm [*odayaka ni*] until his stoic [*sono otokorashii*] end ... I admire the way he died, holding the hands of his family.

Other nurses spoke of how Mr Matsumoto was able to reach out to other patients. One nurse summed up, "In short, he made an impact." Another woman's death discussed in a similar meeting was also seen as being a "good death" by the staff because she had died with her family minister present, while he, her husband, and some of the staff prayed and sang hymns.

The role of organized religion at the Buddhist palliative care ward, called Bihāra, appears to be somewhat different. Hospital director Dr Takashi Tamiya has explained the need for such a place in terms of the underlying assumptions about suffering and death derived from Buddhism that are widely shared in Japanese society (and perhaps especially among elderly rural residents of Niigata who represent an important constituency of the program). In an article introducing the new palliative care unit, Tamiya attempts to differentiate it from the Christian idea of hospice. He explains the name Bihāra is derived from the Sanskrit word "*vihara*," referring to a Buddhist temple or monastery, or to a place to rest or walk to clear one's mind. The founders of this Buddhist palliative care ward chose a Sanskrit word because the term "hospice" has a long history of association with Christianity. Calling this a "Buddhist *hospice*" would be like "grafting bamboo to a tree" (Tamiya, 1994).[7]

Bihāra makes explicit use of various symbols of Buddhism and "Japaneseness" in the physical arrangements of the ward (for example, the Buddhist image in the "chapel" and a rock garden) and in some activities (*sutra* reading). The chaplains directly associated with the hospice are Buddhist priests. Yet the hospice staff at Bihāra and Dr Tamiya himself readily acknowledged that the Christian hospices served as their model for the unit and that they are consciously making it more "Buddhist" and more "Japanese" for the patients' comfort.

Although many Japanese utilize Buddhist services on special ritual occasions, for many a heavy dose of Buddhism is no more reflective of their daily lives than is Christianity. If the main goal of Japanese patients and families in receiving hospice care is pain control, then a secular environment, such as that offered by a palliative care unit at a secular hospital, might be just as satisfying. Due to the principle of separation of church and state in Japan's constitution and legal system, public hospitals do not support chaplains' services, and thus full hospice service which includes spiritual care is not available in the same way. In such units, concern for spiritual care is voiced, some counseling may be offered, and the patient's own clergy person is welcome as a visitor to the unit. Such a style is perhaps more consistent with the secularized world views of many contemporary Japanese, but compromises the full effect of the hospice ideal in the practice of palliative care in Japan by minimizing the provision of "spiritual care." Just what constitutes an ideal environment for spiritual care in Japan undoubtedly varies with the values and priorities of the patients, families, and staff involved.

Changing views of the relationship between the individual and the family

The British ideal of hospice care is predicated on an assumption of individual autonomy and interests, supported by family. Hospice philosophy insists that patients are informed about the nature of their illness and are active participants in decisions about the care they receive. It advocates that patients should spend their last months or days in a manner of their choice, consistent with their own way of living. Although these values may be readily accepted by many contemporary Japanese, the interpretations they are given in hospice practice are derived from historical patterns of social relationships quite distinct from those of the Anglo context in which hospice originated (see, for example, Charlton et al., 1995). This can be seen in particular in the role that family plays in hospice practice, particularly concerning practices of disclosure of diagnosis and informed consent for treatment. The family also serves as an information provider. Since ideal care is defined in hospice as allowing the patient to die according to the way he or she lived (a "Tanaka-san *rashii* way"), deep knowledge of the patient's values, personality, and daily habits are important, and this knowledge is thought to be best interpreted to staff by family members (Long, 1999).

Widespread knowledge of the concept of informed consent and the valuing of disclosure of a poor diagnosis to the patient are quite new to Japan. (See, for example, the arguments of Yamazaki, 1990.) Previously, physicians deemed it unethical to reveal a diagnosis to the patient that left little room for hope. Family members accepted that it was their role to hear the news and to protect patients from it since they were already weakened. Although the results of recent opinion polls report that the large majority of the Japanese public now would want to be told a diagnosis of cancer, the practice of disclosure has been slower to change. In part this is due to the ambivalence exposed in response to a second question: most people still would not inform a close family member of a terminal cancer diagnosis. (See Long and Long, 1982; Long, 1999; Elwyn et al., 1998; Kashiwagi, 1995, 1996, 1997; Kōseishō, 1995; Suzuki, Kirschling, and Inoue 1993; Yanagida, 1996.)

How is it possible to practice hospice care in such an environment? In theory, Japanese hospices assert that patients should know the nature of their disease and their prognosis, and the nature of the care that will be provided in hospice. In practice, they do not always insist on full disclosure as a prior condition to admission.[8] Hospice staff believe that it is possible for patients to be informed gradually, and will allow this in certain circumstances, such as a very elderly widow whose children believe that she could not cope with such news. For the most part, however, hospice patients have been told their diagnosis and poor prognosis, in part because the staff is trained to provide the emotional and spiritual support to patients and families which most physicians and nurses claim they are not. (See Long, 1999, regarding the question of coping and disclosure.) Even so, the family remains a significant part of the decision-making team (Fetters, 1998). For example, in a deteriorating situation, the patient may be consulted about increasing his or her sedation, but the family is likely to be fully informed about the physician's recommendations prior to the patient's participation. The family plays a dual role. They are expected to represent the patient's interests to the staff, and to help interpret the patient's abilities, wishes, and personality. Family are also counted on to assist in implementing what the staff believes to be the best treatment, including gradual disclosure when the patient is not initially aware of the terminal diagnosis.

Physician leadership and the question of trust

The premise of hospice care is team work. The team consists of professional staff from various disciplines, the patient, and the family. Yet this team cannot function effectively when communication is poor and trust lacking. It is likely to be nurses and volunteers who do the most to establish this rapport, but physicians are seen as the team leaders, recognized as having specialized knowledge of how best to control the patient's physical pain, but also setting the tone for the relationships among staff, family, and patient. Although the input of other staff members, especially the patient's main nurse, is considered critical, the physician generally remains the ultimate decision-maker regarding treatment. While families and patients are consulted, they are often asked to concur or to "Leave it to us. We will do our best."

The ambiguity of the physician-patient-family decision-making situation is mirrored in the relationship between physicians and other professional staff. In contrast to regular Japanese wards, hospices have regular, formal channels in place for interdisciplinary communication. At least in the hospice setting, nurses, volunteers, dieticians, therapists, and others appear to have the respect of physicians for their own special expertise that they bring to the care of the patients. Nonetheless, physicians remain in charge in the day-to-day decisions on the ward. This is in part an impact of the physician's presence, mandated by the Ministry of Health and Welfare regulations of 1990; it thus reflects the institutional bias of Japanese hospice care, resulting in team care, but teams with clear leadership from physicians in contrast to home-based hospices in which the physician's role is more limited.

There is additionally ambivalence about staffing because of the difference between the minimum staffing requirements of the Ministry of Health and Welfare regulations and the appropriate level of staffing to meet the needs of patients. The officially sanctioned ratio of two registered nurses for every three patients is insufficient for adequate inpatient hospice care even with the assistance of volunteers. In the experience of Seirei Hospice for example, a ratio of at least one registered nurse per patient is necessary to meet patients' needs. Yet increasing the number of registered nurses will increase costs to the institution which receives the same per diem amount regardless of how many additional nurses are hired. This forces the institution to choose between financial loss or decline in hospice services.

Regulations concerning physicians' qualifications and the educational goals of hospice also are contradictory. The Ministry regulations require that there be a full-time physician exclusively engaged in palliative care on the ward, yet at this time Japan has no system for recognizing who is a qualified palliative care specialist. Most gain their expertise through advanced training in a university department such as anesthesiology, internal medicine, or psychiatry and then because of their own interests, begin to study hospice care through independent study and rotations through palliative care wards.

Hospices are thus faced with a contradiction between the need to train staff and educate the public on one hand, and ideal patient care on the other. These educational goals come into conflict when hospices must deal with requests from professionals, journalists, students, and others to observe or to do training rotations there. Accommodating too many such visitors disrupts the routine of the ward, creates greater commotion, and depersonalizes care whereas good patient care requires a great deal of calm, knowledge, and attention to the individual patient's needs. Yet if requests for training or observation are denied, the administration misses the educational opportunities these represent. The compromise is to limit the numbers of observers at any given time, to screen them, and to be certain that they are aware of hospice rules and routines at the start.

Good care versus good financing

Japanese government policy has supported the development of hospice as an alternative model of end-of-life care and has instituted minimum standards to assure its quality. All indications are that the government was truly interested in improving end-of-life care rather than in saving money. Yet some of these regulations and financing decisions are inconsistent with high quality hospice care, and the standards set seem to many hospice advocates to be insufficient.

The space requirements, for example, are so minimal that wards and rooms which only meet the minimum requirement are extremely cramped, making it difficult to create a comfortable milieu for patients and care providers. Moreover, the size of rooms other than patient rooms, such as the family room and kitchen, are not defined and may be so small as to be inadequate.

Of even greater concern is the issue of private rooms in which people might spend their last days. Hospice or palliative care wards are expected to maximize their number of single rooms to achieve a more appropriate environment to prepare for death and for private family interaction. Yet the institution cannot claim the extra charge for a private room for more than 50 percent of the total rooms. This creates a conflict between the hospice ideal of creating comfortable facilities for all patients or maintaining the economic stability of the institution. Since patients must pay the extra charge for the private room out-of-pocket, there has been increasing concern that only the wealthy will be able to afford hospice care, contradicting the hospice philosophy that every person should be cared for respectfully and equally until his or her death.

Inconsistencies and the future of hospice in Japan

The inconsistencies and contradictions in trying to implement ideal hospice care are not a matter of cultural lag regarding practices such as disclosure of a terminal illness as some authors have suggested. Even if full disclosure were widely practiced and room sizes doubled, hospice practice would not suddenly become simple. Decisions at the individual and societal levels must be made in an atmosphere in which "right" answers may not exist due to ambiguities created by multiple meanings and values in daily life and in policy. But this does not mean that the outlook for hospice care in Japan is dim.

Institutional hospice care

Leadership on these issues has been taken by the Japanese Association of Hospice and Palliative Care Units, an organization founded in 1991 to promote the quality of end-of-life care and to educate the Japanese public about the concepts of hospice and palliative care. Initially, five licensed institutions came together with the encouragement of the Ministry of Health and Welfare. By 1998, membership had grown to 40 institutions that accounted for 705 beds for care of terminally ill patients.

There are, however, other programs which are not part of this organization and which are a cause of concern to the Association. Believing that the standards established by the 1990 Ministry of Health and Welfare regulations are too lenient, the Japan Association of Hospice and Palliative Care Units in 1997 issued its own more detailed guidelines designed to assure high quality palliative care (Zenkoku Hosupisu Kanwa Kea Byōtō Renraku Kyōgikai, 1997). These guidelines insist, for example, on team decision-making, on the use of care plans, on offering bereavement services to families, and on having an internal assessment procedure. (See Appendix 2 for a translation of these guidelines.)

In the process of writing these guidelines, a number of interesting discussions took place which recognized that hospice practice must be adapted to local conditions while at the same time attempting to educate and persuade the public to achieve conditions closer to the ideal.

Hospice care, for example, should be available to any person who is dying and wishes such care. Yet this option is not open to everyone. Only patients who are terminally ill due to malignant neoplasms or AIDS are eligible for hospice according to the 1990 Ministry of Health and Welfare regulations. Japanese hospice advocates find this limitation undesirable, but recognize that such discrimination based on disease may be a necessary compromise in the real world of limited medical and welfare resources.[9]

The Ministry regulations, moreover, do not provide a definition of "terminally ill." Although some physicians argued for a clear-cut six-month prognosis for eligibility, others claimed that it was too difficult to clinically define the terminal stage of each patient, and no effective parameters exist to make an accurate estimate of disease prognosis. They concluded that there is no clinical evidence for meaningfulness of a definition of terminal as a life expectancy of six months or less. The Association guidelines thus adopted the purposely ambiguous language, "after it has been established that there is no hope for cure." Nonetheless, a six-month prognosis remains an informal working definition for many hospice practitioners.

A second issue which the Association guidelines have chosen to leave unresolved is whether full disclosure of the diagnosis must be a requirement for admission. There was general agreement that under ideal conditions, the patient him- or herself requests admission based on an understanding of his or her disease, its prognosis, and the nature of hospice care. They also recognized that, in reality, Japanese families often present a different situation. Frequently, family members request admission for the patient without his or her full understanding and even in cases of adequate disclosure, patterns of family decision-making remain common (Fetters, 1998; Long, 1999). Patients may defer to the opinions of family members out of concern for the interests of the family as a whole or because passivity is an expected part of the sick role in Japan. Since the goals of hospice include calm and reconciliation rather than developing assertiveness, it seemed best to the Association members composing the guidelines to use the phrase "patient and/or family members" to indicate the decision-making unit rather than "the patient" alone. But they also included wording that insists that "At the patient's request, appropriate explanation will be given," so that gradual disclosure is encouraged.

The third major issue that faced the guideline authors was that of the extra charge for a private room. Although Japanese universal insurance coverage is excellent, no plan covers the private room surcharge. Some hospices charge as much as Y35,000 per day for a private room, imposing an enormous economic burden on patients and families. Such charges mean that patients with low incomes are unable to be admitted even when they would benefit from hospice care. This economic discrimination conflicts sharply with a fundamental principle of hospice, that all patients receive care who need and want it. On the other hand, the private room surcharge is an important source of revenue for the institution. Unable to rely on private donations to support hospice, they are dependent on the extra fee to maintain economic viability. Only two of thirty-six institutions licensed by the Japanese government were not charging an extra fee for a private room in 1998. The Association guidelines nevertheless include the wording, "has no reason to discriminate against patients based on the patient's economic status" as a reminder of the ideal that every patient will receive equal and respectful care.

Home hospice care

As noted above, the evolution of home hospice care was much slower than institutional-based hospice practice. There is no national-level association of home hospice care teams, and no official reports concerning their overall activities exist, although local organizations collect their own data.

We can classify existing home hospice teams into three categories:

The annex type   This refers to home services established as an annex to a hospice ward. In these situations, visiting nurses of the host hospital join the hospice ward care team or nurses of the hospice ward take part in home care for the hospice's patients.

The cooperation type In some places, a hospice ward staff cooperates with independent hospice care nurses' teams to provide home care for hospice patients who have been discharged from the ward or for patients who anticipate future admission.

The network-type This is the least institution-oriented type of home hospice care. Private practitioners interested and trained in hospice care do home visits in conjunction with hospital visiting nurse teams and/or independent nurses from a home nursing station.

The vast majority, estimated at more than 90 percent, of home hospice care teams fall into either the annex type or the cooperation type categories. This means that hospice and palliative care wards continue to play an important role in home hospice care and that most home hospice care teams will be able to obtain immediate support from hospice and palliative care wards. Patients can request admission when their symptoms can no longer be controlled at home or when family members become too exhausted to continue to care for them. Thus the institutional ties characteristic of the annex and cooperative types of home hospice care provide reassurance for patients, families, and care providers (see Nihon Hosupisu Zaitaku Kea Kenkyūkai, 1995).

Recent changes in policy have led to increased interest in the network type of home hospice care. Organizations such as the Japanese Hospice and Home Care Study Group founded in Kōbe in 1992 and the Home Hospice Association in Tokyo established in 1995 seek to expand home care for dying patients.[10] They are active in educating the public as well as medical and welfare professionals by publishing journals and newsletters, offering public lectures and symposia, and sponsoring patient and family support groups. They encourage the participation of professionals, volunteers, and lay people with interest in end-of-life and caregiving issues to join, and membership fees support their educational activities. Care activities, however, are now covered through the universal medical insurance system. Increased reimbursement for physician house calls has recently made it financially viable for physicians to spend time seeing patients in their own homes. Other policy changes now allow visiting nurses and other professionals to work independently out of home nursing stations or physician offices and receive reimbursement for physician-prescribed activities. The plans for the new long-term care insurance (*kaigo hoken*) will aid in coordinating medical with social welfare services for older patients in the future. (See Chapter 4 by J. Campbell in this volume.)

Despite these increased incentives, the home hospice movement has not grown as rapidly as some had expected. For example, at Seirei, the number of patients has grown steadily but not dramatically since its inception (Appendix 1, Table 7.9). This may be due to lack of interest or training on the part of health care professionals and to continued preference for institutional care. Many Japanese homes are too small to comfortably accommodate a hospital bed and other necessary equipment,[11] and some family members are unable to provide the necessary support for the patient due to their own ill health or employment. Nonetheless, most people indicate a preference to die in the familiar setting of their own home and it seems likely that as home care technology develops and knowledge of palliative care increases, all types of home hospice care will be in greater demand.

Health policy implications

This chapter has suggested several significant policy implications regarding hospice care. In particular, the insufficiency of private rooms in institutional hospices is a barrier to the provision of ideal hospice care, and yet is in some way consistent with Japanese lifestyles and values in a crowded, sociocentric society. Moreover, the requirement that the private room surcharge be paid by the patient establishes a two-tier system of hospice patients according to socio-economic status. The government must also expand the qualifications for eligibility to include people who are terminally ill but have diseases other than cancer to create greater equality of access to hospice care.

Different cultural values such as the importance of family in decision-making, different physical environments, and different government policies toward end-of-life care result in the adaptation of the hospice concept from its origins in Great Britain to its new home in Japan. In this chapter, we have pointed to a number of inconsistencies and problems in Japanese hospice care. Between the ideal and the realities lie Japanese policy and Japanese values, and in both of these there is ambivalence about how to best provide end-of-life care. People express a respect for a basic right of people to die in their own manner in a dignified human way, but few are willing to "give up" on the promises of technological marvels. The problem is not cultural lag or cultural difference. These are dilemmas about where to draw the line, where to stop aggressive treatment, how to balance suffering with burdening others. It is no wonder that it is difficult to define "terminal," raising our awareness of how arbitrary are policies and regulations that fix care decisions on uncertain life expectancies.

Decisions about where to put financial and manpower resources are no less unclear. Aggressive and high-tech medical treatments and research have made dramatic changes in our expectations about how we will live our lives, but they have been less considerate of the issue of how we die. Hospice promises to combine high-level technological knowledge with intensive, low tech hands-on care in order to offer new possibilities for end-of-life care. Some of the ambivalence of meaning and policy decisions will be resolved over time as definitions are worked out, new policies established, and public expectations continue to change. But to understand hospice practice we must also recognize that ambivalence at the individual and societal levels are an inherent part of the work of caring.

Notes

1. Vital statistics provide the following picture of this change: Shortly after the end of World War II in 1947, 91 percent of deaths took place in the home. By 1977 when the hospice movement was just beginning in Japan, less than half did so, at 49 percent. By 1995, only 20 percent of deaths in Japan took place in the home (Kashiwagi, 1997, p. 9).
2. In terms of absolute numbers, deaths from cancer in 1995 were nearly four times the number for 1951, while over the same period the overall death rate declined by 25 percent (Kōseishō, 1997, pp. 408 and 424).
3. For examples, see *Asahi Shimbun*, 1971; *Asahi Shimbun*, 1977, November 14, Evening ed., p. 1; 1977, November 26, p. 12; *Kōbe Shimbun*, 1977, August 11, Evening ed., p. 1; *Yomiuri Shimbun*, 1977a. Recent surveys suggest a continued lack of trust in physicians, for example during the long national "debate" about whether to recognize brain death as the legal definition of death. Although some have argued against such recognition for cultural reasons, it appears that the majority of ordinary people question whether or not physicians would implement such a policy *impartially* (*Asahi Shimbun*, 1996, October 1), indicating a lack of trust in physicians in general.
4. This influence is evidenced by the large numbers of requests these hospices receive for information and for physicians, nurses, and other professionals to observe and/or do rotations there. During interviews at the Bihāra unit in Niigata and in a new palliative care ward at a secular hospital in Kōbe, a number of physicians and nurses gratefully acknowledged this influence and assistance in unsolicited comments. See also published comments by the founder of the Bihāra Palliative Care Ward in Tamiya, 1994.
5. This amount was originally set at Y24,000 per patient per day regardless of the actual cost of care. In 1998 it had increased to Y38,000 per patient per day of hospice stay. Although the costs to the patient vary somewhat with their particular medical insurance plan, those under 70 generally pay about 20 percent of the fees. Those 70 years or older pay only Y1,000 per day of hospice or hospital stay. No plan covers the extra charge for a single room. However, a national catastrophic insurance system provides reimbursement upon request for expenses over Y63,600.
6. The staff also seemed to act on goals that were more "typically Japanese," namely the expression of gratitude and the maintenance of a cheerful (*akarui*) attitude, as in the quotation below.
7. Tamiya (1994) also states that Bihāra is founded on Buddhist principles which are independent of hospice: 1) It is a place where those who recognize the transience of life can quietly focus on the true self and be watched over. 2) It is a place where medical care revolves around the axis of the patient's wishes ... 3) It is a small community founded upon Buddhism, gathering together people who have been made aware of how precious is the life they desired (but patients and their families are free to hold any beliefs).
8. Estimates of the proportion of patients who do not know their diagnosis when admitted to a hospice range from 30–50 percent (Suzuki, Kirschling, and Inoue, 1993) to 40 percent (Voltz *et al.*, 1997) to 20 percent (Dr Chihara).
9. It may also reflect a bias of medical practitioners to treat cancer patients less aggressively than non-cancer patients with the same statistical prognosis (regarding Japan, Fetters, personal communication; for US, see Danis *et al.*, 1996).
10. *Taiingo no Gan Kanja Shien Gaido* (Guide to Support for Cancer Patients after Discharge), published by the Kōbe-based group, lists thirty-eight hospice and palliative care units and twenty-three such patient and family support groups in 1995. See also Zaitaku Hosupisu Kea Moderu Kenkyū Jigyō Hōkokusho, 1994.
11. In a scene in the film *Kazoku Gāmu* (Family Game), a young housewife tearfully seeks an older woman's advice on caring for her dying father-in-law. Her greatest worry is that if the father-in-law dies in their small apartment, there will be no way to get his corpse into the tiny elevator of the high-rise complex.

Appendix A

Statistical portrait of Seirei Hospice

Table 7.1 Staff members

4	doctors
22	registered nurses
3	nurses-aids
1	clerk
1	clinical social worker
1	chaplain

Table 7.2 Structure of the hospice ward

single-storied, with total 2133.0 m² area
- 27 patient rooms with 1 bed each (19.0 m²/room)
- 3 Japanese-style rooms for family members (16.0 m²/room)
- 1 small family kitchen for common use (10.0 m²)
- 1 bathroom with special equipment for patients who cannot bathe by themselves (24.0 m²)
- 1 relatively large lounge (98.0 m²)
- 1 chapel where a short worship service is held every morning (98.0 m²)
- 1 doctors' room (34.0 m²)
- 1 nurses' work room (44.0 m²)
- 1 nurses' lounge (29.0 m²)
- 1 lecture room for visiting trainees (60.0 m²)

Table 7.3 Annual change in the number of patients (newly admitted inpatients)

Apr. 1981 – Mar. 1982	37
Apr. 1982 – Mar. 1983	51
Apr. 1983 – Mar. 1984	63
Apr. 1984 – Mar. 1985	73
Apr. 1985 – Mar. 1986	55
Apr. 1986 – Mar. 1987	63
Apr. 1987 – Mar. 1988	56
Apr. 1988 – Mar. 1989	68
Apr. 1989 – Mar. 1990	69
Apr. 1990 – Mar. 1991	88
Apr. 1991 – Mar. 1992	104
Apr. 1992 – Mar. 1993	111
Apr. 1993 – Mar. 1994	148
Apr. 1994 – Mar. 1995	142
Apr. 1995 – Mar. 1996	130
Apr. 1996 – Mar. 1997	133
Apr. 1997 – Sept.1997	92
Total	1,483

Table 7.4 Distribution of patients according to gender and age

Age	Male	Female	Total	Proportion (%)
Younger than 10	1	0	1	0.1
10–19	4	1	5	0.3
20–29	3	2	5	0.3
30–39	24	34	58	3.9
40–49	70	81	151	10.2
50–59	145	124	269	18.1
60–69	220	186	406	27.4
70–79	193	173	366	24.7
Over 80	111	111	222	15.0
Total	771 (52.0%)	712 (48.0%)	1438	(100%)

Table 7.5 Distribution of patients according to disease

Name of disease	Number of patients	Proportion (%)
Stomach cancer	302	20.4
Lung cancer	230	15.5
Colo-rectal cancer	210	14.1
Breast cancer	124	8.4
Pancreatic cancer	76	5.1
Liver cancer	73	5.1
Bile duct, gall bladder cancer	58	3.9
Cervical cancer	44	3.0
Esophageal cancer	43	2.9
Malignant lymphoma	32	2.1
Ovarian cancer	32	2.1
Others	258	17.4

Table 7.6 Distribution of patients according to religion

Name of religion	Number of patients	Proportion (%)
Buddhism	552	37.2
Christianity	147	9.9
Shinto (domestic)	65	4.4
Others	85	5.7
No religion	634	42.8
Total	1,483	

Table 7.7 Duration of hospice stay from the last admission to patient death

Duration	Number of patients	Proportion (%)
Less than one month	549	40.7
Less than 2 months	319	23.6
Less than 3 months	164	12.2
Less than 4 months	106	7.9
Less than 5 months	62	4.6
Less than 6 months	39	2.9
Less than 12 months	79	5.8
Over 12 months	31	2.3
Total number of patients	1,349	

Table 7.8 Trends in the duration of hospice stay

Year	Mean days	Median days
1981–1993	82	48
1994	51	32
1995	52	29
1996	55	31
1997	39	24

Table 7.9 Trends of patients entering home hospice care at Seirei Hospice

	1993	1994	1995	1996
Number of patients	31	29	35	29
Average distance to patient's residence (km)	22	23	21	16
Average age	70	68	72	68
Hospice ward death	11	10	10	5
Home death	11	8	22	18
Survivor (to next year)	6	11	3	6

Table 7.10 Average duration of home care in the case of patient death

	\multicolumn{4}{c}{Average duration of home care until patient's death or admission}
	In the case of home death		In the case of hospice ward death	
	Days	(n)	Days	(n)
1993	44	(11)	87	(11)
1994	52	(8)	50	(10)
1995	126	(22)	54	(10)
1996	149	(18)	69	(5)
Total	108	(59)	65	(36)

Table 7.11 A comparison between malignant neoplasms and other diseases in home care (Seirei Home Care Team, 1995)

	Malignant neoplasm	Other diseases
Number of patients	35	20
Number of deaths	32	6
Number of survivors	3	14
Average age	68	80
Frequency of doctor's visits (days)	1/6	1/15
Average distance to patient's residence (km)	23	13

Appendix B

Japanese Association of Hospice and Palliative Care Units Standards of Hospice and Palliative Care Programs at Institutions

January 16, 1997

These standards set forth guidelines for mutual cooperation between persons receiving hospice/palliative care and care providers at a hospice/palliative care unit approved by the Ministry of Health and Welfare or a prefectural governor according to "Regulation of Palliative Care Units."

The Principles and Definition of Hospice/Palliative Care

Hospice/palliative care refers to care which is offered by a team consisting of various professionals to improve the quality of life for patients and their family members, and to enable them to live their lives as comfortably as possible as human beings with dignity. Five important concepts are:

1 The hospice program affirms individual life and respects "the dying process," which inevitably occurs to every person.
2 Hospice care neither hastens nor postpones death.
3 Hospice care relieves pain and other burdensome physical symptoms.
4 Hospice programs assess and respond to psychological and socioeconomic needs and support patients seeking the meaning of their lives (spiritual care).
5 Hospice programs provide support to family members in their struggle while their loved one is alive and after his or her death.

Standards of hospice/palliative care at institutions licensed by the Japanese government

At institutions providing hospice/palliative care programs, staff must first comply with applicable local and national laws and regulations governing the organization.

Patients and their family members

1 The patient/family is a unit of care.
2 Each patient/family will be looked after respectfully, recognizing their own beliefs and/or value system.

Requirements concerning admission

1 Patients with malignant neoplasm or AIDS referred by a physician after it has been established that there is no hope for cure.
2 The patient and/or family members requests his or her admission to a hospice ward.
3 On admission, it is desirable that the patient understands the name and condition of his or her disease. At the patient's request, an appropriate explanation will be given.
4 The staff will not discriminate against patients based on the patient's economic, social, or religious status. It must be acknowledged that the patient may live alone, have low income, or believe in a particular religion.

Care program

1 A care program will be provided at the request of the patient/family members.
2 Accurate and current records on the care and treatment offered to all patients/families will be maintained.
3 Informed consent concerning symptom control and care is an essential requirement.
4 A care program for family members and loved ones should be available before the patient's death.

Palliation of pain and other symptoms

1 Every effort will be made to control pain and other burdensome symptoms with appropriate treatments.
2 Symptom control will be carried out under mutual agreement, assessing the physical, psychological, and social needs of both patients and family members.

3 Pain control and palliation of symptoms will be supplied referring to standardized books listed at the end of this document.

Care team workers

1 The care team consists of such professionals as physicians, nurses, social workers, and volunteers, positioning patient/family members at the center of the team.
2 Team members respect each other's roles, exchange views on an equal footing, provide mutual support, and hold the concept and the goal of hospice/palliative care in common.
3 The care team will hold regular training programs and audits to help team members become increasingly effective.

Volunteers

1 A volunteer will be considered one of the team members and an essential care provider.
2 Volunteers take part in the care team of their own accord, and will be expected to know their role on the team and to take reasonable responsibility for their own activities.

Bereavement services

1 Bereavement services will be available from the time the patient begins medical treatment to support his or her family members and other loved ones.
2 When family members or other loved ones are in morbid grief, sufficient consultations by specialists will be available.

Quality assurance and activity assessment

1 The treatment and care given to patients and family members will be reviewed and assessed.
2 The direction of the care team and the overall care program will be reevaluated.
3 The assessment and reevaluation will in principle be the responsibility of each institution.
4 A special committee consisting of several members of this Association and additional external representatives will be established. The committee will be able to advise any institution based on an examination of its Quality Assurance and Activity Assessment.

Revision of these standards and establishment of a special committee

1 These standards may be revised in accordance with the rules of this Association.
2 The details of the Committee for Quality Assurance and Activity Assessment will be laid down separately.

References to Appendix B

Ministry of Health and Welfare and the Japan Medical Association, eds. *Medical Care Manual for Terminally Ill Cancer Patients.*
World Health Organization, Ed. *Cancer Pain Relief.*
World Health Organization, Ed. *Cancer Pain Relief and Palliative Care.* WHO Technical Report Series, No. 804.

References

Asahi Shimbun. (1971). I (Medicine). Special series, October 19–December 31.
Asahi Shimbun. (1977, November 14)
Asahi Shimbun. (1977, November 26)
Asahi Shimbun. (1996, October 1)
Blackman, S. (1997). *Graceful exits: How great beings die.* New York: Weatherhill.
Char, D.F., Tom, K.S., Young, G.C., Murakami, T., and Ames, R. (1996). A view of death and dying among the Chinese and Japanese. *Hawaii Medical Journal, 55,* 286–190.
Charlton, R., Dovey, S., Mizushima, Y., and Ford, E. (1995). Attitudes to death and dying in the UK, New Zealand, and Japan. *Journal of Palliative Care, 11,* 42–47.
Danis, M., Mulran, E., Garrett, J.M., Stearns, S., Hanson, L.C., Slifkin, R., and Churchill, L. (1996). A prospective study of patient preferences, life-sustaining treatment and hospital cost. *Critical Care Medicine, 24,* 1811–1817.
Elwyn, T.S., Fetters, M.D., Gorenflo, D.W., and Tsuda, T. (1998). Cancer disclosure in Japan: Historical comparisons, current practices. *Social Science and Medicine, 46,* 1151–1163.
Fetters, M.D. (1998). The family in medical decision making in Japanese perspectives. *Journal of Clinical Ethics, 9,* 143–157.
Field, M.J., and Cassel, C.K. (Eds.). (1997). *Approaching death: Improving care at the end of life.* Washington, DC: National Academy Press.
Japan statistical yearbook (Nihon tokei nenkan). (1998). Tokyo: Sōrifu, Tōkeikyoku.
Kashiwagi, T. (1995). *Shi o manabu* (Learning about death). Tokyo: Yūgaikaku.
Kashiwagi, T. (1996). *Shi ni yuku kanja no kokoro ni kiku* (Listening to the hearts of dying patients). Tokyo: Nakayama Shoten.
Kashiwagi, T. (1997). *Shi o mitoru igaku* (Medicine that cares for the dying). *NHK Ningen Daigaku,* January–March.
Kitagawa, T. (1995). *"Ima" nani o suru beki ka: Pīsu Hausu Byōin ni okeru borantea katsudō* (What should be done "now"?: Volunteer activities at Peace House Hospital). *Kango, 47,* 42–47.
Kōbe Shimbun. (1977, August 11).
Kōseishō (Ministry of Health and Welfare). (1995). *Makki iryō o kangaeru* (Thinking about terminal care medicine). Tokyo: Daiichi Hōki.

Kōseishō (Ministry of Health and Welfare). (1997). *Kokumin Eisei no Dōkō* (Trends in Public Health), *44*, 9. Tokyo: Kōsei Tōkei Kyōkai.

Long, S.O. (1980). Fame, fortune, and friends: Constraints and strategies in the careers of Japanese physicians. Unpublished doctoral dissertation, University of Illinois, Urbana-Champaign.

Long, S.O. (1997, September). Reflections on becoming a cucumber: Images of the good death in Japan and the US. Paper presented at the Center for Japanese Studies, University of Michigan.

Long, S.O. (1999). Family surrogacy and cancer disclosure: Family-physician negotiations of an ethical dilemma in Japan. *Journal of Palliative Care 15*, 3, 31–42.

Long, S.O., and Long, B.D. (1982). Curable cancers and fatal ulcers: Attitudes toward cancer in Japan. *Social Science and Medicine, 16*, 2101–2108.

Nihon Hosupisu Zaitaku Kea Kenkyūkai. (1995). *Taiingo no gan kanja shien gaido* (Guide to support for cancer patients after discharge). Osaka: Purimedosha.

Ohnuki-Tierney, E. (1984). *Illness and culture in contemporary Japan*. Cambridge: Cambridge University Press.

Paton, L. & Wicks, M. (1996). The growth of the hospice movement in Japan. *American Journal of Hospice and Palliative Care, 13*, 26–31.

Seirei Fukushi Jigyōdan (Social Welfare Association). (1990). *Seirei rokujūnen no ayumi* (Sixty years of progress at Seirei). Hamamatsu: Seirei Sābisu.

Smith, W.J. (1985). *Dying in the human life cycle: Psychological, biomedical, and social perspectives*. New York: CBS College Publishing.

Sonoda, K. (1988). *Health and illness in a changing Japanese society*. New York: Columbia University Press.

Suzuki, S. (1985). *Shi o dakishimeru (*Embracing the soul*)*. Tokyo: Ningen to Rekishi Sha.

Suzuki, S., Kirschling, J.M., and Inoue, I. (1993). Hospice care in Japan. *American Journal of Hospice and Palliative Care, July/August*, 35–40.

Tamiya, T. (1994). *Bukkyō rinen ni tatta kanwa kea byōtō Bihāra* (Bihara palliative care ward built on Buddhist principles). *Kōsei Fukushi*, No. 3, 2–6.

Tsuneto, A. (1996a). *Kanwa iryō no rekishi to genjō* (The history and current state of palliative care). *Seishin Igaku, 51*, 1831–1835.

Tsuneto, A. (1996b). *Zenjinteki kutsū to chīmu iryō* (Pain of the whole person and team medicine). *Seishin Igaku, 51*, 2235–2240.

Voltz, R., Akabayashi, A., Reese, C., Ohi, G., and Sass, H.M. (1997). Organization and patients' perception of palliative care: A crosscultural comparison. *Palliative Medicine, 11*, 351–357.

Woss, F. (1993). Pokkuri temples and aging. In M. Mullins, S. Shimazono and P.L. Swanson (Eds.), *Religion and society in modern Japan* (pp. 191–202). Berkeley: Asian Humanities Press.

Yamazaki, F. (1990). *Byōin de shinu to iu koto* (Dying in a Japanese hospital). (Y. Claremont, Trans., 1996). Tokyo: Shufu no Tomo.

Yanagida, K. (1996). *"Shi no igaku" e no nikki* (Diary of the coming of "medicine for dying"). Tokyo: Shinchōsha.

Yomiuri Shimbun (1977a). *Iryō o dō suru* (What shall we do with medical care?). Special series, July.

Yomiuri Shimbun (1977b). *Kokumin wa "kusurizuki" ja nai* (We're not a nation of "medicine-lovers"). April 4, p. 14.

Young, R., and Ikeuchi, F. (1997). Religion in "the hateful age": Reflections on pokkuri and other geriatric rutials in Japan's aging society. In S. Formanek and S. Linhart (Eds.),

Aging: Asian concepts and experiences past and present (pp. 229–255). Wien: Der Österreichischen Academie der Wissenschaften.

Zaitaku Hosupisu Kea Moderu Kenkyū Jigyō Hōkokusho (Model Home Hospice Care Research Association). (1994). *Zaitaku hosupisu kea no nozomashii arikata ni tsuite* (Desirable home hospice care). Tokyo: Sōgo Kendo Fukushi Zaidan.

Zenkoku Hosupisu Kanwa Kea Byōtō Renraku Kyōgikai (Japan Association of Hospice and Palliative Care Units). (1997). *Kanwa kea byōtō shōnin shisetsu ni okeru hosupisu kanwa kea puroguramu no kijun* (Standards for licensed hospice and palliative care programs).

8 Policies and practices near the end of life in the US

The ambivalent pursuit of a good death

David Barnard

> There is no such thing as a natural death: nothing that happens to a man is ever natural, since his presence calls the world into question. All men must die: but for every man his death is an accident and, even if he knows it and consents to it, an unjustifiable violation.
>
> Simone de Beauvoir, *A Very Easy Death*, 1965

> The patient and family need a doctor who respects their expertise and can help them clarify and choose what they want, yet who is authoritative, helping to bring clarity and control by saying, "Let's keep trying" or "Let's face the music, it's time to stop."
>
> J. Andrew Billings, *Outpatient Management of Advanced Cancer*, 1985

In the United States, public demand for improved care near the end of life is at an all-time high. After many decades of resistance, academic medicine and professional organizations have begun to respond to this demand. Major medical groups, including the American Medical Association, the American Geriatrics Society, and the American College of Physicians have recently issued calls for a greater emphasis on education for palliative care. The American Board of Internal Medicine (1996) has published a special report, *Caring for the Dying: Identification and Promotion of Physician Competency*, that is specifically aimed at residency programs in Internal Medicine. A National Consensus Conference on Medical Education for Care Near the End of Life, held in May, 1997, brought together palliative care specialists, medical educators, and representatives of major clinical specialties from across the entire spectrum of American medicine. In June, 1997, the distinguished Institute of Medicine of the National Academy of Sciences issued an authoritative and influential report, *Approaching Death: Improving Care at the End of Life* (Field and Cassel, 1997). Major foundations such as the Open Society Institute, through its Project on Death in America, and the Robert Wood Johnson Foundation, through initiatives such as "Last Acts: Care and Caring at the End of Life" and "Promoting

Excellence in End-of-Life Care," are devoting millions of dollars to research and innovation designed (in the words of the Project on Death in America's mission statement) to "transform the culture and experience of dying."

For all of this emphasis on improved care of the dying, however, the American approaches to the subject are full of contradictions. Consider, for example, that:

- America is repeatedly described as a "death denying society," with death relegated to dark and hidden corners of the culture, much as Victorian society dealt with sex. Yet the popular media, especially newspapers, television, and cinema, have saturated the public consciousness with explicit depictions of death. Bookstore shelves sag beneath the weight of personal narratives by people suffering and dying from cancer and AIDS.
- Public opinion polls consistently show that an increasing majority of Americans would prefer to die at home. Yet the proportion of deaths in America that actually occur at home has remained constant, at approximately 25 percent, for several decades. Approximately 55 percent of deaths occur in hospital, with nearly 20 percent now occurring in nursing homes, the fastest growing location of death in the United States (Brock and Foley, 1996).
- Polls demonstrate that approximately 85 percent of Americans believe that "living wills" or "advance directives" are valuable for communicating their preferences for life-sustaining treatment should they lose the ability to communicate near the end of life. Yet only 15 percent of Americans have actually prepared such documents, and for those who do have them most empirical studies show that advance directives have very little influence on medical decision-making (Danis *et al.*, 1991; Schneiderman *et al.*, 1992; SUPPORT Principal Investigators, 1995; Virmani *et al.*, 1994).
- The fear of dying in unrelieved pain is by far the most common fear expressed by patients near the end of life. Yet patients and physicians alike often resist the effective use of narcotic pain medications out of ignorance and prejudices against drug use. These prejudices are made concrete through restrictive government drug policies that inhibit physicians from prescribing adequate doses of narcotics for their dying patients (Cleeland *et al.*, 1994; Field and Cassel, 1997; Webb, 1997).

In this chapter I will argue that these contradictions, and several more that I will describe in more detail below, reflect two prominent characteristics of American society. Many Americans place a very high value on *control*, and also lack *widely shared frameworks of meaning* within which to experience death and dying. These characteristics lead in turn to two forms of ambivalence in the face of death, that manifest themselves at the level of social policy. One is the all-out effort to forestall death, followed by an insistence on painless, quick death once curative efforts fail. The other is a view of hospice and palliative care that expects more of them than they can deliver (i.e., the perfectly managed death) even while the society refuses to fund them adequately in the competition for limited health care resources. Care for the terminally ill, in other words, provides an excellent opportunity to observe the interplay between cultural meanings, professional practices, and public policy, which is one of the major themes of this book.

Cautionary note: is there an "American way of death"?

Cultural, ethnic, and socioeconomic diversity in the United States makes generalization about attitudes toward death especially hazardous. Much of what we know about attitudes toward medical care near the end of life reflects the opportunities and experiences of white, English-speaking, middle- and upper-class Americans with reliable access to nearly unlimited medical care. We are only beginning to appreciate the frames of reference of non-English speakers, people of color, and the poor, who are typically more concerned about the risks of *under*treatment than *over*treatment at the hands of the medical profession (Blackhall *et al.*, 1995; Carrese and Rhodes, 1995; Danis *et al.*, 1988; Orona, Koenig and Davis, 1994).

Furthermore, what we most want to know about the experience of dying is what takes place in the private, day-to-day lives of individuals, families, and caregivers. Yet, until recently, vivid and detailed narratives of this kind have been extremely rare in the medical or social science literature (Barnard *et al.*, 2000; Byock, 1997; Quill, 1996). In the absence of other, quantitative forms of empirical data, cases can distort and mislead as well as inform. Nevertheless, cases convey aspects of human experience that go beyond statistics or surveys of patients' and families' needs or preferences when coping with terminal illness (Singer, Martin and Kelner, 1999). In her introduction to one such case-based approach, published in 1997, Joanne Lynn commented on the paucity of such resources for understanding the possibilities for "good dying":

> Our popular culture [Lynn writes] almost completely ignores the life experience of people with serious chronic illness that will end in death. No evening television shows tell the story of old people slowly dying. Even newspaper obituaries tell the deceased's life story only until retirement – and say nothing of the life that was led in the ensuing twenty years, including telling nothing about the dying except its putative "cause."
> (Webb, 1997, p. xvii)

Meaning, control, and the attempt to forestall death

These important qualifications notwithstanding, one prominent theme in the American experience of life-threatening illness is the absence of widely shared frameworks of meaning that help people make sense of death and accept its inevitability. Without such a framework, it is more likely that death will appear as the absolute negation of all human values, and that the power of medicine to forestall death will become the ultimate object of faith and hope. The physician Eric Cassell provides an impressive example of such an attitude in his book *The Healer's Art* (1979). Cassell asked one of his patients, "What is the doctor's job?" She replied:

> To keep me alive – and more. Because especially now, I don't believe in God anymore really and truly. So the doctor's job is one that never existed before – far beyond any of the others. There were some gods who took care of everything, and there was Jesus. ... There was once another world, but since I don't believe in it any more, for me the doctor is now God ... Now there is only the doctor to protect me from the things around us.
>
> (Cassell, 1979, p. 182)

Even in a period when many Americans are more skeptical of their physicians, and of all other official experts, this way of thinking frequently reasserts itself at a time of crisis. The intensity of these feelings is captured by another physician, G. Gayle Stephens (1981), in a review of the book *Heartsounds* (Lear, 1980). Lear's book describes her husband's long, anxious death from heart disease after the relentless application of every form of medical heroics. These people had made medicine their religion. Of them, and of others like them, Stephens wrote:

> Committed to the narcissistic pursuit of pleasure, deconverted from every creed, and having no sense of the past or future, these prototypes of secularity experience illness as an unjustified intrusion into their lives. Having no resiliency against the nonrational elements of life, they turn to the medical supermarket for redemption. When this fails, as inevitably it must, they rail at their doctors and [now quoting Edna St. Vincent Millay] "...the moment it begins to get dark, as soon as it's night, go out and howl over the grave of God."
>
> (Stephens, 1981, p. 16)

Although physicians are frequently accused of urging patients to accept unwanted efforts to prolong life, the actual situation is often the reverse. It is the patient, or the patient's family, who frequently demands that the doctor persist in life-extending efforts long after the doctor has concluded that it is time to stop. In an important book, *The Troubled Dream of Life: Living with Mortality*, Daniel Callahan (1993) captures the profound ambivalence toward death that engenders such behavior:

> Even if we *say* we can accept death, we believe in our hearts that the sting of death can be medically delayed, that fatalism is itself a source of fatality, that death is a kind of human artifact. No less than physicians have we lay people come to believe that part of the success of modern medicine stems from a commitment to a zealous use of technology, a zeal no place better expressed than at the margins and against the odds. We believe as a general

value that one ought, with spirit, to fight death. We may in all sincerity mean it when we say we do not want clearly useless or futile treatment. But that is not of much help when clinical uncertainty or psychological ambivalence are present; then we may waver, unsure of ourselves. We are all co-conspirators with medicine against death, more than we think.

(Callahan, 1993, p. 51)

Callahan's observations are supported by empirical data on the use of advance directives. I have already mentioned the discrepancy between the proportion of people who say an advance directive is important and those who have actually prepared one. There is also evidence that even among people who have thought in advance about limiting life-prolonging treatment, many change their minds and accept (or demand) such treatment when the situation arises. Marion Danis and her colleagues found, for example, that as many as 20 percent of patients in their studies wanted *more* treatment than they had initially indicated, once their illnesses had progressed (Danis *et al.*, 1994). Ashwini Sehgal and colleagues (1992) studied 150 patients dependent on kidney dialysis who had advance directives regarding eventual termination of life-support. Of these, more than 40 percent wanted their care providers to have substantial leeway to override their previously expressed wishes if the providers believed it would be in the patients' best interest to receive more treatment.

It would be a mistake to conclude from these observations that advance planning with patients regarding care near the of life is unimportant. Quite the opposite is true. Indeed, these data suggest that discussions with patients and families should be routine and regular features of professional-patient relationships. Moreover, they suggest that these discussions should be ongoing, throughout the course of a patient's illness, and the discussions should try to ascertain not only the *content* of the patient's values, but also the *intensity* and *stability* of their preferences. Patients' ambivalence regarding the end of life means that more, not less, dialogue is needed to make the most appropriate decisions about life-supporting treatments.

Meaning, control, and the pursuit of the "perfect" death

What should be done when curative efforts fail? As in the case of death itself, the pain, disability, dependency, and anxiety that are often the precursors of death strike many Americans as absolute negations of human value or meaning. Two prominent features of current medical and social practice in the United States suggest that, without a framework of meaning or, in many instances, any social or community network within which to encounter suffering, the goal for many people is to bring as many aspects of the dying process as possible under total control. Thus are the fierce energies that have been aimed at the *avoidance of death* transformed and redirected to the *management and control of dying* (Filene, 1998).

The first example of this desire for control is the American predilection for legal forms and procedures. Though living wills and other advance directives have so far failed to fulfill their promise, they have received enormous attention. In 1990 the US Congress even passed a law that requires health care institutions to offer patients the opportunity to write an advance directive. The emphasis on advance directives as a solution to problems of end-of-life care seems to reflect a hope that bureaucratic strategies can somehow master the otherwise uncontrollable forces of nature. Many patients and families are disappointed, however, when they discover that their advance directives play little or no role in end-of-life decisions after all (SUPPORT Principal Investigators, 1995; Webb, 1997). The uncertainty, mystery, and ambiguity of dying are simply too pervasive to be eliminated through our advance planning. As Callahan comments,

> Many patients and families, lulled by the possession of an advance directive, find to their dismay that it does not do them as much good as they expected. Sometimes doctors just ignore such directives. More often, and more significantly, the nature of the terminal illness makes it exceedingly hard to know when to invoke the provisions of the directive. As one friend tearfully told me, her mother has been suffering for years from congestive heart failure; though advance directives were in hand, they were useless to the patient and everyone around her. The doctors have simply not been able to determine, in crisis after crisis, whether she is dying. Given that uncertainty, the provisions of the advance directive could not be invoked.
> (Callahan, 1993, p. 40)

In this and other cases, the sting of the dying process is not so much death itself as the helplessness of the patient and family in the face of death, despite every effort to assert control.

The second example, ironically, is the hospice movement itself. The proliferation of techniques for pain and symptom control, hospice and palliative care specialists, and the resurgence of interest in "death with dignity" are not, in any simple way, manifestations of the *acceptance* of death as a "natural" end to the life cycle. Rather, they can appear as the persistence of the obsession with control and the intolerance of suffering that characterize the relentless struggle to *prevent* death. The logical endpoint of this tendency is the demand for physician-assisted suicide and euthanasia, both of which aim to eliminate suffering by eliminating the sufferer.

Rising expectations for painless, symptomless death have been accompanied by the further expectation that one's dying can be the greatest, most exalted experience of one's life. This is the expectation for what Robert Kastenbaum (1979) called "healthy dying." Healthy dying would not merely be free of pain, comfortable, and dignified, but it would be "'special,' exalted, fulfilling – something well beyond the ordinary dimensions of daily experience" (p. 203). Timothy Leary, who gained attention in the 1960s for his experimentation with LSD and other psychedelic drugs, provided a vivid example of this trend, which he and others have referred to as "designer dying." Leary invited the entire world to witness his approach to death by videotaping himself and creating a web-site on the Internet. Leary captured the essence of the American quest for the "perfect" death as an antidote to whatever disappointments and shortcomings life itself has provided. "It's a hip, chic, vogue thing to do," Leary told a reporter for the *New York Times*. "It's the most elegant thing you can do. Even if you have lived your life like a complete slob, you can die with terrific style" (*New York Times*, 1995).

Experienced palliative care specialists and hospice workers know that these fantasies and expectations of the perfectly managed death are often unrealistic. Michael Kearney (1996), a palliative care specialist in Dublin, Ireland, relates the story of Anne, a "beautiful young woman" who suffered intense mental and spiritual anguish as she approached her death from breast cancer. Kearney attended Anne with every possible palliative treatment, including the most advanced forms of pain and symptom control, psychological and spiritual support, and anxiety-reducing image-work and visualization techniques. Close to the end, he encountered Anne writhing and twisting restlessly in her bed. Trying to comfort and reassure her with prayers and with his simple presence, Kearney told her, "Anne, it's okay. We are with you. It's okay. It's going to be all right." Anne's response struck Kearney with the force of a blow. As he describes it, "[She] looked at me as if I were a stranger, and clearly and slowly, with the annoyance of one talking to another who despite repeated attempts could not be made to understand, said 'It's *not* all right.' "

Kearney's reflections on Anne's response capture the humbling truth of death's ultimate dominion over even the most expert attempts to tame it. Her words, Kearney comments,

> do not undermine [my thesis] that good palliative care and preparatory depth work can make a real difference to how we live our dying, but they do put these initiatives in a humbling perspective. They are a reminder that despite all we might say and all we might do, the process of dying includes suffering and painful separations and unfinished business. Death cannot be tamed. Death is unknown. Death is other. Death is death.
>
> (Kearney, 1996, p. 128)

Ambivalence and social policy: the case of hospice care in the United States

Profound contradictions and ambivalence characterize attitudes and behaviors toward death and dying for many people in American society. These contradictions manifest themselves not only at the bedside of the critically ill patient, but also – as in the case of living wills and other advance directives – at the level of social policies. Other examples are the discrepancy between people's stated preferences for dying at home and the actual location of most deaths, and between the prominence of fears of unrelieved pain and policies that restrict the use of narcotic drugs. To focus on the policy dimension in more detail, I will now examine the status and prospects of the hospice movement, which for the past thirty years has been the primary societal response to problems in the care of the dying in the United States.

Hospice: definition and goals

The term "hospice" is often used to refer either to a philosophy of care for dying persons, or to a particular mode of delivering such care. As a philosophy, hospice care is dedicated to maximizing a person's comfort, independence, and quality of life when the prolongation of life is no longer a realistic goal. In the United States, Canada, and Great Britain, "hospice care" is often used interchangeably with the term "palliative care," which has been defined by the World Health Organization (WHO) as:

> the active total care of patients whose disease is not amenable to curative treatment. Control of pain, of other symptoms, and of psychological, social, and spiritual problems is paramount. The goal of palliative care is achievement of the best possible quality of life for patients and their families.
> (WHO, 1990, p. 11)

Further elaborating this definition, the WHO states that palliative care

> affirms life and regards dying as a normal process; neither hastens nor postpones death; provides relief from pain and other distressing symptoms; integrates the psychological and spiritual aspects of patient care; offers a support system to help patients live as actively as possible until death; offers a support system to help the family cope during the patient's illness and in their own bereavement.
> (WHO, 1990, p. 11)

Hospice or palliative care has emerged as a specialized field only within the past thirty years. Landmark dates include the opening in 1967 of St Christopher's Hospice in London under the leadership of Cicely Saunders; the opening in 1974 of the first hospice program in the United States in New Haven, Connecticut, under the leadership of Florence Wald; the establishment in 1975 of the first palliative care program in a major academic medical center, at the Royal Victoria Hospital in Montreal, under the leadership of Balfour Mount; the recognition in 1987 of palliative medicine as a medical specialty in Great Britain; and the publication in 1993 of the *Oxford Textbook of Palliative Medicine*, the definitive scientific textbook in the field.

It is noteworthy that the modern hospice movement grew up in the English-speaking countries of the west. Non-western countries such as Japan have also followed the British model. (For a survey of hospice and palliative care around the world, see Stjernswärd and Pampallona, 1998.) While it is beyond the scope of this essay to account for the British origins of hospice care, four aspects of medicine and society in Britain, Canada, and the United States suggest some contributing contextual factors:

- *Medical technology* has blurred the line between life and death, leaving many people attached to invasive mechanical life support and enduring pain, helplessness, and expense throughout their last weeks and days of life, and seeking more comfortable alternatives.
- *Lack of attention to symptom control in medical education and practice* has caused caregivers to concentrate narrowly on the pathophysiology and cure of disease rather than the patient's experience of illness, resulting in a great burden of preventable but unnoticed suffering.
- *A loss of extended family ties and community* has caused the physical and emotional burdens of caring for a dying person to fall more heavily on the members of isolated nuclear families, and particularly on women, leading people to turn to professionals for necessary support.
- *Strained and evasive relationships*, caused by our discomfort around the dying and bereaved, frequently increase loneliness and suffering, making a philosophy of care that emphasizes human contact especially attractive.

Development in the United States

In the decade after the first hospice opened in 1974, the number of hospice programs in the United States grew to 516. Most relied heavily for financial support on private philanthropy and grants. Beginning in 1983, patients over the age of 65 could elect to receive a "hospice benefit" under the federally-financed Medicare program. A patient who has been certified by his or her physician as "terminally ill" – defined as having a life expectancy of six months or less – may waive access to Medicare payment for curative treatments for the terminal illness. In return, the patient receives a package of noncurative medical and nonmedical support services that would otherwise not be covered, or would be provided in an uncoordinated manner. The Medicare hospice benefit is payable as a per diem reimbursement to Medicare-certified hospice providers. It includes nursing care in the home (up to sixteen to twenty hours per week, with temporary 24-hour care available under limited "crisis" circumstances); home health aides; medical appliances and drugs; homemakers, and volunteers for personal and respite care; physician services; short-term hospitalization; physical and occupational therapy; psychological and spiritual support; social services; and bereavement counseling.

Medicare requires hospices to conform to several procedural and staffing requirements in order to receive federal funds. Among the most significant requirements are:

- The full spectrum of services must be available to all patients
- The hospice must have a core, interdisciplinary team made up at least of a physician, a registered nurse, a social worker, and a chaplain or other counselor

- Patients must have an identified primary care provider in the home (usually a family member or someone else who is available on a 24-hour per day basis)
- No patient may be discharged for lack of ability to pay
- No more than 20 percent of the total aggregate number of days of care provided by the hospice may be in inpatient settings

Since Medicare funding became available, the number of hospice programs in the United States has increased dramatically, and Medicare funds account for almost 70 percent of all hospice payments. The balance comes from private insurance, programs for the indigent, and payments by patients themselves. In 1996, according to data from the National Hospice Organization reported by the Institute of Medicine (Field and Cassel, 1997), approximately 2,800 hospices served approximately 440,000 patients. This amounts to roughly 20 percent of the persons who die annually in the United States, and approximately 25 percent of the 1.6 million people who die annually with "hospice-appropriate" illnesses. Approximately 80 percent of patients served by hospices die at home.

Despite the fact that Medicare's hospice benefit allows for six months of care, most patients receive services for a much shorter period of time. According to the most recent data from the National Hospice Organization, the median length of stay in United States hospice programs in 1998 was only 20 days (Russell K. Portenoy, MD, personal communication).

Problematic features of hospice care in the United States

Several additional features of the American hospice movement help explain its relatively minor penetration into the overall system of care for the terminally ill. These features, in turn, are best understood in relation to the contradictions and ambivalence that characterize American society's attitudes toward death and dying.

Dependence on care providers in the home

Both the hospice philosophy and Medicare regulations require that the greatest proportion of care be delivered to patients in their homes. Currently, according to National Hospice Organization data, only 45 percent of US hospices will accept a patient for care if that patient does not have a primary caregiver at home (Kathleen Foley, MD, personal communication). While receiving care at home accords with most patients' stated preferences, it is often impractical. Some people live in unstable or unsafe environments. Some have no family or friends who can take on the hospice- and Medicare-mandated role of "primary care provider." Some families who initially agree to take on these responsibilities become exhausted, frightened, or overwhelmed with the demands of care. To date, however, there are relatively few inpatient hospice facilities with the staffing and atmosphere conducive to optimal palliative care. Moreover, because the cost of an admission to an inpatient facility must be paid by the hospice with the money it receives for the per diem care of the patient at home, hospices have an economic incentive to minimize such admissions.

Underrepresentation of patients with diseases other than cancer

Nationally, approximately 80 percent of patients enrolled in hospice programs have cancer as their principal diagnosis, though this figure varies somewhat by individual hospice. The relatively predictable pattern of death from cancer – gradual deterioration followed by relatively swift decline toward the end – is well suited to the hospice approach. There is time for organizing and implementing a multidisciplinary plan of care. The fear of cancer in the general population, and the long history of denial and evasion in communicating with cancer patients, make the hospice philosophy of openness and concern for psychological and spiritual suffering especially appropriate. At the same time, in light of the six-month prognosis that is a requirement for admission and the generally predictable course of the disease, there is relatively little economic risk to the hospice program in accepting the cancer patient.

Less predictable diseases, with more frequent remissions and exacerbations and greater opportunities to benefit from life-prolonging interventions, fit less well with the economic, philosophical, and practical aspects of hospice care. Consequently, patients with AIDS, chronic obstructive pulmonary disease, heart disease, and many other conditions are underrepresented in hospice programs. In the case of AIDS patients, especially, the frequent lack of dependable in-home care providers has aggravated the problem.

Anti-physician bias

While hospice programs in the US are required to have a physician in the role of medical director, physicians are often marginal to the actual care of patients, except in the relatively few programs that are based in hospitals or academic medical centers. This is in contrast to England, Canada, and Australia, for example, where physicians are more closely integrated into the planning and implementation of care. A practical barrier to physician involvement is the hospice orientation toward home-based care, which is viewed as inefficient and uneconomical by many US physicians. Perhaps more significant, however, are some aspects of the medical profession's attitudes toward incurable illness and death, which have had a great influence on the development of the hospice movement in the United States. Although there are important exceptions, physicians in the United States have tended to view the care of dying patients as an uncomfortable and unrewarding task. Without hope for a cure, many physicians convey to the patient (either directly or indirectly) that "there is nothing more I can do." As a result, for many physicians a referral to hospice is the equivalent of giving up responsibility for the patient's care. The hospice movement in the US defined itself from the outset as a compassionate alternative to the abandonment of patients by these technically oriented, emotionally distant physicians. Many of the hospice pioneers were nurses, motivated (as many still are) by a desire to offer the incurably ill patient superior treatment to what they perceived the patient to be receiving from uncaring or incompetent doctors. This anti-physician bias, built into the history of the US hospice movement, has impaired the development of fully integrated multidisciplinary teams.

The hospice ideology of the "good death"

The publicly stated philosophy of the hospice movement is to respect each patient's unique way of facing death. According to this view, it is improper for hospice workers to impose their own beliefs or expectations regarding the "correct" way to die (International Work Group on Death, Dying, and Bereavement, 1994). In practice, things are often quite different. Despite a stated tolerance for individual uniqueness, many hospice workers either covertly or overtly encourage patients and families to forego life-prolonging measures, in order to facilitate "acceptance" of death (Ackerman, 1997). Hospice workers' anti-physician bias stems in part from their assumption that physicians will recommend more aggressive treatment to the patient, or encourage greater resistance to the disease, than is consistent with the ideology of "acceptance." I have already observed that hospice programs have an economic incentive to minimize their patients' recourse to technology or inpatient care, even when such care could have real benefits. This convergence of ideology and economics may well explain much of the reluctance of physicians to refer patients to hospice programs as early as most hospice workers would consider ideal.

While empirical data on conflict or discord between patients, families, and hospice workers are very difficult to obtain (which in itself may be a sign of hospice programs' reluctance to engage in critical scrutiny of their prevailing ideology), experience and anecdotal evidence suggest genuine tensions between the "hospice way of death" and the needs or desires of significant numbers of patients (Barnard, *et al.*, 2000). A more flexible approach on the part of hospice (with corresponding changes in financing and relations with physicians) will be necessary if hospice care is to be a viable option for a greater proportion of the US population.

The interplay of cultural meanings and public policy in the care of the dying: the marginalization and underfinancing of palliative care

The desire of most Americans for all-out efforts to prevent death, supported by the most advanced (and expensive) medical technology, is in genuine tension with the desire for excellent, well-financed services for the care of the dying. There is no intrinsic or inherent incompatibility between these two goals. Nevertheless, American society has yet to find a way to reconcile them at the level of public policy and the organization of health care services. The contradictions and ambivalence with respect to death and dying in American society have, at the policy level, manifested themselves in two significant problems for end-of-life care in the United States. The first problem is a rigid and unfortunate *polarization* between curative and palliative care in the health care system. The second problem is the *serious underfinancing* of palliative care or hospice services.

Hospice and palliative care have yet to overcome the legacy of opposition to mainstream scientific medicine that characterized their beginnings in the 1960s and 1970s. The growth of rigorous scientific research in palliative care, the publication of textbooks, and the growth of a cadre of palliative medicine specialists with a base in academic medical centers, should ameliorate this problem in the years to come. For the present, however, hospice and palliative care remain at the margins of the American health care system. With their eyes fastened on cure and the conquest of death, patients and physicians tend to ignore or minimize the contributions of the hospice or palliative care approach to critical illness. The rigid ideology of "acceptance" of death, overtly or covertly espoused by many hospice workers, aggravates this problem by making it more difficult to integrate palliative care – with its focus on excellent symptom control and quality of life – into the overall care of the patient while cure or prolongation of life remain the patient's primary goals. The frequent result, even when the patient's disease is very far advanced, is a delayed referral to a hospice program or the half-hearted effort to apply the principles and techniques of palliative care by a physician who has neither enthusiasm nor competence for the task.

The problem of financing is particularly difficult because of one more instance of ambivalence on the part of planners and policy makers in the US health care system. There is no agreement on the part of policy makers whether the primary value of hospice and palliative care is their ability to *improve the patient's and family's quality of life*, or their effectiveness in *reducing health care expenditures*. Despite the claims of their early proponents, hospice and palliative care do not significantly reduce the overall costs of caring for the incurably ill patient. While hospice reduces the costs of care that are attributable to hospitalization and the use of expensive diagnostic tests, these savings are largely cancelled out by labor-intensive nursing and support services. The result is that overall costs are redistributed rather than substantially reduced when significant numbers of people elect hospice care over traditional care near the end of life (Emanuel, 1996; Emanuel and Emanuel, 1994). Moreover, many of the patient-oriented outcome measures of hospice care – e.g., subjective estimates of quality of life, ability to die in one's own bed, etc. – are difficult to measure in the quantitative, economic terms in favor with health care planners and executives of health insurance companies. It is thus by no means clear how hospice and palliative care services will fare under the capitated, pre-paid managed care systems that are rapidly becoming the standard method of insuring access to health care in the United States (Miles *et al.*, 1995; Morrison and Meier, 1995).

At the level of financing of services or research, the desire to forestall or prevent death overwhelms support for hospice and palliative care. Once again precise data are difficult to obtain, but one indicator of the disparity is presented in the Institute of Medicine's report, *Approaching Death* (Field and Cassel, 1997). The report cites a personal communication from an official from the National Institutes of Health (NIH), who estimated that in fiscal year 1996 NIH spent about $70 million dollars on pain research out of an overall budget of *$12 billion* (Field and Cassel, 1997, p. 238). A further indication of the same trend is the allocation of space for the presentation of research at the Annual Meeting of the American Society of Clinical Oncology, recognized as the main forum in the world for dissemination of cancer-related knowledge. According to data presented in the most recent edition of the *Oxford Textbook of Palliative Medicine*, only 7 percent of the space has been devoted to palliative care research, and of that 7 percent almost 70 percent is related to studies of chemotherapy-induced nausea (Doyle, Hanks and MacDonald, 1998, p. 180). Rigorous, well-designed, and well-funded research into the physical, psychological, and spiritual support of the dying is still a minuscule item on the agenda of the American health care system.

While this gross disparity in financial support follows directly from the desire to oppose death that is so prominent in American society, it is not consistent with the equal (if unrealistic) desire to insure a perfectly managed death, free of pain or suffering. It remains to be seen whether American health policy can strike a more appropriate balance between these goals.

Acknowledgements

Symposium on "Care and Meaning in Late Life: Culture, Policy, and Practice in Japan and the United States." Sponsored by the Abe Fellowship Program and the Social Science Research Council, Zushi, Japan, February 26–March 1, 1998.

References

Ackerman, F. (1997). Goldilocks and Mrs Ilych: A critical look at the "philosophy of hospice." *Cambridge Quarterly of Healthcare Ethics, 6*, 314–324.
American Board of Internal Medicine. (1996). *Caring for the dying: Identification and promotion of physician competency.* Philadelphia: American Board of Internal Medicine.
Barnard, D., Towers, A., Boston, P., and Lambrinidou, Y. (2000). *Crossing over: Narratives of palliative care.* New York: Oxford University Press.
Blackhall, L., et al. (1995). Ethnicity and attitudes toward patient autonomy. *Journal of the American Medical Association, 274*, 820–825.
Brock, D., and Foley, D. (1996). Demography and epidemiology of dying in the US, with emphasis on the deaths of older persons. Paper presented at symposium on A Good Dying: Shaping Health Care for the Last Months of Life, Washington, DC.
Byock, I. (1997). *Dying well: The prospect for growth at the end of life.* New York: Riverhead Books.

Callahan, D. (1993). *The troubled dream of life: Living with mortality.* New York: Simon & Schuster.

Carrese, J., and Rhodes, L. (1995). Western bioethics on the Navajo reservation: Benefit or harm? *Journal of the American Medical Association, 274,* 826–829.

Cassell, E.J. (1979). *The healer's art: A new approach to the doctor–patient relationship.* Baltimore: Penguin.

Cleeland, C.S., Gonin, R., Hatfield, A.K., Edmonson, J. H., Blum, R.H., Stewart, J.A., and Pandya K.J. (1994). Pain and its treatment in patients with metastatic cancer. *New England Journal of Medicine, 330,* 592–596.

Danis, M., Patrick, D. L., Southerland, L.I., and Green M.L. (1988). Patients' and families' preferences for medical intensive care. *Journal of the American Medical Association, 260,* 797–802.

Danis, M., Southerland, L.I., Garrett, J.M., Smith, J.L., Hielema, F., Packard, C.G., Egner, D.M., and Patrick, D.L. (1991). A prospective study of advance directives for life-sustaining care. *New England Journal of Medicine, 324,* 882–888.

Danis, M., Garrett, J., Harris, R., and Patrick, D.L. (1994). Stability of choices about life-sustaining treatments. *Annals of Internal Medicine, 120,* 567–573.

Doyle, D., Hanks, G., and MacDonald, N. (Eds.). (1998). *Oxford textbook of palliative medicine* (2nd ed.). Oxford: Oxford University Press.

Emanuel, E.J. (1996). Cost savings at the end of life: What do the data show? *Journal of the American Medical Association, 275,* 1907–1914.

Emanuel, E.J., and Emanuel, L.L. (1994). The economics of dying: The illusion of cost savings at the end of life. *New England Journal of Medicine, 330,* 540–544.

Field, M.J., and Cassel, C.K. (Eds.) (1997). *Approaching death: Improving care at the end of life.* Washington, DC: National Academy Press.

Filene, P.G. (1998). *In the arms of others: A cultural history of the right-to-die in America.* Chicago: Ivan Dee.

International Work Group on Death, Dying, and Bereavement. (1994). *Statements on death, dying, and bereavement.* London, Ontario: King's College.

Kastenbaum, R. (1979). "Healthy dying": A paradoxical quest continues. *Journal of Social Issues, 35,* 185–206.

Kearney, M. (1996). *Mortally wounded: Stories of soul pain, death, and healing.* Dublin: Marino Books.

Lear, M.W. (1980). *Heartsounds: The story of a love and loss.* New York: Simon & Schuster.

Miles, S.H., Weber, E.P., and Koepp, R. (1995). End-of-life treatment in managed care: The potential and the peril. *Western Journal of Medicine, 163,* 302–305.

Morrison, R.S., and Meier, D.E. (1995). Managed care at the end of life. *Trends in Health Care, Law, and Ethics, 10,* 91–96.

New York Times. (1995, November 26).

Orona, C., Koenig, B., and Davis, A. (1994). Cultural aspects of nondisclosure. *Cambridge Quarterly of Healthcare Ethics, 3,* 338–346.

Quill, T. (1996). *Midwife through the dying process: Stories of healing and hard choices at the end of life.* Baltimore: Johns Hopkins University Press.

Schneiderman, L.J., Kronick, R., Kaplan, M., Anderson, J.P., and Langer, R.D. (1992). Effects of offering advance directives on medical treatment and costs. *Annals of Internal Medicine, 117,* 599–606.

Sehgal, A., Galbraith, A., Chesney, M., Schoenfeld, P., Charles, G., and Lo, B. (1992). How strictly do dialysis patients want their advance directives followed? *Journal of the American Medical Association, 267,* 59–63.

Singer, P.A., Martin, D.K., and Kelner, M. (1999). Quality end-of-life care: Patients' perspectives. *Journal of the American Medical Association, 281*, 163–168.

Stephens, G.G. (1981). Doctors at bay. *Continuing Education for the Family Physician, February,* 15–16.

Stjernswärd, J., and Pampallona, S. (1998). Palliative medicine: A global perspective. In D. Doyle, G. Hanks, and N. MacDonald (Eds.), *Oxford textbook of palliative medicine* (2nd ed.). Oxford: Oxford University Press.

SUPPORT Principal Investigators. (1995). A controlled trial to improve care for seriously ill hospitalized patients. *Journal of the American Medical Association, 274*, 1591–1598.

Virmani, J., Schneiderman, L.J., and Kaplan, R.M. (1994). Relationship of advance directives to physician–patient communication. *Archives of Internal Medicine, 154*, 909–913.

Webb, M. (1997). *The good death: The new American search to reshape the end of life.* New York: Bantam Books.

World Health Organization. (1990). Cancer pain relief and palliative care. Technical Report No. 804. Geneva: World Health Organization.

Part III
Assisting in Care
Non-profit organizations and volunteers

9 The development of social welfare services in Japan

Kiyoshi Adachi

Within these pages I will discuss how social welfare has been introduced into Japanese society and how these concepts have been transformed, or "Japanized." In addition, I will summarize the issues related to social welfare which Japan must deal with in the near future. In order to examine how social welfare was introduced into Japan, how it is being Japanized and how current reforms will alter Japan's social welfare system, I have adopted a historical-sociological approach, an investigative study of the conditions under which social welfare has taken root in Japan.[1]

In Japan, the development of the social security system over the years has caused a shift in the fundamental meaning of "social welfare." When the American forces that occupied Japan after World War II (WWII) demanded that the Japanese government implement social security measures, social welfare was understood to mean an absolute minimum level of economic social security, e.g. daily life security, public assistance, and the like. Some years later social welfare developed further and came to include personal social services and social work.[2]

In the 1980s, the issue of Japan's rapidly aging society brought elderly welfare services to the forefront of the social welfare debate, where it has remained to this day. In response to the rapid aging of Japanese society the central government has initiated a set of measures which are commonly referred to simply as "The Welfare Reform." This welfare reform is intrinsically bound to the problems of elderly welfare and care services, in particular to the financial problems caused by this rapid aging of society (for example, the sudden increase in pension and elderly medical payments) and the failure of individual families to provide adequate elderly care.

The introduction of social welfare and its Japanization

Social welfare

According to the research of Takeshi Ishida and his colleagues, the idea of social welfare had never existed until it was introduced to Japan via the direct orders of the general headquarters of the allied powers (GHQ) during the Allied Occupation after World War II. The United States, having investigated the prewar rise of fascism, had come to the conclusion that the establishment of social work and social welfare policies would work to prevent a second occurrence: one of the chief causes of the rise in fascism had been the absence of a social security/social welfare system or an equivalent specialized system to counter poverty and social problems. According to their analysis, the failure of the Japanese government to address the problems of famine and poverty in the countryside had helped to set off a wave of militarism and thus contributed to the rise in fascism. It is obvious that, in the eyes of the United States, social welfare was essential to Japan's democratization (see Ishida 1983, 1984).

From social work to social welfare

To be sure, social welfare-like policies had existed in Japan earlier. Partly in order to propagate the emperor system, the Japanese government introduced a number of so-called "charity policies" during the Meiji era (1868–1912). These evolved into the social work policies of the Taisho era (1912–1926) which attempted to counter poverty and workers' uprisings and thus maintain peace and order. However, it is important to note that, like the emperor system which portrayed the Japanese nation as one big family, the central government designed and implemented these policies as "a dutiful father" protecting its children – that is, the Japanese people. Takeshi Ishida (1983) cites a number of documents and depositions which confirm that Department of Interior and Department of Health and Welfare officials possessed this sort of paternalistic mentality. In guiding the people as a father would guide his children, these officials felt driven by a strong sense of moral duty. Interestingly, this sense was not shared by their Nazi Germany counterparts.

As Japan entered the Showa era (1926–1989), the Japanese government implemented a new series of paternalist policies with the purpose of developing a high-quality military force and reliable labor force. These became the pillar the Ministry of Health and Welfare's war-time policies. The Ministry took an active fatherly role in raising the health and nutrition standards of the Japanese people in order to develop strong soldiers and a strong (primarily female) war-time labor force.

The GHQ's welfare policies

The GHQ pressured the Japanese government to adopt three basic principles of social welfare:

- non-discrimination and equality
- public assistance as a national responsibility
- separation of the public and private sector.

The GHQ's social welfare policies were in line with the innovative nature of the American New Deal, including policies so progressive that they had not been fully adopted in the United States. Had the measures been adopted exactly as they had been proposed, Japan would undoubtedly have very quickly become a welfare state. However, as the newly introduced social welfare concept was unfamiliar to all but a few Japanese, those trying to implement the new policies were faced with a troublesome problem: the shortage of educated and skilled staff at the various welfare offices across Japan.

The Japanization of social welfare

The postwar Japanese government has consistently shown resistance to the concept of a "people's right to social welfare." In particular, it has been unwilling to recognize the people's right to demand services, believing that an expansion of social welfare would result in an "idle citizenry" dependent upon welfare. It is fair to say that the Japanese government has concentrated more on developing the national economy than on elevating its citizens' quality of living. Most industrially developed countries became welfare states under the influence of labor or socialist parties which came to power after World War II. These regimes had placed priority on developing livelihood assistance for their laborers and social security for their citizens. By contrast, the introduction of social welfare legislation in Japan is characterized by the partially forced implementation which took place under the GHQ.

The Japanese government's traditionally paternalistic attitudes toward social security and social welfare policies remained intact. For example, Japan's medical-, welfare- and pension-related policies have been proposed and implemented almost entirely by the Japanese government. The most recent instances of this sort of policy making are the Ten Year Strategy to Promote Health Care and Welfare Services for the Elderly which was introduced in the late 1980s and the Public Long-Term Care Insurance Act of 1997 (*Kaigo Hoken Hō*). Neither the Japanese people nor local governments had anything to do with the decision-making behind either of these two very important social security/social welfare policies.[3]

The postwar Japanese approach to social welfare, though different from that of other developed nations, has been called successful by some. John Campbell, an American scholar who has done much research concerning Japanese medical and welfare policy, has underscored the advantages of the Japanese government's approach to policy-making (Campbell, 1996; Ikegami and Campbell, 1996). The welfare ministry bureaucracy, employing its ability to plan for the long term and supported by the widely shared perception that Japan is a paternalist nation by nature, took the leading role in developing Japan's medical, social security, and social welfare policies.

As the Japanese government's method produced successful, far-sighted policies, it is only natural that the results of their efforts should be favorably critiqued. However, this sort of policy development has made the Japanese people and local governments excessively dependent upon the national government with regard to social security and social welfare. Such a welfare system is highly susceptible to the undulations of the national economy. There is no guarantee that medical- and welfare-related policies for the elderly will not be curtailed or otherwise suffer the effects of a drastic change in the nation's overall direction.

The Japanization of social welfare organizations

The GHQ laid the foundation for Japan's social welfare policies. However, a system was needed to implement those policies – the development of this system is a most curious example of the Japanization of social welfare.

Social welfare councils

The GHQ demanded that Japan clearly acknowledge its national responsibility for social welfare and establish a single, nationwide governmental organ specialized to the task of implementing social welfare policy. Despite financial and personnel inadequacies, Japan drew up plans for private social welfare organizations based upon America's Social Welfare Council, a body which had been evolving together with American community-chest fundraising since 1910. Japan's central government created the Japanese version of the Social Welfare Council by redesigning preexisting community organizations; at this time there were no private organizations specializing in welfare services in the communities. For example, they created the Central Social Welfare Council by unifying the Compatriots' Aid Organization, the Servicemen's Aid Organization and the Japan Social Work Society. These social welfare councils have thrived under the bureaucratic guidance they received.

However, the same bureaucratic involvement has obfuscated the line separating the governmental and private sectors. According to Daisaku Maeda, a full half of the directors of county and city social welfare councils were either mayors or regional office chiefs. For many years, most of the directors of local social welfare councils were mayors, upper-level bureaucrats, or chairman of local assemblies. These people convened regularly but their committee meetings did not bear many concrete results. In Japan there has never been a community-based social welfare system; the social welfare councils developed in compliance with orders from above (Maeda, 1990).

Social welfare corporations

A sort of Japanization may also be observed in the development of social welfare corporations. The GHQ stipulated that the Japanese government should not directly fund privately operated social welfare organizations as it had in the past. This restriction was written into the Japanese Constitution as Article 89 which reads, "No government money or other property shall be expended or appropriated for the use, benefit or maintenance of any religious institution or association, or for any charitable, educational or benevolent enterprises not under the control of public authorities."

However, these organizations have been and continue to be managed under the control of the central government. They must abide by a host of stringent government-authored legal restrictions and are dependent upon central government funding via a system of "welfare placement by commission," whereby the government commissions welfare projects to them. Although social welfare corporations are technically private enterprises, very few have been able to design welfare projects independent of the government due to the tight restrictions on them.

Furthermore, even though social welfare corporations are technically allowed to create separate services using nongovernmental funds, very few have managed to do so because of the time and energy needed for government-commissioned projects. Moreover, the government is able to exert influence over the hiring and decision-making processes of the social welfare corporations. This blurring of the line between public and private creates an environment which is conducive to corruption and other problems.

In this respect, the Japanese model of the social welfare corporation is significantly different from that of America, where the private sector is much more clearly separated from the governmental sector. Reform may be on the way. The Reform of Basic Structure of Social Welfare, a section meeting of the central government sponsored by the Central Social Welfare Advisory Committee, is currently debating ways to reform the part of the Social Work Law that deals with social welfare corporations.

The Japanization of volunteerism

The concept of "welfare volunteer" has been adopted by Japan, but not before going through the Japanization process.

The area commissioner and community welfare commissioner

If welfare volunteers may be defined as people who do social work or social welfare work without pay, the Area Commissioners of Japan's Taisho period may be described as Japan's earliest welfare volunteer.[4] They were government-appointed, unlike their western counterparts, and contributed to the Japanization of welfare services. They also illustrate the problem points of the process. The post of Area Commissioner was established as a result of the Rice Riots of 1919 as an attempt by the government to deal with the rising number of impoverished people becoming concentrated in Japan's urban areas as a result of capitalist development.

Peace-keeping and social work policies previously introduced by the government at the national level had not been sufficient means for coping with the problems of the day. Therefore, the central government decided that the best way for dealing with community problems was to commission the voluntary position of Area Commissioner to local men of high standing in the various communities across Japan. The Area Commissioner was an unpaid honorary post, and as such, there were no personnel costs. This is one of the reasons it was very quickly adopted throughout the nation.

After the end of World War II the Japanese government considered reinstating the Area Commissioner system. However, the GHQ, intent on breaking up the Imperial Rule Assistance Association (the political organization created by the Japanese government in 1940), demanded that the system be abolished on the grounds that a more decisive line needed to be drawn between the government and private sectors. In the end, as there was a shortage of qualified specialists and no possibility of introducing government employees into the social welfare sector, the Japanese government successfully negotiated with the GHQ for the creation of a new post similar to that of the Area Commissioner, the Community Welfare Commissioner. Like their predecessors, these new commissioners were volunteers. They would go on to play an important auxiliary role in the implementation of social security policies.

The first Community Welfare Commissioners had little understanding of postwar social welfare concepts. Rather, they believed public assistance to be an expression of the "nation's mercy" and made such payments based on the Meiji/Taisho paternalistic traditions. Naturally, their pension payment practices fell under heavy criticism from the GHQ. In the eyes of one GHQ dignitary:

> When a Community Welfare Commissioner gives public assistance to a person, he considers it a personal, emotional act, as if he were giving out a personal present. It is common and natural for a Community Welfare Commissioner to say, "I gave them assistance because I felt sorry for them." This is a paternalistic, feudalistic way of thinking.
>
> (Ishida, 1983)

Ishida further notes that

> The Japanese government used the Community Welfare Commissioners and social welfare councils to introduce into the community a system which was half governmental and half private. It came to be co-opted by the community's men of high standing and was run by rules which differed from community to community.
>
> (Ishida, 1983: 225)

Still, the volunteer services of the commissioners were instrumental in establishing post-war social welfare policies. The Community Welfare Commissioner system is still in place today. The Commissioners investigate their community's welfare needs by conducting surveys to determine the number of bed-ridden elderly in their community. They also provide private support for local government welfare offices.

Citizens' participation programs in reformist local governments

Before the mid-1960s, most of Japan's local governments had conservative politicians at their helm. Then, from the latter half of the 1960s until the 1970s, Japan saw a rise in reformist local governments. During this time period, a number of local government heads began to actively promote citizens' participation. A vigorous debate regarding the necessity of citizens' participation in the decision-making process at the local level ensued. In the end, however, reformist local governments lost support before much social welfare reform could take place. Little mention was made of the role of citizens' participation in social welfare.

Social welfare reforms of the 1980s

A major overhaul of the Japanese social welfare system was initiated in the 1980s. This large-scale reform was triggered by the following:

- The government grant reduction proposed by the Second Extraordinary (Ad Hoc) Administrative Research Council of 1981
- The 1986 reduction of national grants and transfer of government welfare offices to the municipalities
- The 1989 decision to implement the Gold Plan
- The 1990 revision of eight welfare laws
- The 1992 revision of the Social Welfare Act.

Reform is based on the concepts of deregulation of social welfare services, decentralization, privatization and the introduction of a sophisticated supply system (Ōmori, 1989, 1990; Furukawa, 1995). It also draws from two different schools of thought. One, welfare policy reexamination theory, was put forth in response to the current economic recession. It proposes funding reductions, deregulation, self-reliance, an emphasis on family-based welfare services, the revitalization of the private sector and the introduction of the market mechanism. In contrast, welfare policy reform theory is advanced by social welfare scholars. It advocates development of a plan to meet home care needs, decentralization, the introduction of policies pertaining to at-home specialized staff, NPO-based welfare services and the granting of permission to those wishing to engage in "paid volunteer" welfare services.

According to social welfare scholar Kōjun Furukawa (1997), this plan for welfare reform, should it be fully implemented, represents a new social welfare paradigm. The most important elements of this paradigm are universalization (whereby social welfare recipients would no longer be limited to the impoverished), pluralism (whereby nonprofit organizations would be able to provide welfare services together with governmental offices and social welfare corporations), decentralization (whereby the power to make decisions regarding social welfare services would be transferred to the local governments) and regionalization (whereby at-home welfare services would be developed alongside institution-based services). As decision-making powers are increasingly transferred to local governments, Japan would seem to be moving toward a less centralized system. Yet this represents only a limited paradigm shift since it is the national government itself which has established to whom it will relinquish its power. Muneyuki Shindō (1996), a scholar of public administration, insists that the welfare reforms of the Ministry of Health and Welfare are not true decentralization but "regulated decentralization." Nonetheless, under this reform plan some changes have already taken place. For example, the majority of welfare services for the elderly and handicapped are now managed directly by local governments, in contrast to the old system which delegated administrative functions from the central government to local governments.

Recent social welfare reforms

Katsuhiro Hiro (1981) and Kōjun Furukawa (1997) have identified a number of motivating forces behind recent welfare reform: the end of the Cold War, the rise of a new conservatism, increased fiscal restrictions due to low economic growth, a rise in the standard of living, the breakup of the traditional family structure,[5] a diversification and elevation of social service needs, changing values and a maturation of social security policies. The observations of Hori and Furukawa are, for the most part, appropriate. However, they have failed to note the contribution made by citizens' groups demanding a more independent welfare service system. According to my research (Adachi, 1998), citizens' groups all across the country petitioned strongly for welfare reform through the 1980s. The result of that movement is the system known as "community-based home care services." Petitions and other movements made by these citizens' groups played an indirect but important role in instigating the current welfare reform.

Grassroots community organizations as providers of home care services

From the 1980s, citizens' groups nationwide began developing small mutual assistance groups to deal with the scarcity of home care services for the elderly who live alone or who need support. These groups usually operated on a membership basis, sending out home helpers who would provide services in return for a small gratuity. The "community-based at-home welfare services" that they provided marked the birth of what can be called the "paid volunteer citizens' mutual aid groups."[6] At first, participants in these groups provided only basic home helper services such as shopping, cleaning, laundry, and meals preparation. But in response to changing welfare needs, they now often perform more care-oriented services such as nursing, hand-feeding, and sponge-bathing.[7] At the end of the 1980s there were only 120 such organizations but this number had grown to 1,180 by 1997. An estimated 80,000 people are reported to be involved in welfare activities in this sector.

It should be noted that although these citizens' mutual aid groups are on the rise, citizens' participation in the decision-making process of welfare policies is not. However, the emergence of these groups has allowed communities to express their welfare needs and their dissatisfaction with the status quo. It has also provided citizens with a new tool for resolving their own problems.

The community's increased interest in social welfare is rooted in the rise of nuclear families, smaller family units and the family's increasing inability to provide care for the elderly in their households. Until the 1980s, most people in Japan associated social welfare with social security or with nursing homes for the elderly. Since then, however, social welfare has come to mean home care services for the elderly. Middle-aged housewives in particular see at-home welfare services as an answer to the rising problems of elder care in their homes and neighborhoods.

According to research that I undertook in conjunction with the National Social Welfare Council (Adachi, 1993), more than 90 percent of the people who took part in home care services were housewives. Most of those surveyed were between their late forties and sixties in age. The most common motivation for participating in the home care services was "an interest in social welfare." My research shows that housewives who have finished raising their children and thus have time on their hands are at the heart of the grassroots welfare volunteer movement. These women recognized early on that their immediate family, friends and neighbors would soon be facing a crisis. Who would care for the increasing numbers of elderly among them? They didn't have to imagine the problems that they themselves would be facing in their old age; their future welfare needs were reflected in the elderly people all around them. Because they saw social welfare as intertwined with the futures of their own families, these housewives have begun participating in community volunteer activities such as citizens' mutual aid groups which provide home care services.

Volunteerism in Japan

The National Social Welfare Council's National Center for the Promotion of Volunteerism conducted a survey in 1990 which found that approximately 4,110,000 people are participating in volunteer activities of some kind. This is by no means a small figure, but it should be noted that volunteer activities in Japan have various limitations. In Japan, the activities of grassroots nonprofit organizations were never considered an essential element of society. Only government-run activities have been taken seriously. Grassroots organizations could receive the accreditation, acknowledgment and approval of the government, but only provided their activities supported the government's own projects. The establishment of public corporations by individual citizens has been subjected to a host of ministerial restrictions. Establishment of a nonprofit organization is said to be more difficult in Japan than in any other developed country. As a result, the great majority of Japan's citizens' groups and volunteer organizations remain unauthorized groups called *nin'i dantai* (literally "arbitrarily established organizations").

These organizations have non-existent or weak structural and fiscal foundations and are not accredited. Their inability to accept government-commissioned work makes it very difficult for them to engage in cooperative social welfare projects with the government. This is also responsible for the short-lived and limited nature of Japan's volunteer activities. The Great Hanshin Earthquake of 1994 turned public attention to volunteer organizations. A number of volunteer organizations played an important relief role immediately after the earthquake hit, and were also instrumental in the revival and reconstruction of the devastated Kōbe and surrounding areas. Media attention made it widely known that these organizations had no official legal standing and had experienced difficulty continuing and developing their activities, and many people came to believe that governmental restrictions on volunteer organizations should be lifted. This led to the enactment of the Nonprofit Organization (NPO) Act in 1998 which makes it possible for nonprofit organizations to acquire the status of juridical persons – that is, to become incorporated, accredited nonprofit organizations. Members of welfare volunteer organizations and citizens' mutual aid organizations may now become eligible to accept central government-commissioned projects by incorporating and by procuring care insurance licensure as individuals.

With the NPO Act, Japan is one step closer to forming a new welfare services partnership between the public and private sectors. The recently enacted Public Long-Term Care Insurance Plan will help in defining the nature of that new relationship.

Public Long-Term Care Insurance

The welfare reform that began in the 1980s is epitomized by the Public Long-Term Care Insurance Plan (*Kaigo Hoken Hō*) which was introduced in 1997. Its chief characteristic is in its message: public long-term care insurance is not only for a small minority of impoverished people but rather something to be used for all people as they enter old age. In other words, utilizing long-term care services is not accepting charity; it is taking advantage of a privilege shared by all citizens. (See Chapter 4 by J. Campbell, this volume).

The Public Long-Term Care Insurance Plan is designed to provide care for the elderly via a new type of social insurance. It is important to note that the Plan provides the legal basis for the shift from a government-based welfare system to a more plural one which would include both private and nonprofit service providers. Political scholars Masaru Nishio (1975) and Wataru Ōmori (1974) have pointed out the significance of particular clauses contained in America's Community Action Program, part of the Economic Opportunity Act of 1964, which call for the "maximum feasible participation" from the community with regard to the planning, decision-making and implementation of community programs. In Japan, there had never been legal grounds for citizens' participation in social and community welfare programs. The establishment of the Public Long-Term Care Insurance Plan and the NPO

Act will not generate a sudden quantitative and qualitative increase in citizens' participation in social welfare programs, but it does provide the legal grounds for such participation.

Participatory welfare services

The grassroots community organizations that began providing home care services in the latter half of the 1980s instigated a movement within the Japanese government which has been dubbed the participatory welfare system. For example, local governments have developed *fukushi kōsha*, welfare-oriented public corporations. These organizations have begun government-initiated welfare service projects which closely resemble those of the grassroots community organizations. The government is responding to volunteer groups as indicated in documents published by the Central Social Welfare Advisory Committee, an advisory council to the Ministry of Health and Welfare.

In statements regarding its medium- to long-term plans for promoting volunteerism, the Committee expressed hope that more people (particularly housewives) will choose to take part in volunteer welfare services and thus help the nation meet the increased welfare needs generated by the rapid aging of society. At this point in time, the government's view on participatory welfare is not what the participation scholars of the 1970s had demanded, a system whereby citizens participate in the planning and decision-making processes of policy-making. Rather, it is a system whereby the citizens may provide manpower for welfare service providers and assist them in addressing the escalating and diversifying welfare needs of the community.[8] Noaki Tanaka (1998) has noted that although this government-led limited type of participation could be considered an example of citizens' participation, it is necessary to develop a home care service system which is led by the citizens themselves. These groups typically have no more than twenty members. Social welfare corporations and large welfare nonprofit organizations such as the Sawayaka Welfare Foundation and the Wonderful Aging Club (WAC) are now attempting to avoid this problem that the smaller community groups are experiencing by appealing to the Japanese people's historical sentiments regarding *tonari gumi*-related mutual aid – that is, Japan's traditional concept of volunteerism.

The welfare NPO – its establishment and future developments

Until now, the Japanese government has controlled the reform of the welfare system. However, it seems likely that citizens' participation in general and particularly citizens' participation in social welfare services will gradually become more prevalent. We must turn our attention to the direction that community welfare services will take after the Public Long-Term Care Insurance Plan and the NPO Act come into full effect. These laws will give private volunteer organizations official status and make it possible for them to work cooperatively with the government (Adachi, 1998). As many as one-third of the grassroots citizens' mutual aid groups may be transformed into nonprofit organizations for the provision of welfare services.[9]

Although there are still many problems with the long-term care insurance system that must be resolved,[10] when the Public Long-Term Care Insurance Plan is fully implemented, private welfare nonprofit organizations and corporations will for the first time be able to enter the home care service sector. As we have seen, this does not mean that citizens will be participating in decision-making. However, it does mean that private welfare nonprofit organizations will become integral elements in the community welfare providers system.[11]

Citizens' groups will have limited roles as community welfare providers initially; there is little doubt that in time they will take on more vital tasks such as care planning and needs assessment. Private volunteer organizations and welfare-oriented nonprofit organizations can help bridge the distance between the central government's welfare services and the welfare needs of the people. We may even see the growth of citizens' participation in areas previously tightly controlled by the government such as decision-making regarding the assessment of general welfare needs, evaluation of insurance-based welfare services, and policy decision-making.[12]

Japan's NPO Act is very different from its American counterpart. The Japanese Act has been established as a special law within the civil code. It seriously limits the activities of nonprofit organizations. Accredited organizations which obtain official NPO status are not eligible to receive tax benefits as they do in the US; the Japanese government has put off discussion of this issue to a later date. Accreditation by the government thus means only that the organization may accept public insurance funding and government-commissioned welfare projects. By contrast, if a volunteer group were to establish itself not as an NPO but as a social welfare corporation, it would be eligible for generous tax breaks. Unfortunately, in reality this option is not open to most private volunteer groups because it requires very stringent evaluation by the Ministry of Health and Welfare. In addition, social welfare corporation status requires that the corporation possess land or comparable fundamental assets.

Compared to social welfare corporations, organizations which become accredited NPOs through the NPO Act will have a much more difficult time financially due to the lack of tax considerations. However, the welfare NPO is capable of providing new, sophisticated social welfare services because it has the independence of a private organization and the pioneering spirit and flexibility of a volunteer organization. These services differ greatly from the government-affiliated welfare services in that they are more personal in nature and more precisely suit the welfare service needs of today's Japan. For this reason, there is little doubt that the welfare-oriented NPOs will change the face of community-based and home care services.

Japanese society is now changing dynamically as it grapples with the problems introduced by a decreasing child population and rapidly aging society.

Undoubtedly, the welfare reform will not come to a conclusion in its present form but will continue to develop and to be an important policy issue. Until recently, Japan's welfare reform has amounted to little more than government-led "regulated decentralization." Still, Japan's social welfare system is sure to move slowly toward a model in which the local rather than the central government will be in control. It is too early to tell whether or not the transfer of power will continue even further to a point where citizens' groups will be holding the reins. However, there is no doubt that the Japanese people have never been as ready as they are now to take on that challenge.

Notes

1 This paper is in part based upon academic discussions that were held under the auspices of the Japan Foundation US-Japan Center's Abe Fellowship program and in which I participated. I would like to thank my friend Tony Laszlo, Tokyo-based journalist, who did a splendid job in translating this paper from the original Japanese into English.
2 It is personal social services and social work, not economic social security, that are central to the day care center-based juvenile welfare services and the elderly welfare services of special nursing homes for the elderly.
3 During the heyday of the reformist local authorities in the 1960s and 1970s some local governments tried their hand at designing social welfare policy independent of the central government. Minobe Ryōkichi, a governor of Tokyo during this period, is one of them. His experiments resulted in a social welfare policy much more progressive than that of the central government.
4 Some scholars trace Japanese volunteerism back to Buddhist activities of the Nara Period (710–784). Others say the mutual aid activities of the *goningumi* policies (a system in which community members formed small groups to aid – and inform upon – each other) which began in the Tokugawa period (1603–1867) are the first examples of volunteer activities. However, the Buddhist activities should be classified as Buddhist missionary work rather than volunteerism. Likewise, the "volunteer groups" of Tokugawa were actually formal groups created by the Tokugawa government to facilitate tax collection. In fact, the area commissioners of the Taisho period were Japan's earliest welfare volunteers because they were the first to engage in social welfare work on a gratuitous basis.
5 Japan's traditional family system has recently undergone radical changes due to two factors. First, the move toward the nuclear family: it had been standard practice for children to live together with and care for their aging parents; these households are becoming increasingly rare. Second, the move toward smaller families: Japan has one of the lowest birthrates in the world. Japanese families, struggling to adjust to these shifts, also must cope with the new challenges brought on by Japan's rapidly aging society.
6 The National Social Welfare Council uses the following categorization: organizations managed by the social welfare council, government-involved organizations (welfare public corporations), citizens' mutual aid organizations, organizations managed by cooperative associations and workers' cooperatives. They have determined that there are certain problems with the term "citizens' participatory model" and have stated their preference for the term "citizens' mutual aid." See Tanaka (1998).
7 While a person engaged in home helper services does not need special credentials, those providing care services must take home helper training courses and obtain the required certification.
8 Okamoto (1987) was quick to bring attention to this problem and criticize it. Takegawa (1996) pointed out the fact that, as interest in participation ebbs among academics, participatory welfare services are being discussed more and more among those who are actually providing welfare services.

9   The exact number is still unclear; I am making this estimate based on interviews conducted with the leaders of the Sawayaka Welfare Foundation and the Long-Life Social and Cultural Association.
10 Furukawa (1996) has pointed out that when the medical and nursing professionals make decisions concerning accreditation of public long-term care insurance or the formulation of care plans, they effectively exclude the welfare professionals from the decision-making process. As a result, Furukawa says, the social aspects of long-term care, a point of great importance to social welfare scholars, is largely ignored (Furukawa 1996, 34). This is an example of the "medical model vs. living model" conflict that has concerned scholars for some time.
11 Organizations involved in community-based at-home welfare services (e.g. the Sawayaka Welfare Foundation, Long-Life Social and Cultural Association, etc.) have expressed great interest in the NPO Act and have actively promoted it. See Tanaka (1996).
12 Under these circumstances it is possible that citizens' participation in community welfare programs will not progress. However, if that is the case, the reason citizens' participation was not realized will be vigorously debated among social welfare scholars.

References

Adachi, K. (1993). *Jūmin sankagata zaitaku fukushi sābisu katsudō: Ninai te no ishiki* (The consciousness of volunteers who participate in home care services in Japan). *Gekkan Fukushi, 76*, November, 54–57.

Adachi, K. (1998). *Fukushi shakai ni okeru borantea katsudō to NPO* (Home care service volunteer activities and NPOs in Japan). In K. Aoi, A. Takahashi, and K. Shoji (Eds.), *Fukushi shakai, kazoku, shiminundō* (Welfare society, family and citizen's movements). Chiba-ken, Matsudo-shi: Azusayama Shuppansha.

Campbell, J. (1996). *Nihon seifu to kōreika shakai* (The Japanese government and the aging society). Tokyo: Chūō Hōki Shuppan.

Furukawa, K. (1995). *Shakai fukushi kaikaku* (Social welfare reform). Tokyo: Seishin Shobō.

Furukawa, K. (1996). *Kōteki kaigo hoken to fukushi manpawā mondai* (Public long term care insurance and lack of manpower in social welfare). *Jurist, 1094*, 32–41.

Furukawa, K. (1997). *Shakai fukushi no paradaimu tenkan* (Paradigm change in Japanese social welfare). Tokyo: Yūhikaku.

Hori, K. (1981). *Nihongata fukushi shakai ron* (The Japanese model of the welfare society). *Kikan Shakai Hoshō, 17*, 1, 37–50.

Ikegami, N., and Campbell, J. (1996). *Nihon no iryō* (The Japanese medical system). Tokyo: Chūō Kōronsha.

Ishida, T. (1983). *Kindai Nihon ni okeru 'shakai fukushi' kanren kannen no hensen* (The concept of 'social welfare' in modern Japan and its transformation). In Ishida T. (Ed.), *Kindai Nihon no seiji bunka to gengo shōchō* (Political culture and symbols of modern Japan). Tokyo: Tokyo Daigaku Shuppankai.

Ishida, T. (1984). *Nihon ni okeru fukushi kannen no tokushitsu* (The characteristics of the social welfare concept). In Tokyo Daigaku Shakai Kagaku Kenkyūjo (Ed.), *Fukushi Kokka 4* (Welfare States, 4). Tokyo: Tokyo Daigaku Shuppankai.

Maeda, D. (1990). *Chiiki fukushi no hattatsu* (The development of community welfare). In W. Nogami (Ed.), *Chiiki fukushi ron* (Community welfare). Tokyo: Aikawa Shobō.

Nishio, M. (1975). *Kenryoku to sanka* (Political power and participation). Tokyo: Tokyo Daigaku Shuppankai.

Okamoto, E. (1987). *Borantea katsudō no bunsuirei* (A crossroad of volunteer activities in Japan). In K. Oda, and I. Matsubara (Eds.), *Henkakuki no fukushi to borantea* (Social welfare and volunteers in a period of change). Tokyo: Minerva Shobō.

Ōmori, W. (1974). *Gendai gyōsei ni okeru 'jūmin sanka' no tenkai: 1960 nendai Amerika ni okeru 'katsudō jigyō' no dōnyū to henyō* (The development of citizens' participation in local administration: Introduction and transformation of community action programs in the 1960s in the US). In K. Taniuchi, B. Ari, Y. Ide, and M. Nishio (Eds.), *Gendai gyōsei to kanryōsei* (Modern administration and bureaucracy). Tokyo: Tokyo Daigaku Shuppankai.

Ōmori, W. (1989). *Shakai fukushi ni okeru shichōson no yakuwari* (The role of towns and villages in social welfare). *Shakai Fukushi Kenkyū, 46*, 10.

Ōmori, W. (1990). *Jichi gyōsei to jūmin no genki* (Citizens and self government of towns and villages). Tokyo: Ryōshō Fukyūkai.

Shindō, M. (1996). *Fukushi gyōsei to kanryūsei* (Welfare administration and bureaucracy). Tokyo: Iwanami Shoten.

Takegawa, S. (1996). *Shakai seisaku ni okeru sanka* (Citizens' participation in social policy). In Shakai Hoshō Kenkyūjo (Eds.), *Shakai fukushi ni okeru shimin sanka* (Citizens' participation in social welfare). Tokyo: Tokyo Daigaku Shuppankai.

Tanaka, N. (1996). *Shimin shakai no borantea* (Volunteers and civil society). Tokyo: Maruzen.

Tanaka, N. (1998). *Borantea no jidai: NPO ga shakai o kaeru* (The volunteer era: NPOs changing Japan). Tokyo: Iwanami Shoten.

10 The accountability dilemma

Providing voluntary care for the elderly in the US and Japan

Yuko Suda

Japan experienced a drastic change in social welfare and health care for the elderly in the 1980s. For years, almost all social and health services had been provided through the government, but the system was not flexible enough to respond to changing needs of seniors and their caregivers. In the 1980s, Japanese volunteers undertook the leadership to change the situation. They designed new social welfare and health care services with the goal of providing services of good quality, while retaining the role of advocate for seniors and their caregivers. The efforts of these volunteers have been boosted by a wide range of public support, especially after Japanese society recognized the contribution of volunteers in the turmoil of the Great Hanshin Earthquake. This led to the passage of the Nonprofit Organization (NPO) Law in the Diet. The process of establishing an NPO system in Japan is continuing as people gradually become aware of serious dilemmas and problems in Japanese voluntary activities. Some people are concerned that Japanese NPOs might be abused by the government to organize voluntary organizations for the purpose of implementing *Kaigo Hoken* (Long-Term Care Insurance). Other people are afraid that some for-profit organizations might use NPOs as channels to recruit seniors as customers of their businesses.

On the other hand, in the US, twenty years had passed since the independent sector for volunteer activities was established, based on the NPO system. Japanese scholars and policy makers saw the American voluntary sector as providing a wide range of social and health services while having a strong impact on the society through sophisticated advocatory activities. It was expected that we Japanese would have much to learn from the more experienced way that Americans organized volunteer activities to create a supportive social environment for seniors.

What I observed in the US, however, was that the American voluntary organizations were struggling for survival while they were suffering from the dilemmas and limitations stemming from the existing NPO system. The American NPOs were expected to be accomplishing visible achievements cost-effectively in a short space of time. The expectation seemed to increase the demand for professionalization or commercialization of their activities, which deprived lay citizens of opportunities to take leadership. In addition, the NPO system seemed to be helpless in resolving the unequal treatment suffered by low-income seniors.

Each country seems to have unique problems in its NPO activities stemming from the differences of its stage of development and of their social and cultural context. At the same time, some common issues are observed as well, which seems to suggest that there are some universal dilemmas which voluntary organizations must face when they try to function as established service providers. An accountability dilemma seems to be one of those universals and it is the focus of this study.

Discussions regarding accountability have just begun in recent years in the US and no consensus on the definition of the word has yet been established. In reviewing discussions by American scholars for this chapter, fifteen different definitions were identified, varying from information release on the organization's financial condition to the conscientiousness of an organization. In this chapter, the word "accountability" is used to mean how voluntary organizations fulfill expectations of those who are associated with the organization's activities.

Even within one organization, different kinds of accountabilities occur. Cooper (1996) charted accountabilities of a voluntary organization along with the order of relationship among the key actors and stakeholders of the activities (Figure 10.1) (Cooper, 1996). Within the organization, the board (administrators of the organization) is required to be accountable to the staff and volunteers who are associated with the agency. The board sets the goal which reflects on

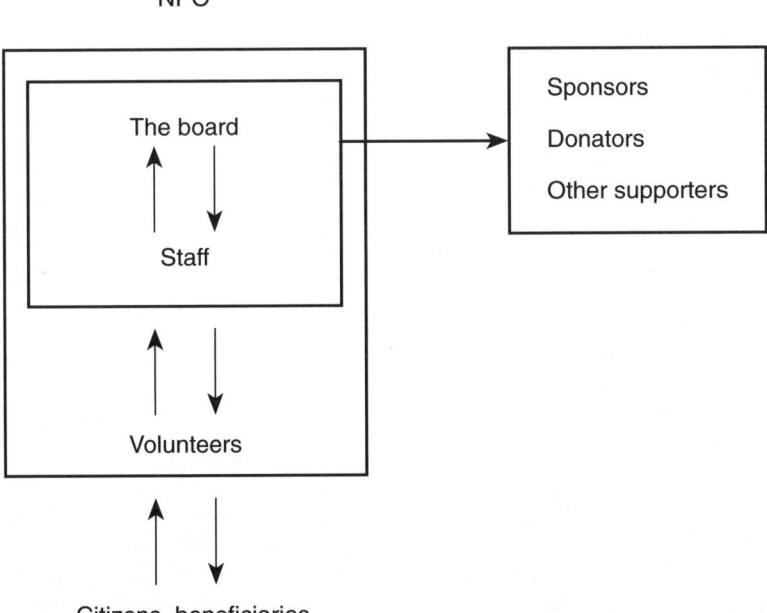

Figure 10.1 Accountability along with the order of relationships among the key actors and stakeholders

the mission statement and assures necessary resources to accomplish the goal. The staff owes accountability to the board to implement their plans. The board and the staff are held accountable to volunteers who are supporting their activities. The board and staff provide necessary support such as insurance coverage, supervisory services, and so forth. Volunteers are held accountable to the board and the staff to accomplish the assigned task. As to relationships outside, the organization is accountable to sponsors, donors, and other supporters to assure that those people's benevolence is reflected in daily operations. The organization is also held accountable to citizens and beneficiaries for the mission of serving the public and preserving the public trust.

When one organization is required to be accountable in multiple ways, the organization is under "multiple accountabilities". When the multiple accountabilities interfere with each other and the organization's daily operation is confused or disturbed because of it, the situation is understood as the problem of "the accountability dilemma."

In the activities of NPOs which provide human services such as in-home help services or meal services, the accountability dilemma stems from the two contradictory expectations from clients: one is to perform as a service provider, and another is to perform as an advocate for clients.

In order for an organization to function as a service provider, the organization would need to have such provisions as:

- standardized delivery mechanism to reduce costs
- well-structured job assignment
- routine operation of programs
- program evaluation
- often an exclusive contact with one funding source
- systems for speediness
- often hierarchical decision-making.

On the other hand, in order for an organization to function as an advocate, the organization would need characteristics such as:

- organizational independence
- closeness to the socially disadvantaged
- representative structures
- willingness to spend a large amount of time in consciousness-raising dialogue.

Obviously, it is extremely difficult to maintain these two contradictory characteristics within the same organization. Edwards and Hulme (1996) described such an unreasonable expectation of voluntary activities as the illusion of "the magic bullet."

In order to project the future role of service-providing NPOs in the care for the elderly, it seems to be important to examine how the accountability dilemma is experienced in service-providing NPOs, and how the NPOs are responding. In addition, special attentions needs to be paid to volunteers, since volunteers seem to share important roles in advocatory activities.

Based on these interests, this chapter focuses on American and Japanese NPOs which are providing in-home help services for the elderly, and:

- examines how the issue of the accountability dilemma is experienced in the NPOs
- compares how roles as service providers and as advocates are fulfilled, and what kind of roles volunteers undertake in the process
- draws implications for future roles of NPOs in the care of the elderly.

Methodology

Subjects

Two voluntary organizations which were providing in-home help services in the Tokyo metropolitan area in Japan participated in this study.

Organization A   Initiated by three housewives in the Tokyo metropolitan area. Fifty-five volunteers (including the three leaders) provided fifty seniors living in their community with a wide range of in-home help services such as home making, grocery shopping, respite care, cooking, and so forth.

Organization B   Initiated by a resident of the Tokyo metropolitan area. Fifty-two volunteers provided approximately sixty seniors living in their neighborhood with a wide range of in-home help services as in Organization A.

Two 501(c)(3) organizations (see Appendix 1 for an explanation of codes) which were providing in-home help services in St Louis, Missouri, provided the American data.

Table 10.1 Background information on organizations in study

	Japan				US	
Organization	A	B	I	II	Auxiliary I	Auxiliary II
Number of clients (approx.)	50	60	500	150	—	2,000
Number of employees	0	0	170	45	2	2
Number of volunteers (members)	55	52	15	1	124,600	300

Organization I Located on the north side of St Louis city, the organization was initiated eleven years ago by a resident who, at the time of this study, was the executive director of the organization. It provided approximately 500 seniors with four kinds of in-home help services: basic care (home making), personal care, advanced care, and respite care services, under contract with the Missouri State Division of Aging. Fifteen volunteers were associated with this organization.

Organization II The organization was initiated by a self-employed business person in the 1970s; since then the business person has been serving as the chair of the board. They were providing approximately 150 seniors with the same kinds of in-home help services as Organization I provided under contract with the Missouri State Division of Aging. One volunteer was associated with this organization.

Since very few volunteers were involved in service provisions of these 501(c)(3) American organizations, additional observations were conducted in the following organizations which were organizing volunteers to support seniors:

Auxiliary Organization I A 501(c)(3) organization, this organization was initiated by a retired school teacher as a grass-roots activity, which expanded nationwide. The activities of a branch of the organization located in a suburb of St Louis were observed. A wide range of services such as insurance programs, recreational programs, and educational programs were provided.

Auxiliary Organization II This 501(c)(3) organization on the north side of St Louis was initiated by a Protestant church. Its yearly budget was over $1 million, 84 percent of which was made up of the governmental funds. The total number of employees was over 500. They allocated two employees to a program for seniors, in which 300 seniors were organized as volunteers to provide case management services to over 2,000 frail seniors living in the St Louis area.

Data collection

The information on the Japanese organizations was collected through participant observation, interviews of the board, staff and key volunteers, and through questionnaire surveys. The study period was from August 1991 to April 1993 (Asakura, 1993; Asakura, 1994; Asakura *et al.*, 1992; NPO Study Group, 1992).

The information on the American organizations was collected through participant observation and interviews of the board, staff and volunteers. Since the number of volunteers involved in in-home help services was few, a questionnaire survey was not conducted. The study period was from August 1993 to December 1997.

Some definitions

Volunteer

In both the US and Japan, the word "volunteer" has different meanings depending on the context. Few differences were observed between the US and Japan in terms of the strictest definition of "volunteers." The definition in both countries would be those who voluntarily take part in activities for public benefits without receiving any kind of financial reward, except the reimbursement for the actual expenditures such as the cost for transportation.

However, the reality of "volunteers" is more diverse in both countries. For example, in Japan, some "volunteers" receive stipends from the organization they are associated with, and the amount per hour is sometimes higher than the minimum wage. Some Japanese "volunteer" groups even charge their clients for the services they provided. These volunteers are called *yūryō* (paid) volunteers, while some Japanese scholars argue that *yūryō* volunteers should not be considered as volunteers at all.

In the US, anyone who receives more than 100 dollars per year is technically considered an employee according to the regulation of the Internal Revenue Service (IRS). Interestingly, however, in some NPOs that I visited, some workers are called volunteers even if they are receiving more than the limit.

Theoretically, the boards of American voluntary organizations are also volunteers. According to the IRS's 501(c)(3) regulations, NPOs cannot be owned by individuals but only by the board. At least two-thirds of the board members must be volunteers who do not receive financial rewards. No qualifications are required to serve as a board member. However, the board members are not usually called volunteers. In addition, the boards of many American voluntary organizations are largely comprised of those who have professional backgrounds in areas related to the organization's activities, and some of them receive substantial financial reward for their services.

This chapter focuses on volunteers in voluntary in-home help service organizations for the elderly who are called volunteers regardless of whether or not the individual is paid. Board members are not included as "volunteers."

Nonprofit organization

In this study, the word "nonprofit organization" is used to describe an organization which is neither governmental nor for-profit, and provides social and health care services for the elderly based on private and voluntary activities among citizens. NPOs are also called voluntary organizations.

The definition of NPOs has involved wide-ranging discussion, including issues such as the legal system's regulation of corporate bodies, the tax system, and the notion of public benefits. In the United States, the system of 501(c)(3) organizations in the IRS code provides the standard definition of NPOs. Japan, on the other hand, just recently passed a bill which gave legal recognition to nonprofit organizations, but this law defined NPOs separately from existing nonprofit organizations operating for public benefits. (See Appendix 1.)

Results

Japanese Organizations A and B

The Japanese organizations did not require any qualification to become a volunteer. The majority of the volunteers were upper- to middle-class well-educated housewives in their forties. Organization A had 55 volunteers, 23 (69.7 percent) of whom were in their forties. Seventeen (51.5 percent) volunteers graduated from junior or four-year colleges, and 26 (78.8 percent) volunteers were homeowners. In Organization B, all volunteers were housewives, and 18 (34.6 percent) were in their forties and 17 (32.7 percent) were in their fifties. Thirteen (25.0 percent) had received professional training or licenses in the past such as nurses, licensed care workers, social work, teachers, and nutritionists.

These organizations were charging clients 650 yen ($5.00) per hour for the services they provided, which was the primary funding source for support of their activities. Organization A maintained their office space and hired part-time staff with support from a wide range of grant programs. The fee collected from clients was spent as payment to volunteers. When volunteers were asked about the average income from their activities, 85 percent of them did not answer. According to the leader of the organization, they are receiving "probably 3,000 to 4,000 yen a month." Organization B saved 150 out of the 650 yen for administrative expenditures, and the rest was paid to the volunteers as stipends. The average income that the volunteers received from their activities was 5,150 yen per month. Forty percent of the volunteers did not respond to this question.

In both organizations, volunteers were undertaking major roles in all tasks. A volunteers' meeting was held every week and serious discussions continued for hours. Important decisions such as the amount of fees, cases to be accepted or rejected, organization development plans, and so forth, were made by a vote of all volunteers including leaders who initiated the organizations. The care plan for each client was designed by volunteers who had professional backgrounds. The administrative work was primarily conducted by the leaders, but some roles such as accounting, publishing newsletters, answering telephone calls, and cleaning the office were shared among other volunteers taking turns. Organization A had a paid staff whose role was to assist the leader and other volunteers to carry out these tasks.

These organizations responded to complaints and problems among volunteers or from clients by discussing the issues together. Professional supervision was not available. Three (8.6 percent) volunteers in Organization A and four volunteers (12.1 percent) in Organization B felt that they did not have enough skills to respond to clients' needs. Compared to the study on in-home help service workers of nine organizations (three governmental, one voluntary, and five for-profit organizations) in Tokyo, in which 26 (4.9 percent) among 528 workers answered that they did not have enough skills to respond to clients' needs, volunteers in Organizations A and B seemed to have less confidence about their skills (Asakura,1993).

When asked why they were participating in these activities, Japanese volunteers expressed their decreasing trust in the government. Since the *Rōjin Fukushi Hō* (Law for the Welfare of the Elderly) was enacted, the government has been almost the only source through which the majority of Japanese seniors were able to access social welfare and health services. This Japanese social welfare system succeeded in responding to primary issues among seniors such as hunger and poverty, but it also created a government-dominant relationship over seniors and their caregivers. There were extremely limited opportunities for service users to choose services. The procedure was bureaucratic and differences in individual needs were not given sufficient consideration. Information was not fully disclosed and service users were granted limited opportunities to communicate with the service provider, the government. A leader of Organization B stated:

> I personally have difficulty trusting the government. I never felt that they listened to us, ordinary citizens. When I tried to talk to a director in City Hall, he was horrible. He almost said that we, ignorant housewives, could do nothing. He said, "Why don't you stay at home? Let us help you." Who do they think they are? And, you know, those who make laws and run the services for seniors are caught up with political games and bureaucracy. They don't know what's really going on among seniors and their caregivers. We need to let them know what we want and what we need.

Another motivation observed among Japanese volunteers was the serious concern about the security of the existing governmental service system. They realized that the existing system was struggling with the rapidly increasing number of older people. Volunteers feared that the existing system might not function in the future, and that they, who would be probably left after their husbands' deaths with insufficient pension coverage because of the lack of employment history, might not receive necessary support from anywhere when they reached retirement age. A volunteer in Organization A stated, "We need to work together to improve the social environment for the future. We cannot rely on our children or the government any more. We have to help ourselves." Another volunteer in Organization A stated,

> If the government cannot do everything, we have to find our own way. Aging is a normal part of life, and it seems to be more natural to me that we overcome difficulties of aging by helping each other, instead of buying services from companies or asking the government for help.

Leaders of the Japanese organizations emphasized the importance of mutual help. They stated that the ultimate goal was to create a social environment where anyone could feel comfortable to age, and that his goal should be accomplished by the collective effort of the service-providing volunteers and seniors who are receiving services.

Charging seniors a fee seemed to be a device to maintain this egalitarian relationship. Universal pension coverage made it possible for seniors to pay. The charge prevented them from being humiliated by the thought that they were relying on the mercy of others. Interestingly, both organizations were charging service-providing volunteers a membership fee as well. The leader of Organization B stated:

> Our goal is to create a community where everybody helps each other as a family. We, volunteers and seniors, are equal as members who work together to accomplish the goal. It makes more sense to me that every member makes the same contribution to support the activities.

Outreach was an important issue for the voluntary organizations' claim that they were the ally of seniors and their caregivers. The existing governmental system functioned on the basis of *shinsei shugi* (principle of application) in which services were not provided unless seniors claimed the need for services. On the other hand, Organizations A and B outreached to seniors in need. Organization B was especially aggressive in this effort, very often beyond differences of social and economic class. They visited seniors' houses which were so filthy that even professional social workers hesitated to visit, cleaned the dirtiest parts of the house, such as the toilet, and tried to establish rapport with their clients. They did not charge the clients regardless of the hard work until the clients agreed to join their activities as members. A volunteer commented:

> I am not doing all these tasks for the purpose of recruiting a new customer. I am doing this because I believe this senior needs help and he will feel much more comfortable once he accepts our help. I am trying to convince him to accept for his own benefit.

They were also actively reaching out to a wide range of residents in order to recruit younger volunteers. One time, they visited over 400 houses, but no new members were recruited. According to a leader, "Recent young wives are interested in pursuing either a career or personal comfort. They are not coming to take care of messy seniors for nothing."

Another struggle was in legitimating their activities in the society. Japan had operated with only two sectors: the government and the for-profit sector. Japanese volunteers appealed for a comprehensive legal system which would provide voluntary organizations with legal status and a wide range of support such as tax exemption. In the meantime, they tried to overcome the widely accepted negative assumptions about their activities, that volunteers and their activities were not dependable.

Organization B was trying to operate in a professional manner. Many volunteers responded to as many requests as possible from each client. Volunteers very often had to stay at clients' houses longer than scheduled, which made it difficult to assign more than one case to a volunteer a day. The leaders intended to manage volunteers' schedules professionally, and to provide care more efficiently. They invited a successful small business owner and learned marketing and financial management skills. The leaders proposed to members that they consider their relationships with clients as contractual relationships. By encouraging volunteers to be compliant with the exchanged contract, leaders tried to clarify the tasks to be accomplished and the hours to be spent for each visit. These efforts seemed to confuse some volunteers in Organization B. In a volunteers' meeting, one volunteer expressed a strong concern that the organization was too business oriented. On the other hand, a more business-minded volunteer complained that the performance of volunteers who were merely motivated by benevolence was too "amateur."

In a questionnaire survey, twenty-seven (81.8 percent) volunteers in Organization B stated that establishing their organization as a service provider through financial independence and gaining a certain legal status was necessary, two (6.1 percent) opposed the idea, and four (12.1 percent) did not answer. At the same time, twenty-nine (87.8 percent) volunteers answered that they should provide whatever care they could even if it was not part of the contract "because they were volunteers" (Asakura, 1993). One volunteer stated:

> Recently, the people in the office intervene a lot with the relationships between me and my clients. They tell me to report everything I do for my clients, and then, they tell me not to do so much for them. I am here to help seniors in their predicament. I am happy to do anything, as much as I can. I bought cakes the other day with my own money and ate them with one of my clients. What's wrong with that? But the people in the office didn't like it. They have to understand that we are all volunteers. They are not my boss or employer. They cannot tell me what to do.

Organization A was struggling with the conflict between its lobbying activities and its role as a service provider. Organization A, as a pioneer in a voluntary service provision, was actively involved in the movement to establish an NPO Law which would provide numerous voluntary organizations with legal status and a wide range of support. At the same time, they were developing their own business for the purpose of maintaining their financial independence as an organization. They initiated a for-profit corporate body, through which they exchanged contracts with other organizations to provide in-home help services. They also sold original products such as slippers and purses especially designed for seniors through the for-profit organization. The profit from these activities supported their in-home help service program. It seemed that the more they succeeded in their business and in-home help services, the more lobbying activities became a burden to some volunteers. One active volunteer complained:

> We are doing great. I made more than 20,000 yen ($150) last month by providing in-home help services. We can do more. We should concentrate on the service-providing part. Once people realize that we are good, the government will naturally start thinking about giving us a certain legal status and support. The leader is seldom in the office. She is busy with the NPO thing. She told us the other day to collect people's names who would support the legislation. I know it's important, but collecting people's names does not bring us any money. We cannot have a bankruptcy to make the law thing happen. I am afraid we might be missing a great opportunity for success by distracting ourselves with the political matter.

American Organizations I and II

American Organizations I and II were operating in-home help services under contract with the Missouri State Division of Aging. The care plan for each client was designed by the Division of Aging in detail, such as "sending a basic care worker two hours a day, three days a week, to clean the house and do errands." The role of in-home help service organizations was to implement the plan. Little autonomy was granted to each organization. The executive director of Organization I, who was also the founder of the organization, stated:

> One day they told us to stop sending our worker to an old lady's house. They said the lady could get around by herself and she did not need our help. But the lady had a stroke and her mind was not right. She could not cook, she could not clean the house, she even forgot to eat. I told them that. But they cut our services. We cannot send our workers for nothing. I feel sorry for the lady, very nice lady, but we can't help her.

Neither of the two organizations was marketing or outreaching to seniors in the community for recruitment of new clients. Referrals from the Division of Aging were the primary source of clients.

In both American organizations, basic and personal care workers constituted the majority of workers. According to the standard of the Division of Aging, in-home help service organizations were required to provide twenty hours of training to the basic and personal care workers. One hundred and sixty five out of 170 workers in Organization I, and 147 out of 150 workers in Organization II were basic or personal care workers who had completed the training and were working at the minimum wage. The majority of these workers had received a twelve year formal education. These workers were considered part-time workers, not volunteers, although the minimum wage was almost the same amount as the stipends Japanese volunteers were receiving.

The board of Organization I was comprised of two church priests in the community, three residents over 60 years old and a nurse who was a friend of the executive director. The board seemed to be inactive. The program was operated in accord with the complex regulation of the Division of Aging. As long as their contract continued, its financial condition was stable. Interactions with other organizations were not necessary. The executive director took strong leadership in daily program operations, and the role of the board was to approve the plans presented by the executive director.

Organization I seemed to maintain a volunteer spirit primarily because of the personality of the executive director. The executive director and founder stated:

> We have been here for eleven years. We are helping people, and we are doing very well. But we still have a lot of people on the street. I don't like to see people starving. I said to my girls [workers of the organization], "This is the time I need your help." I started a food pantry. We make money from in-home help services and spend that profit for the food pantry. I go anywhere to buy food, diapers, anything. My girls help me. No, they don't get paid. The girls help me as volunteers when I do the food pantry stuff.

Fifteen employees of Organization I were involved in the food pantry program as volunteers. One volunteer stated:

> I was a single mother living on welfare. I struggled. Every morning I woke up and thought, "How can I feed my babies ?" I came to this food pantry and Ms R [the executive director] told me I could get a job from her. I clean houses, cook, and do grocery shopping for sick old people. Ms R helped me get off welfare. That's why I decided to help her when she started this food pantry.

Although the volunteers were active based on their strong attachment to the executive director, few interactions among volunteers were observed. The volunteers usually did not see each other in the work of in-home help services, since they worked individually according to an assigned schedule. When they held a fashion show for the purpose of raising funds to support the food pantry, each volunteer came whenever convenient to her, accomplished the task assigned by the executive director, and left.

During the interview of the leader of Organization I, a telephone call came from a client. The client was complaining that the house chore worker had not shown up yet. When asked about the workers' compliance with working conditions such as working along with schedules and code of ethics, the leader sighed and said,

> Some workers are responsible and dependable, and others are not. Some girls are, ah, you know? The workers themselves have so many problems. [For example,] a son was sent to a jail, a husband hits her, somebody at home is sick, the worker does not have money to catch the bus to come to work. I tell them to hang in there. But some girls are not ready to work.

Organization II seemed to be solely focused on providing services cost-effectively. The chair of the board who initiated the organization stated,

> This business is really good. The government gives us about twelve dollars per hour. We just pay the minimum wage to workers, then half of the money from the government comes to us. Look. Now we have three computers, forty-five workers, one full-time and two part-time staff in the office. We will move to a new office soon. There are a lot of nonprofit organizations which close their business because of financial problems. I would suggest starting this business in order to save their organizations.

The chair of the board undertook major roles in program operation and organization management such as organizational development, future plans for the organization, supervising staff and care workers, designing and supervising workers' training, and so forth. The board was comprised of the chair of the board and representatives of seniors in the community. The representatives of seniors seemed to be highly admiring of the chair of the board. They did not raise questions or express opposition in the board meeting.

The only volunteer in Organization II was a retired accountant who was providing the bookkeeping service. He came to the office twice a week, worked for a few hours, and left. No interactions were observed between him and clients. He stated,

> After I retired, I found that I had a lot of free time. It was fun to hang around with my wife, to travel with my friends, but I sometimes got bored. The chair of the board of this organization is a friend of mine, and when he asked me to help his business, I thought it was pretty neat. I spend my time for something meaningful, and his business goes well. Everybody is happy.

It seemed that he had a good understanding of the organization to the extent that he needed as an accountant. However, he did not express any interest in in-home help services or social problems among clients beyond that.

American Auxiliary Organizations I and II

Auxiliary Organization I is a membership organization for seniors. Based on the good reputation that the organization operated for the benefit of seniors, members purchased a wide range of products from the organization such as insurance policies, mutual funds, mail-order pharmaceuticals, auto rentals, auto club memberships, major credit cards, and hotel discount packages. Major for-profit companies provided the products and services, and they paid the organization a percentage of their sales in return for the use of the organization's name and reputation. These programs were developed and operated by paid professional staff in the office. The role of members was to pay the membership fee and contact the office when they wanted to purchase products.

Many of the board members were professionals in marketing and other for-profit businesses, professionals of social and health services and other related areas. Some of the board members received a large financial reward for their contributions to the organization, which became a large scandal in 1993.

Events seemed to be almost the only occasion when members interacted with each other. When the Missouri Botanical Garden in St Louis offered free admission to senior citizens, members of Auxiliary Organization I volunteered to set up a booth and hand out information on its programs for the purpose of recruiting new members. One senior couple who were helping with the event came from a suburb of St Louis. The wife explained:

> The kids have gone, and they have their own lives. We are supporting ourselves and enjoying our retirement life. This organization gives us a lot of information. If you want to go to a show in Las Vegas, you can get a discount. You pay a little bit of a membership fee, and you save money. You can buy health insurance, car insurance, traveling package, anything, for a good price! I want people to know that if we get together, if we combine our resources, we can help each other.

In addition to selling products, this organization exerted influence on the policy-making process based on its vast network of members nationwide. It lobbied the government to increase the budget for social welfare and health services for seniors. Members participated in these lobbying activities by endorsing written petitions to the government or by sending donations to support the activities.

While maintaining a wide range of influence as a successful voluntary organization for seniors, Auxiliary Organization I was also exposed to serious criticisms. This organization was taxed on advertisement revenue from its magazine and on income from its money market funds and credit cards. But its pharmacy, auto club, and insurance profits were not taxed. For-profit organizations which were providing similar services to seniors claimed that they were put under "unfair competition." They questioned why such organizations as Auxiliary Organization I should be exempt from taxes when virtually identical companies not affiliated with "the nonprofit giant" must pay taxes to provide the same services. It was also pointed out that the products Auxiliary Organization I was selling were inferior to other organizations' products. A newspaper article criticized such activities by nonprofit organizations:

> The commercialization of nonprofit activities is a disturbing trend, because it squanders the organization's most valuable asset, the public trust. In the long run, the nonprofit sector is jeopardized. The mere perception that a charity is hocking its halo – its good name – for profit will scare donors away. They won't contribute to a charity that prefers to sell its services instead.
>
> (DiLorenzo, 1996)

Auxiliary Organization II operated over twenty programs which were supervised by five program directors who had doctoral or master's degrees in the area of social work. The board was comprised of representatives of residents, for-profit organizations in the neighborhood and some scholars. The board was not active. It seemed almost impossible for board members, who came to the organization only once a month for a couple of hours, to comprehend all of the issues related to the wide range of activities of the organization.

One of the programs of Auxiliary Organization II was to provide volunteer case management services for seniors. The program office was located in an economically struggling neighborhood. Two staff members were assigned to the program operation. Seniors who were financially struggling could not afford services on the market. These seniors also tended to be left out of useful information networks. Many of them did not have telephones at home, could not afford newspapers, and did not have access to "the information highway." Auxiliary Organization II organized relatively healthy and active seniors in the community and trained them to function as volunteer case managers for the poor and frail seniors. The role of the volunteer case managers was to distribute useful information to their members and to make referrals to existing community resources when necessary. One volunteer case manager stated:

> I am helping three seniors. One is a lady down the street, and the other two are a couple. I feel so sorry for that lady. Her son is living with her but he is not working. When I visit her, she always cries and says, "Oh, I am so happy that you came. I am sitting alone here all day long. Nobody visits me. Nobody." I have good heath. I can get around still. I am blessed, so I want to help somebody like her.

Interactions among volunteer case managers seemed to be few. Most of them came to the monthly meeting individually, received the training, and left as soon as the meeting was over.

This program was struggling with a decreasing number of participants. Its support from the state government was cut and the stipends provided to volunteer case managers stopped. The director explained that the program itself did not provide any substantial services but tried to utilize the existing community resources to the maximum, and it was extremely difficult to prove the positive outcome of such activities. The program was eleven years old and volunteer case managers who used to be active had become frail. New members were seldom added and participants at monthly meetings were decreasing, which made it difficult for the staff to update the information on frail seniors assigned to volunteer case managers. It was said publicly that 300 volunteer case managers were assigned to 2,000 frail seniors in the St Louis area. However, when I randomly sampled fifty volunteer case managers from the name list, six (12.0 percent) had moved and twenty-four (48.0 percent) were not active. As to the frail seniors, among the 100 who were randomly sampled, sixty-four (64.0 percent) had died or moved, twenty-four (24.0 percent) were still living in the community but not in touch with the volunteer case managers, and only twelve (12.0 percent) were receiving volunteer case management services in the way that the program was designed.

Implications for the future

Experiences of the accountability dilemma

Japanese voluntary organizations observed in this study seemed to consider the accountability dilemma as a meaningful challenge stemming from the limitation of existing systems. This motivated them to seek a new system which would enable them to fulfill both roles at the same time, the role of service providers and the role of advocates for seniors and their caregivers. They approached the challenge by professionalizing the organization's management, by introducing the concept of "contract" to relationships with their clients, and by exploring opportunities to generate surplus for the purpose of securing financial stability. At the same time, they tried to strengthen their function as advocates by introducing the decision-making system involving all volunteers related to their activities, or by charging a membership fee to both clients and service-providing volunteers. These efforts, however, were creating identity confusion among volunteers. For example, it was observed that some volunteers considered their service-providing activities as "business", while other volunteers defined themselves as "volunteers" based on sympathy toward clients. A relatively high number of volunteers expressed anxiety about their skills as in-home help workers. In addition, the majority of them hesitated to report the amount of financial reward from their service-providing activities while none of them complained about the amount. These facts seemed to suggest that many Japanese volunteers devoted themselves to in-home help services with stoic attitudes while uncertain whether they were sufficiently qualified as professional workers. These volunteers' reluctance to determine their identity as one or the other seemed to be the reflection of the accountability dilemma that the Japanese organizations were experiencing.

In the US, on the other hand, the dilemma of fulfilling two different accountabilities seemed to be resolved by assigning different roles to different organizations. In-home help service organizations seemed to concentrate on the role of service provider, while others were functioning as advocatory organizations without providing instrumental services. The agony of the accountability dilemma as was observed in the Japanese organizations was not observed inside the American organizations, which suggests a distinct difference between the NPO activities of the two countries.

Cost-effectiveness as service providers and the role of volunteers

The belief seemed to be widely shared both in the US and in Japan that providing human services through NPOs was more cost-effective than governmental services. However, several studies on NGOs have reported that voluntary grassroots activities were not necessarily cost-effective compared to governmental programs (Edwards and Hulme,1996). A simulated application of game theory also showed that the cost performance of American voluntary service-providing organizations would not be improved in the current system where voluntary service-providing organizations operated as subcontractors of the government (Gates and Hill, 1995). The observations in this study also suggest the complexity of the issue.

It was commonly observed both in the US and Japan that service-providing volunteers or in-home help workers were receiving extremely small financial rewards. As mentioned before, many Japanese volunteers hesitated to be considered professional workers and did not expect to be paid as such. Many of them spent hours providing services without requesting payment from their organizations. The total financial reward that most of the Japanese volunteers were receiving was not enough to support themselves. In the US, volunteers were not directly involved in the service delivery process. NPOs achieved low-cost service delivery by hiring unskilled workers at the minimum wage, which also did not provide enough financial support to lead a decent life. Considering the low morale and the insufficient skills of the workers, American voluntary organizations seemed to sacrifice the quality of care for the sake of the organization's financial performance. These facts suggest that even if existing NPOs both in the US and in Japan were achieving low-cost performance, it did not necessarily serve as the proof of NPOs' good performance; rather it might just suggest the unique working conditions of their volunteers or workers.

Some dilemmas were observed among NPOs in terms of efficiency as well. The Japanese NPOs were providing services by organizing volunteers. However, organizing volunteers was energy and time consuming. Each volunteer had different schedule and working condition. Coordinating volunteers and clients' needs required elaborate work, and even then some volunteers would cancel appointments with their clients at the last minute. In addition, as was observed in Organization B, volunteers did not necessarily comply with the policies of leaders because of their identities as "volunteers." It seemed to be extremely difficult for an organization to achieve efficient service delivery in such a situation. On the other hand, in the US, in addition to the low morale observed among not a few workers, many other workers were those who had difficulties in obtaining other jobs because of their insufficient social skills. These facts suggest the difficulty for an organization to provide services efficiently while maintaining a certain quality in services.

Performance as advocate and the role of volunteers

The word "advocate" seemed to have different implications in the voluntary activities of the US and Japan. "Advocate" in Japan meant that volunteers, most of whom were in their middle age, interceded on behalf of seniors. On the other hand, in the US, advocatory activities were performed by seniors themselves who claimed or defended their interests through voluntary activities such as with Auxiliary Organizations I and II. The similarity of the advocacy activities of the two countries was that both of their activities seemed to stand upon traditional values, but the values themselves were challenged because of multiple changes in society.

Japanese voluntary in-home help service organizations were trying to encourage volunteers' participation by emphasizing "mutual help." The "mutual help" implied an intergenerational network of reciprocity. Japanese volunteers reinterpreted the service – provider/service-receiver relationship as an egalitarian one in which members of the younger generation and seniors helped each other toward the ultimate goal of creating a community which would function like a family. These voluntary organizations' activities were considered innovative, yet their assumption seemed to be based on the very traditional notion of "obligation" and "taking turns" in intergenerational relationships. The difference was that they extended the traditional notion which was applied among family members to the larger community.

Hashimoto (1996) stated that such a Japanese intergenerational relationship was supported by their concept of fairness. Younger family members undertook the role of taking care of old parents, which was "fair" since the old parents had taken care of their old parents when they were younger. Younger family members would expect their children to support them when they became old and frail. According to Hashimoto, the key to continue this intergenerational fairness game depended on whether the younger generation agreed to join the cycle of "taking turns," creating the uncertainty among Japanese seniors about their aging process.

The NPO-based support system in Japan seemed to hold the same "uncertainty" as long as they stood upon the traditional value of intergenerational fairness. As a result of multiple changes in the Japanese society, younger generations have been resigning from or unable to participate in the intergenerational fairness game at the family level. Would it be possible for Japanese NPOs to attract younger generations against the trend? The example of Organization B, which was struggling to recruit younger volunteers, suggests that Japanese NPOs are seriously challenged in integrating younger generations into their activities.

Similarly, the US seemed to be facing the challenge of the generation gap. In the American in-home help service organizations observed in this study, a very limited number of volunteers were associated with the in-home service organizations. Even when there were volunteers, they were not directly involved in service provision and they had no influence on the decision-making process of the organization. Decreased involvement of volunteers in service providing NPOs was, in fact, a large trend. A survey on the distribution of volunteers reported that fewer than 10 percent participated in the activities of 501(c)(3) organizations which were providing human services (Hodgkinson *et al.*, 1994).

In addition to the low involvement of volunteers, there seemed to be very little room for service-providing NPOs to represent the interest of their clients.

Their flexibility is limited because of their contracts with the government. The episode in which Organization I was required to terminate services serves as a good illustration that clients' needs were sometimes ignored because of the system. In addition, as Organization II showed, some organizations consider in-home help services as a great business opportunity. They exhibited no interest in advocacy for the elderly. These facts suggest that American service-providing NPOs were not necessarily actively involved in the role of advocate.

In the advocatory organizations observed in this study, seniors who were participating in the activities seemed to function more as "consumers" than "advocates." For example, members of Auxiliary Organization I seemed to be more motivated by the benefit they received from the organization, than in contributing to the common goal. The situation of Auxiliary Organization II suggests other difficulties advocatory organizations face, such as the existing evaluation and funding systems which were not necessarily supportive of advocatory activities, and the increasing frailty among senior members and the difficulty of recruiting new members.

A decrease in volunteers and citizens' involvement in communities seemed to be a general trend in the US. Putnam (1996) states, "Americans today are significantly less engaged with their communities than was true a generation ago." By examining the data of the past sixty years, Putnam found that the reason lay in "the generation effect." He indicated that those who were born in 1930s created "Civic America" through active involvement in social issues, but that lifestyle and values were not passed on to later generations.

The difficulties of advocatory activities observed among American NPOs in this study might be a reflection of such a general trend in the US. In the past twenty years, American NPOs have grown in number, organization size, and size of budget, but not in the number of volunteers. The existing American NPOs, like their newer Japanese counterparts, face the challenge of transforming themselves to fit a changing society.

Challenges for the future: establishing a philosophy of "care" and "the role of citizens"

In the Japanese NPOs observed in this study, there seemed to be two contradictory forces: one to pursue cost-effectiveness and the other to interfere with the effort for cost-effectiveness. The value which "interferes with the effort for cost-effectiveness" was not clearly defined, but it seemed to be vaguely suggested in some volunteers' statements such as, "Because we are volunteers."

This contradiction was not identified among the American NPOs observed in this study. However, considering that the system of delivering services through NPOs was chosen at the beginning of this century as an alternative to establishing a welfare state, it seemed obvious that the American NPO system incorporates multiple values as well. That decision is based on the social and cultural assumptions among American people, such as the belief in social Darwinism, discomfort with centralizing authority and resources, and the reluctance of the government to intervene in the "natural" social process of survival in the guise of social welfare (Hall 1992). Obviously, some philosophical factors were involved in the decision which laid the seed of multiple accountabilities.

The existence of multiple values in both the US and Japanese NPO activities suggest the complexity of "care" and "voluntary activities of citizens." "Care" should be more than "delivering services," and "voluntary activities of citizens" should be different from other organized activities such as for-profit or governmental activities. Such complexity seems to be experienced more as a stress than of the fruitfulness of human life, as the necessity to support an older population with the institutionalized system has increased, and from which complexity the issue of the accountability dilemma seems to be stemming. In other words, the issue of the accountability dilemma in our modern society seems to be the reflection of the value conflict between the society's needs and the reality of an individual's human life.

As our societies change, the meaning of "care" and the role of citizens must change as well. The value conflicts mentioned above seem to be a necessary part of the process. One of the greatest challenges is how voluntary activities can find a way to establish common ground for older and younger generations to collaborate with each other. Where value conflicts occur, a high level of energy is involved. When the different generations find channels to communicate with one another, the value conflict can serve as an opportunity to create a new meaning of "care" and a new definition of the role of citizens.

It is difficult to predict the future. What seems certain is that the solution for the accountability dilemma does not lie in technical matters such as how to manage an NPO or whether volunteers should or should not be paid. Rather, the accountability dilemma should be understood as part of a process of creating an alternative culture of "care" and the role of citizens in contemporary society.

Appendix 1: background information on nonprofit organizations

The US

In the US, the law generally provides for two types of organizations, other than governmental entities – the for-profit organization and the nonprofit organization. In order to receive a legal status as a nonprofit organization, the organization needs to be registered as such at the state level. A wide range of nonprofit activities are provided with tax exemption benefits by the federal tax law. There are 29 codes to sort tax-exempt activities: 501(c)(1) – 501(c)(25), 501(d), 501(e), 501(f) and 521.

Literally speaking, all nonprofit organizations should comprise the nonprofit sector, regardless of whether they have the tax-exemption benefits. However, the term is used, in many occasions, only for 501(c)(3) and 501(c)(4) activities. The nonprofit sector is also termed the "independent sector," "philanthropic sector," "private sector," "third sector," and "voluntary sector" (Hopkins, 1994; Hodgkinson et al., 1996).

Table 10.2 Activities of 501(c)(3) organizations, US

1	The relief of poverty
2	The advancement of religion
3	The advancement of education
4	The advancement of science
5	Lessening of the burdens of government
6	Community beautification and maintenance
7	The promotion of health
8	The promotion of social welfare
9	The promotion of the arts
10	The promotion of environmental conservancy
11	The promotion of patriotism
12	The promotion, advancement, and sponsorship of recreational and amateur exchanges
13	Care of orphans
14	The facilitating of student and cultural exchanges
15	Maintenance of public confidence in the legal system

The 501(c)(3) organizations are charitable institutions (Table 10.2). Nonprofit organizations which provide social welfare and health care services for the elderly are usually categorized under this code. They are the only group of tax-exempt organizations that may receive tax-deductible contributions from individuals and corporations. Charitable organizations may not be owned by individuals or exist for the purposes of making a profit. They may not collect taxes to implement programs as in government, and excess revenues may not be distributed to individual owners as in business organizations. Charitable organizations are also limited in their ability to lobby for social or legislative changes.

The law defines 501(c)(4) organizations as social welfare organizations which primarily work for public benefit and but have no restrictions on the amount of lobbying in which their organizations can engage. Because of their freedom to lobby, they may not receive contributions that are tax-deductible.

Japan

Japan does not have other sectors besides the government sector and the for-profit sector. There exist nonprofit activities for public benefit, but they are regulated by different laws depending on their activity areas. They do not comprise an independent sector as does the American nonprofit sector. For example, private schools operate under the regulation of the *Shiritsu Gakkō* (Private Schools) Law, private social service agencies operate under the *Shakai Fukushi Jigyō* (Social Services) Law, religious organizations fall under the *Shūkyō Hōjin* (Religious Corporation) Law, and health and medical service organizations are provided with a special legal status of *Iryō Hōjin* (Corporation for Health and Medical Services). Most other nonprofit activities for public benefit are regulated by the *Kōeki Hōjin* (Organizations for Public Benefits) Law.

The primary problems of this existing system are as follows.

First, the fact that Japanese nonprofit corporations are regulated by different laws decreases the flexibility of their activities. When the Great Hanshin (Kobe) Earthquake occurred in 1995, many existing nonprofit organizations were not able to provide support because of restrictions from governmental regulations. For example, a nonprofit corporation for international volunteer exchange was not allowed to join the rescue activities for the victims because the purpose of their activities was international, not domestic.

Second, a large endowment (generally more than $1 million) is required to receive the legal status of nonprofit corporation. Many small- to medium-sized voluntary organizations are not able to afford this. The Nonprofit Organization (NPO) Law which passed the Diet in 1998 does not require such an endowment. In addition, the law seems to provide more flexibility to the activities of each organization. However, the law does not provide any tax benefits. The implicit purpose of the law may be related to *Kaigo Hoken* (Long-Term Care Insurance) which passed the Diet in 1997, which will increase greatly the demand for in-home helpers. Under the NPO Law, small to medium voluntary groups will be able to provide social and health care to the elderly under contract with the government and ensure a sufficient supply of care workers.

Without tax benefits, the NPO Law was not appealing to other voluntary organizations not related to health and social care for the elderly, such as organizations for cultural activities, environmental issues, and so forth. Many of them had been seeking legal status, but it appears unlikely that Japanese NPO status can bring any benefits to such groups.

References

Asakura (Suda), Y. (1993). Fukushi seikyō katsudō no genjō to kadai: Shimin shutai ni yoru kōreisha fukushi iryō shisutemu no kanōsei ni kansuru kenkyū (A study on the possibility of voluntary organizations as social and health service providers: Challenges of co-op movements in social services, The Co-op Institute Bulletin). In Seikyō Sōgō Kenkyūjo (Ed.), *Seikatsu kyōdō kumiai kenkyū hōkoku ronbun shū* (Compilation of research reports of the Association of Co-ops) (pp. 5–39). Tokyo: The Co-op Institute.

Asakura (Suda), Y. (1994). Home help services (in-home help service providers). In I. Takagi. and E. Horikoshi (Eds.), *Seikatsu o yutakanisuru rōdō no hakken* (The work to increase the quality of life: Public services and workers) (pp. 235-255). Tokyo: Dai-ichi Shorin.

Asakura (Suda), Y., Inuzuka, H., Suzuki, K., Seto, M., Hagiwara, N., Yumoto, H., and Watanabe, G. (1992). *Jiritsu to kyōsei wo mezashite: Kusa no ne katsudō no kadai to tenbō* (Toward independence and collaboration: The future of the grassroots movement in Japan). Tokyo: Toyota Foundation

Cooper, T. (1996). *The responsible administrator: An approach to ethics for the administrative role*. San Francisco: Jossey-Bass.

DiLorenzo, T. (1996, August 17). Hocking the halo: Are America's charities for sale? *The Washington Times*.

Edwards, M., and Hulme, D. (1996). *Beyond the magic bullet: NGO performance and accountability in the post-Cold War world*. West Hartford, CT: Kumarian Press.

Gates, S., and Hill, J. (1995). Democratic accountability and governmental innovation in the use of nonprofit organizations. *Policy Studies Review, 14*, 1–2.

Hall, P., (1992). *Inventing the nonprofit sector*. Boston: The Johns Hopkins University Press.

Hashimoto, A. (1996). *The gift of generations: Japanese and American perspectives on aging and the social contract*. New York: Cambridge University Press.

Hodgkinson,V., Weizman, M., and the Gallup Organization, Inc. (1994). *Giving and volunteering in the United States*. Washington DC: Independent Sector.

Hodgkinson, V., Weizman, M., Abrahams, J., Crutchfield, E., and Stevenson, D. (1996). *Nonprofit almanac: 1996–1997*. San Francisco: Jossey-Bass.

Hopkins, B.R. (1994) *Nonprofit law dictionary*. New York: John Wiley & sons, Inc.

NPO Study Group (NPO Kenkyu-kai: Awano, S., Mashiko, D., Asakura [Suda], Y., Murakami, Y., Hayasaka, S., Yaginuma, N., Komatsu, K., Kim, A., and Nishi, Y.). (1992). *Shimin katsudō ga sodatsu shakai kankyō o tsukuru tame no chōsa* (The social system to support voluntary activities). Nara, Japan: Networking Kenkyūjo (Networking Institute).

Putnam, T. (1996). The strange disappearance of civic America. *The American Prospect*, Winter, 34–48.

Part IV
Coordinating and caring
Family caregivers

11 Variations in family caregiving in Japan and the US

Ruth Campbell and Berit Ingersoll-Dayton

In Japan and the US, as in most countries, the family is the main provider of care for the elderly (Maeda and Nakatani, 1992). However, the concept of family care may be interpreted differently in each country. What is meant by family? Which family members provide care? What are the expectations of family members with respect to caregiving? Answers to these questions vary according to cultural background and personal history.

If the family is indeed the primary source of care for the elderly, it follows that government policy should be directed to support and supplement the family's efforts at care. Determining what is meant by family, what is meant by caregiving, and who should provide care seems vital to successful policy. Moen and Forest (1995, p. 82) encourage policy makers to examine "families and the lives of their members in terms of stability and change over time and across generations, as well as within their particular social and historical contexts." Understanding the varying expectations for family caregiving is a crucial ingredient in the development of policies and services that are culturally relevant. In this chapter, we will explore variations in living arrangements and perceptions of caregiving among Japanese and Americans.

Previous research

An examination of existing research on this topic suggests that Japanese and Americans have different views of what is meant by family caregiving, which family members provide care, and differing attitudes and expectations of the roles of family members in giving care. Japanese tend to equate family caregiving with living together in the same household while Americans are more likely to give care to a parent living separately. In the US, only 13 percent of men and women over age 65 live with relatives while 53 percent of elderly Japanese are living with their children (American Association of Retired Persons, 1997; Kōseishō, 1997). In fact, census reports in Japan categorize the elderly living with their spouse as elderly "living alone," but similar reports in the US view couples-only households as elderly "living with family." Japanese often express surprise when told that Americans also are the primary support for their elderly parents since they know that elderly Americans are much less likely to be living with their children. Thus, when using the term "family," Japanese and Americans may be talking about different concepts of care.

In addition, there are differences in relation to *who* is expected to be the care provider. In Japan, daughters-in-law are more involved in caring for elders whereas in the US, daughters are more likely to provide care (Brubaker and Brubaker, 1992; Ikegami and Yamada, 1996). The tensions in these individual roles and how they relate to other family members are quite different in both countries and the meaning attached to family care stems from the cultural perceptions given to these respective family roles. In the US, the initial research (Brody, 1990) on caregiving focused primarily on daughters, "the sandwich generation," even though spouses provide much of the care to the elderly and over longer periods of time. In Japan, the *yome* (daughter-in-law), usually the wife of the eldest son, is frequently the symbol of caregiving. Home helpers, for example, are said to be in the role of the *yome* and policy makers assert they do not intend to replace the *yome* with public services. However, the proportion of daughters-in-law providing care to the elderly has been decreasing, while that of daughters, although still considerably lower than daughters-in-law, has been increasing. In both countries, spouses, if available, are the preferred caregivers. Given that women are more likely to outlive their husbands, for elderly males the wife is usually the major caregiver (Sodei, 1998).

There is also evidence from existing research indicating that Japanese and Americans have different attitudes about caring for the elderly. For example, based upon survey data, Japanese often report more negative feelings than Americans about the current and future state of family care for the elderly. In a US-Japan study of three generations of women, the Japanese were less likely than the Americans to think that old people could depend on their grown children, that adult children should be expected to help and stay in contact with their parents, and that help should be forthcoming from grandchildren as well (Campbell and Brody, 1985). Another cross-cultural study compared people over age 60 in Japan and the US as well as several other European and Asian countries. Surprisingly, the Japanese felt more uneasy about "the children not caring about me," than did the Americans. Only 24 percent of Japanese *never* felt uneasy about their children caring about them as compared to 74 percent of Americans (Policy Office for the Aged, 1991).

Part of the explanation for these differences in attitudes can be attributed to differing concepts of security. Hashimoto (1996) talks about the sense of security as being central to expectations for support in old age. She sees this sense of security conceptualized differently in Japan and America. Japanese prefer a "protective" approach focused on care provided by children because it promotes a sense of certainty. Americans equate security with the ability to maintain autonomy and choose from multiple options, what she calls the "contingency" approach. Hashimoto states:

> For the Japanese, the open-endedness of the American practice does not create a sense of security, because it promotes uncertainty; by the same

token, the predictability of the Japanese practice does not foster a sense of security for the Americans, because it offers no choices.

(Hashimoto 1996, p. 152)

Elderly Japanese may be less certain about the care they hope to receive because their expectations rest on plans which they fear their children will not fulfill. Americans expect less and tend to rely on their own ability to cope with whatever occurs.

Finally, the expectations of family members about the nature of the caregiving role may be different. Japanese caregivers tend to put a greater emphasis on "physical comfort, the avoidance of conflict in providing care and the totality of the caregiving experience" (Long, 1996, p.161). Although the stigma of nursing home care is present in the two countries, it is probably stronger in Japan where daughters-in-law frequently feel pressure from other family members to avoid institutionalization and continue, despite hardships, to care for their in-laws at home. About 6 percent of the over-65 population in both countries are in institutions, but the type of institutions they are in reveals the stigma of placement in a nursing home. Japanese are more likely to prefer long-term hospitals, even though there are often eight beds in a room, because they are part of the medical system. Patients can be admitted in a "normal" way as anyone ill might be and then the stay can be extended almost imperceptibly into long-term care.

Hospitals are also more numerous and easier to enter than nursing homes. In nursing homes, admission must be approved by the local welfare office, engendering a feeling of shame for middle-class Japanese who historically considered welfare services only for the poor. There are often long waiting lists for nursing home admission, especially in urban areas. Three quarters of the population 65 years and older who are institutionalized in Japan are in hospitals (Ikegami and Yamada, 1996). In contrast, in the United States, 5.5 percent of those 65 and over are in nursing homes and a negligible 0.1 percent in long-term general and special hospitals (US Bureau of the Census, 1992).

Changes in the caregiving arena may be imminent in both countries. In Japan, the new Long-Term Care Insurance Act, *Kaigo Hoken Hō*, passed in November 1997 to be implemented in the year 2000, represents an attempt to help all families, regardless of composition or living arrangements. This long-term care insurance system represents a major change from the past where community services were largely designated for specific groups such as those living alone and those who were bedridden. Often, working women who sought help for their parents or in-laws who were living with them were told to quit their jobs and take care of their parents. Home help was reserved for those living apart from their children (Campbell, 1998).

In America, the movement by states towards Medicaid "waivers," which allow payment for community services at a somewhat lower level than Medicaid payments to a nursing home, wins approval from older people who prefer to stay in their own home and from politicians who want to save costs. At the same time the average length of stay for older people in hospitals is slightly over a week, a decrease of 6.8 days since 1968 and 3.3 days since 1980 (American Association of Retired Persons, 1997). Elderly people in need of care can now stay in the community longer but the strain on the family to provide assistance has also increased (Aneshensel *et al.*, 1995).

With economic pressures on both the medical care system and the long-term care system as well as longer life expectation, anxiety about who will provide care will continue to be felt by family members and the elderly themselves. It is important, therefore, to consider the way cultural patterns affect how family members perceive their roles and deliver care to their elderly relatives.

Older couples' experience with caregiving

To explore further the meanings given to family care in both countries and their potential impact on policy, we analyzed the narratives of older American and Japanese couples who spoke to interviewers about their marriages and family relationships. The interviewers encouraged the couples to discuss their own views of family relationships by providing only minimal guides for these narratives. This study is described in greater detail in previous articles (Ingersoll-Dayton *et al.*, 1996; Ingersoll-Dayton, Campbell, and Mattson, 1998).

A total of twenty-four couples were interviewed. The eleven Japanese couples lived in a large city in Japan and the thirteen American couples lived in a small Midwestern city. The couples were purposively selected to obtain variability in relation to age, race (for the Americans), health and socioeconomic status. The Japanese couples (ranging in age from 54 to 77) were younger than the American couples (ages 62 to 89), mirroring the differences in the elderly populations in the two countries in the early nineties. The Americans averaged fourteen years of education and the Japanese averaged twelve years. The major cultural variations were reflected in the fact that most of the Japanese marriages had been arranged and the Japanese women were less likely to have worked outside the home than were the American women.

Though not asked directly about their concept of family caregiving, the couples spoke about the various stages of their marriages, encompassing care of parents, children, friends and extended family. In this chapter, we will focus on three topics that were illuminated by our discussions with these older married couples: current living arrangements and expectations of care, variations in the nature of caregiving, and caring for extended family and non-relatives. We will provide illustrations from the couples' narratives but will change their names and other identifying information to maintain confidentiality.

Current living arrangements and expectations of care

Although we usually think of Americans as having more options than Japanese in terms of where and with whom they live, a careful examination of our interview data shows a variety of living arrangements among the Japanese couples and more homogeneity among the American couples. At the time of the interview, all of the Americans lived only with their spouses in their own homes or rented apartments. Most of them had at least one child living within an hour's distance. One couple had moved to live near their daughter, two blocks away. Out of twelve couples (one couple was childless), only three had no children living in the area.

Among the Japanese, the situation was more varied. Three couples lived with their married sons, two couples lived with their divorced daughters and grandchildren, four couples lived by themselves (all had daughters living separately) and two lived with their unmarried sons. One couple who lived with their son's family also lived next door to their daughter's family. In all cases, the adult children were living in their parents' houses, not the other way around.

Of the five couples who lived with their children, three were living in the traditional oldest son, daughter-in-law and grandchildren household, one was living with an unmarried son, and another was living with their oldest daughter who was divorced. There was a sense that these arrangements could change and that the choice of who to live with depended on traditional norms such as gender and being the eldest child, as well as compatibility, children living abroad for business, and daughters returning home because of divorce.

Americans: a preference for pairs

For the Americans, the choice of whom to live with was not in doubt. Living together as a couple was so obvious that it was not mentioned as a conscious choice and living with children did not come into consideration. In fact, children seemed tangential to their current lives. In the Smith family, the elderly wife talked about visiting her son and daughter-in-law in another state: "The kids would like us to come but ten days is fine." Mrs Smith felt that her daughter-in-law was such a perfect housekeeper that she was uncomfortable in her house. On one visit, they were scolded for drinking the wrong milk. Apparently, their daughter-in-law labeled one carton hers and one carton her husband's and the older couple was to drink from their son's carton.

Perhaps the American perception of living arrangements with children was summed up best by Mrs Thomas when she talked about her developmentally disabled son, a child who did not fit the norm. She said, "Your other kids go away from you, but this child really doesn't leave home. We are still very important to him."

Since most of them were in fairly good health, the American couples did not seem to think beyond the current time. When the couples infrequently talked about their own care needs, it was clear that they expected care from each other. If they looked toward their children for care sometime in the future, they did not discuss it. With a few exceptions, most of the couples did not anticipate relying on their children.

One couple who illustrated this pattern, the Kleins, had taken care of her mother and both of their fathers. Mrs Klein was now caring for her husband who had Parkinson's disease and died not long after our interview.

Their easy joking manner with each other was in contrast to the sad stories they told about taking care of their elderly parents. When they were asked if they would expect their children to do what they did for their parents, Mrs Klein answered, "No, I know my children won't." Her husband agreed, "Absolutely not. Our kids are very affectionate but I don't think they could possibly do this sort of thing. My son couldn't, I know he can't. His schedule is such that he couldn't possibly." Mrs Klein explained that both their son and daughter worked. "It's a whole different world. I was home, and I could do it," she said.

In the few instances in which couples depended upon their children, there was a tendency to view daughters as the more reliable source for care. The Saunders had moved to their daughter's community to be nearer to her. Mrs Saunders explained, "We wanted to be close to our daughter because we had both been in the hospital quite a bit. And she was going back and forth a lot. She did more than our son who lived ten miles away." Mr Saunders pointed out that their daughter had the freedom of movement that he (their son) didn't have: "He had to attend to business. She didn't." Mrs Saunders countered that her daughter had always been more available to her parents. In contrast, their son visited only two or three times a year and called on Mother's Day.

Most of the American couples tended to look to their children for emotional support rather than physical care. For example, in the Johnson family, the older couple talked about the pleasure they derived from their relationship with their son and his wife. They had provided their daughter-in-law with considerable encouragement throughout her education and now felt that their son and daughter-in-law provided them with a similar kind of emotional support. The wife said, "There was a real support here with [her son and daughter-in-law] that we could really count on."

Japanese: a range of options

Though the Japanese couples seemed to anticipate a need for care and planned for it by having their adult children live with them or by building an addition to their house for them, they also spoke frequently about their children's independence.

One couple, the Tomitas, lived separately from their only child, a daughter. The couple was accustomed to their daughter's independence since she had worked for a Japanese company in the United States before her marriage and then continued to live there for several years with her husband and children.

This couple also illustrates a situation which will become more common in the next generation of Japanese elderly – an increase in one-child families (Ogawa and Retherford, 1996). Since she is their only daughter, the Tomitas were happy when she married because their family would expand. She spoke about the pressure her son-in-law was under to take care of both sets of parents since he is the oldest son and her daughter is the only child. The Tomitas felt somewhat uncomfortable about this because, as they put it, "we gave our daughter to (the son-in-law's) family." Traditionally, after marriage, the bride moved into her husband's house, becoming officially a part of his household rather than the one in which she was born. The bride's parents would only see their married daughter a few times a year. This custom has changed considerably in recent years with daughters maintaining much closer relationships with their own parents, even when they are living with their in-laws. Ironically, in an attempt to be a good son-in-law, the Tomitas' son-in-law insisted on taking his in-laws to *karaoke* because he had done so with his parents. The couple related, "We both hate *karaoke* so we tried to refuse but he said he brought his parents to *karaoke* so he felt he had to bring us. He takes care of us and his parents very well."

The fluidity of the Japanese couples' living arrangements reflects the changes in family structure such as the increasing divorce rate. Three of the Japanese couples had daughters who were divorced. The Akiyamas had worked together in a butcher shop for many years. Their daughter was married a short time and they had been in favor of her divorce because they considered her husband a spoiled child who gambled a lot. After her divorce, the daughter lived with her boyfriend in the Akiyama's house until they recently moved out to their own apartment. The young couple continued to come back several times a week and it was clear that her older parents enjoyed having their daughter and her boyfriend around the house whether they were living with them or not.

The impermanence of what used to be a permanent arrangement, that is living with the oldest son and his family, is seen in two families. In both cases, decisions about living arrangements changed in the face of personality clashes. In the Tanaka family, the mother-in-law admitted to losing her temper with her son's wife and so her son's family moved out. Mrs Tanaka explained that her son had intended to live with his wife and child in his parents' home. However, conflict erupted between the mother and her daughter-in-law. The older woman observed:

> Although I never intended to make so much noise by complaining, when she bathed the baby I would tell her not to rest him in the bathtub since the bottom is cold. After I went downstairs, she said, "How can the bottom of the tub be cold when it's filled to the brim with hot water?" She was young, you see, and everyone went over to her side. Even if I insisted that I was correct, all the men in the family would still be on her side. As you see, sometimes conflicts arise and I lose my temper.

Another couple, the Suzukis, also experienced clashes with their older son, his wife, and their adult grandchildren. The two families lived in separate quarters in the same house, each with their own entrances, but the inter-generational struggles made the older couple feel as if they were living with strangers. Mrs

Suzuki was confined to a wheelchair and he provided all her care, taking her to a day care center a few times a week. He, more than his wife, was very bitter about his relationship with his son's family.

Mr Suzuki's main conflict was between his ideal of what a traditional family should be and the reality he experienced. His expectations were the traditional ones: that the two families would function as one with the daughter-in-law providing constant help and support. His estrangement from his daughter-in-law meant that he had to assume the role of the sole caregiver for his wife. He described his wife as exclusively dependent on him, "She can't do anything without me now. So I take care of her breakfast, lunch and supper, and cook rice, then care of her body then cleaning of our house and doing the laundry. I studied a lot about cooking." Because of the frequent family conflicts, he said, he became sick and was hospitalized. When he was in the hospital, his daughter-in-law took care of his wife. Mr Suzuki said, "I don't know how she did it. I doubt she did it with love."

Mr Suzuki rarely saw his son and complained that his son only did what was best for himself. For example, he asked his son not to park his car at the entrance to the house because it made taking the wheelchair in and out more difficult, but his son refused unless his father would agree to pay for another parking space. The grandchildren, although they live next door, did not stop and say hello to their grandmother. He described his feelings of separation from his son's family, "The worst thing is that the one home became two homes. I thought it was one home until now. But it became two homes. Living in the same house, our hearts completely became two."

Variations in the nature of caregiving

Among both the American and Japanese couples, we heard the refrain that times had changed and families were no longer caring for their parents as they did in the past. However, the differences between the past and present seemed more dramatic for the Japanese than for the Americans. For example, although the length of time people spend in caregiving has increased in both countries with the advent of longer life expectancy, the change has been faster and more dramatic in Japan where fifty years ago people were more likely to die of tuberculosis (TB) and thus require fewer years, if any, of caregiving by their children.

As expected, many of the Japanese couples had lived with their parents or parents-in-law in contrast to the Americans who lived independently. As Kobrin (1976) points out, coresidence in America has declined over the past fifty years and the extended family has been more myth than reality in American history. In Japan, however, the tradition of the oldest son marrying and staying in the family household, with his wife providing most of the care of the aging parents, has been firmly established. There was built-in flexibility so that if there were no sons, a son-in-law or another distant relative could be adopted into the family, thereby insuring the continuance of the family name and the *ie* (traditional inter-generational household). As coresidence declined and values changed (Ogawa and Retherford, 1996), many older Japanese feel as if the ground rules are changing and life in old age has become less secure.

For our Japanese couples, the experiences of living with parents varied considerably. For some couples, these inter-generational living arrangements contributed to marital disharmony that drove the wives to contemplate divorce. For other couples, such arrangements resulted in reciprocal help giving such that daughters-in-law helped their mothers-in-law and the mothers-in-law enabled the daughters-in-law to work by sharing in child rearing (Morgan and Hirosima, 1983; Ogawa and Retherford, 1996).

The American daughters, on the other hand, received little help from their parents in child rearing. In fact, they often kept the failures of their children a secret from their parents, preventing help that might have been forthcoming. Although both Japanese and American women spoke of isolation in the early years of marriage, often due to the husband's absence from household life, conflict between husband and wife was more openly discussed by the Japanese and conflict between parents and children was more likely to be discussed by the Americans.

Americans: caring after an illness

Most of the American couples had not been deeply involved in the daily care of their parents. In some cases, parents cared for themselves until they died and several had parents who died at a fairly young age. Of those who took care of parents, some helped financially, others provided long-distance support to siblings who provided care, and others placed their parents in nursing homes when they needed extensive care, frequently after brief stays in their own homes. In all cases, care was provided only after an illness and the parents' poor health precipitated the move. When a move occurred, it was generally the older parent(s) who moved rather than their adult children.

In one family, Mrs White moved her mother from another state. She then moved her to three different nursing homes, finding problems with all of them until she was finally satisfied. Mrs White also viewed the care of her mother as a way of teaching her children about aging, but her efforts backfired. As she said, "... In certain ways, it was interesting, (but) they kind of resented this because they were still needing a lot of attention."

Most of the American couples, like the Whites, did not actually live with their parents. Only three of the couples had lived with their parents, two of whom were African American. These two couples described their caregiving experiences very positively. The Bakers, for example, came from the South. Mrs Baker was raised by her grandparents who still lived in the South and when they became ill, she traveled back and forth from her Midwestern home to take care of them. Mr Baker's sister and other relatives took care of their baby while she was gone. "Then," Mr Baker said, "after her grandmother died, her grandfather came and lived with us. I liked that a whole lot better."

Mr Baker talked about how much this elderly man contributed to their household. He said:

> So he was home but he still did some work. When I bought the place in Highland Park there was lots of things that needed to be changed around there and I didn't have to say anything. He just take over and just go ahead. He was in very good health until it looked like all at once, it just "boom," he was gone.

The other African American couple, the Mortons, took care of Mr Morton's parents who moved from the South to live with them. Mrs Morton reminisced:

> I think one of the other high points in our life was when [her husband's father] had a stroke and we built two rooms on the back and they moved in here with us ... and it was such a pleasure having them here. The stroke had affected Papa's speech ... His eyes would light up and you could understand just from his expressions ... He loved to play checkers. He could get all the kids to play with Gramps.

The third couple who had parents living with them were the previously mentioned Kleins whose experience was more demanding. Her mother had a serious neurological illness that left her bedridden. Mrs Klein regarded this as one of the major changes in her life. She had to nurse her mother through "thirty-three months of horrible, agonizing problems." Mrs Klein felt she had not been the same since and traced the beginning of her chronic problems with depression and claustrophobia to this "heart-wrenching" experience of caring for her mother. For her husband, the experience was sad but he was affected mainly in changes made to the house as they turned one of the rooms into a nursing room for her mother. Mr Klein remarked, "I didn't give it a second thought." They both attributed their willingness to give care to family tradition. "It didn't occur to you that there was any alternative. I mean this is what you did." But they added that at that time the nursing homes were bad and there were no viable services to help.

Japanese: caring over the long haul

Most of the Japanese women had lived with their mothers-in-law since their marriage. Some women found themselves embedded in relationships that were interdependent and, in some ways, eased their responsibilities and provided affection that substituted for their husbands' lack of warmth. Others were enmeshed in relationships that were exhausting, demeaning, and left them lonely and isolated.

The Satos illustrate an enmeshed family unit. When she married, Mrs Sato moved in with her husband's family: his mother, aunt and uncle, younger brother and a maid who had been the brother's baby-sitter. Her husband was largely absent due to work commitments and her relatives ruled her life. Her husband's aunt, who was living with them, determined when they would have a child and insisted that Mrs Sato have an abortion because they felt there was not enough money to support a child.

Mrs Sato's mother-in-law was a very religious person, an active leader in the Tenrikyō sect of Buddhism for more than 60 years, and interfered in all aspects of the household. When the children had a fever, she interpreted it as a will of God and that they had to spend money as quickly as possible. "Even for a low fever, she would insist that we see the doctor. And it was not easy to hide it from her so that even in benign cases when we thought that just a rest at home could help cure the fever ... it was not funny for us."

Caring for this mother-in-law was especially difficult and illustrates the communal nature of caregiving and the fear of what others might say about the caregiver. A few months before her death, her mother-in-law decided to move in with her sister both because she feared being a burden to her son's family and because she wanted to help her sister whose son was in trouble because of his alcoholism. In order to help her sister, she devoted herself to praying along with fasting to stop him from drinking. Mrs Sato pleaded with her to eat because it was clearly harmful to her already weak condition. She explained:

> And you know in my position, the death of my mother-in-law due to fasting could be easily blamed on me by other people. It was very difficult for me to bring her to my view. I tried to convince her that when she does not eat with us, her son may think that I am refusing to give her food. I wanted to do everything I could because I knew that my husband's wish was to assist her until her last day ... I was so concerned by that attitude and by the interpretation our relatives and my husband's young brother would make of that behavior. But ... my brother-in-law knew very well the character of his mother and didn't blame me for that kind of attitude. She stopped us from buying some food pretending that it was luxurious and a waste of money. We had better use that money to fulfill the wishes of God. Even when relaxing all together in some park, you still felt the weight of the big problem we had in our family. Really, if you look at those pictures of that period you will have the impression that everybody had a shrunken face.

During the early years of her marriage, Mrs Sato had considered divorce but realized she had no way to support herself. It was not until her mother-in-law died, that her relationship with her husband improved. Mr Sato felt pulled between his responsibilities to his family and to his wife. He explained that, "Really for me, my deep feeling was the same from the beginning. It was just a problem of form you know, I had to care about people around me."

The more reciprocal nature of the embedded relationship is apparent especially in relation to the Tanaka family. Mrs Tanaka, a teacher, said her mother-in-law thought highly of her career. At first, after her marriage, her mother-in-law wrote her a letter, asking her to quit her job because at that time it was unusual for a married middle-class woman to be working. But after thinking about the importance of her daughter-in-law's profession, she reconsidered, tore up the letter, and strongly supported her daughter-in-law's career.

The mother-in-law moved in with the Tanakas because she was not getting along with the wife of her oldest son. She quickly became an important source of support. Mrs Tanaka said, "Both my sons turned out to be kind children, thanks to the influence of Grandmother. I am really grateful. Things would have been terrible if I had to work and look after the children at the same time."

This mother-in-law's death is described quite differently from that of Mrs Sato. Mrs Tanaka explained:

> The last year of her life, she said, "I am old. I can no longer do any more work. I am leaving all the work to you." But she carried on. She was in a terminal state for about two weeks. Three days before she died, her two daughters came and everyone stayed together in the house. She was very happy. She would suddenly open her eyes and say, "The flowers in the garden are in full bloom. They are really beautiful." I thought it was a loss that I didn't give birth to a daughter. The daughters were all there. Grandmother was so happy. She was such a fortunate lady.

Caring for extended family and non-relatives

One of the frequently cited differences between the Japanese and American elderly is that Americans have wider support networks of friends and neighbors than do Japanese (Policy Office for the Aged, 1991). Among our couples, however, it was striking that the Japanese wives had cared for an extended network of family and friends during their marriage. A few Americans, too, brought non-family members into their home but this was largely voluntary – hospitality to foreign students, helpful interactions with previous spouses, or frequent contact with siblings.

Americans: voluntary caring

The Morton family gladly welcomed a variety of young people into their family. "As Christians," Mrs Morton said, "We found ourselves having to reach out and the young people came from the South and were lost in this Northern environment." She vividly remembered the meals she cooked for these young students and described the resulting benefits for her own family, "We actually found that with all the various ones that have been part of our household, and we had all races, that we got far more probably than what we felt we gave."

The Johnsons had also taken in many students to live in their home. At various times they had students from Mexico, Germany, and Kenya. They had also had African-American students from the inner city. Mrs Johnson reminisced:

> They found out that neither of us had ever tasted chitlins. And so they made a point of coming out again and preparing the chitlins and giving us a chitlin dinner. The smell of it was absolutely awful, and they said themselves, they can't stand the smell. But the taste was delicious.

In addition, the Johnsons provided support to Mr Johnson's ex-wife. He said, "She felt that she could depend on us more than she could on anybody she knew. It was strange. It really was, but it was gratifying too."

Japanese: obligatory caring

The Japanese caregiving experiences were generally involuntary or at least not at the wife's invitation but at the husband's. When the Yamadas were married, Mrs Yamada moved into her husband's house and took care of his brothers and sisters. "My husband's youngest brother is two years older than our daughter." She also took care of a stream of young people from the country who came to the city to work in her husband's company. Mrs Yamada described a typical day:

> I woke up at 5:00 a.m. to make six lunches. I made them breakfast and let them take their lunch. After that there were many things to do like washing ... When I finished all household affairs it was about midnight. I had to prepare for the next breakfast ... our children grew up with them, with many brothers. There were always eight or nine people in our house.

She thought that the experience was good for her own children who "grew up freely. I saw their parents who left their children to us. I was very sorry for them. I could understand their feelings well because I also have children. That's why I thought I should take care of them heartily."

The couple who worked together as butchers, the Akiyamas, extended themselves to care for the children of relatives. Mrs Akiyama came from the countryside as a young girl to work at her uncle's shop. There she met and married her husband. Besides continuing to work in the butcher shop, Mrs Akiyama took care of her uncle's children along with her own so that these children and her children grew up together almost as one family. Employees were also part of their lives and they described people sleeping everywhere with little privacy. The atmosphere, however, rather than oppressive, often sounded like a party with people playing games and drinking late into the night.

Another couple, the Tanakas, cared for teachers associated with Mr Tanaka's school. Mr Tanaka, a former science teacher, said, "We took care of many teachers. I let them stay here for three months to half a year." Mrs Tanaka also took care of all the animals that were in her husband's school. Although she adds that her husband was "a person who lives for society," it appeared that much of his work was done by his wife. At one point when her husband's brother's business failed, his family moved in with them. "I had three babies," she said, "but I brought up six."

The Japanese census since 1920 has defined the household as a group of people who share a house and a livelihood. It may include non-relatives, domestic servants, employees who are living together and does not include family members who are living apart (Sodei, 1998). Although this caring for extended family and friends was an important role for Japanese women in the past, it is clear that with increasing mobility and industrialization this pattern is changing. The older couples' children were having fewer children and fewer relatives living with them. In addition, the affluence of the Japanese society necessitated less need for sharing scarce household resources with non-family members, employees, and students.

Implications for programs and policy

This analysis of the older couples' interviews begins to address the questions posed at the beginning of this chapter. Several findings emerge from these interviews as particularly salient. First, the Japanese couples experienced considerably more fluidity in their living and caring arrangements than did the American couples. Second, the American couples generally provided care to elderly parents only after a health care crisis whereas Japanese couples participated in reciprocal intergenerational help-giving over the course of their marriage. Third, both Japanese and American couples, particularly in the past, had expanded their caregiving network to include extended family and friends.

The experiences of our informants provide several recommendations for policy and program development. As suggested by our study, policy makers must know more about families and their caregiving needs to develop programs that are congruent with current expectations. A crucial step is to collect data that will be useful in policy development. Asking questions that address the fluidity of family living arrangements is important. Such questions also need to address the complicated patterns of family relationships that are emerging. While divorce is more common in the United States, we are seeing an increased incidence of divorce in Japan as well. For example, even in our small sample, it was striking that a fourth of the Japanese couples had divorced children living with them. These parents appeared to welcome their divorced daughters and their children back into their homes. These newly emerging patterns of family relationships will have an impact on family caregiving. For example, adult children who are divorced may be responsible for multiple sets of parents – their parents, in-laws, and former in-laws. Policy makers in Japan and the United States need to be aware of such trends in family caregiving.

Dramatic changes in Japan, such as the decline in coresidence and the increase of women in the work force, have already led to new policy initiatives.

Coresidence, with women primarily staying at home, previously formed the basis of a "Japanese-style" welfare system in which all the responsibility for care fell on the family. The Gold Plan (Ten Year Strategy to Promote Health Care and Welfare Services for the Elderly) introduced in 1990 and revised in 1994, was a comprehensive policy mandating and expanding such services as home helpers, day care centers, and short-stay respite facilities as well as institutional care. The Gold Plan, and the new Long-Term Care Insurance Law passed in 1997, illustrate Japan's decision to make services for the elderly one of their top national priorities.

In the United States, legislation has been developed to address the needs of the elderly, such as Medicaid waivers which permit Medicaid benefits to be used in the community instead of solely in nursing homes, but such programs tend to be inconsistently implemented across states. Although Japan had been behind the United States in developing community care services for the elderly until about 1990, since then, needed services for the elderly and their families have been expanding rapidly, although they are still not sufficient to meet the growing needs. When Long-Term Care Insurance begins in 2000, the resources invested in this area should increase very substantially.

What implications do these newly converging policy changes have for families such as the ones described in this paper? In the US, the government will intervene during crises for relatively short periods and families take over much of the burden. In Japan, although the family will certainly maintain a sense of responsibility for elderly parents in most cases, the expanded framework of services should be able to assume some of the actual burden of caregiving. It is interesting that the Japanese experience of care "over the long haul," as described in this chapter, may lead to more concerted efforts to influence public policy whereas the more "crisis-oriented" American experience has not produced a unified ground swell for a comprehensive national policy of relief for caregivers. In the United States, the emphasis on the individual leads Americans to assume their situation is unique to their family whereas in Japan the more institutionalized role of family care and the daughter-in-law's responsibility, in particular, makes it seem more like a societal problem. American policy makers should look to Japan and make the needs of the frail elderly a top priority, with a comprehensive plan for services that are equitably distributed throughout the country.

US planners should also consider Japan as they examine models of respite care. For example, short-stay programs which offer a week or more of respite care in a nursing home or hospital are widely available in Japan, as they are in many European countries. The need for available respite care when the caregiver becomes ill or needs a break is an important option, especially among elderly spouses caring for each other, such as the ones described in our study.

Japan, in turn, may want to look to the United States as they consider new housing alternatives for the elderly. Government-supported housing has not been a major program in Japan. Despite the steady decline of elderly living together with their adult children, the widespread image that "normal" older people are living in three-generation households has been one factor inhibiting much policy development in this area (Campbell, 1992). Nonetheless, the varied living arrangements illustrated by our Japanese respondents indicates the shifting values in Japanese society from shared households to "shared togetherness" (Elliott and Campbell, 1993).

Americans, both in the public and private sectors, have developed innovative housing opportunities for the elderly including senior subsidized housing, assisted living, small group homes for people with dementia, and continuing care retirement communities. Although the emphasis in American society is on the elderly remaining independent, experience in the past two decades with "independent" housing has taught planners that additional services such as meals and home care are necessary if people are to realistically "age in place." In dealing with these problems, both the United States and Japan could usefully learn from Scandinavian countries, where housing as a focus for caregiving has been most highly developed.

The stories of our couples as well as the findings of other researchers (Moen and Forest, 1995) indicate that the meaning of family and the nature of caregiving is changing. Instead of posing the artificial notion of "family" care vs. institutional care, policy makers need to recognize and support the variety of patterns of caring in the United States and Japan. As both countries face the challenges of a graying population, each can learn from the other concerning policies and programs that strengthen the different patterns of family care and enhance the vitality of the family in continuing to care for its elderly members.

References

American Association of Retired Persons. (1997). *A profile of older Americans*. Washington, DC: American Association of Retired Persons.
Aneshensel, C.S., Pearlin, L.I., Mullan, J.T., Zarit, S.H., and Whitlatch, C.J. (1995). *Profiles in caregiving: The unexpected career*. San Diego: Academic Press.
Brody, E.M. (1990). *Women in the middle: Their parent care years*. New York: Springer.
Campbell, J.C. (1992). *How policies change: The Japanese government and the aging society*. Princeton: Princeton University Press.
Campbell, J.C. (1998). Financing the ideal long-term care system through social insurance. *The Keio Journal of Medicine, 47*, Supplement 2, A49–A50.
Campbell, R., and Brody, E.M. (1985). Women's changing roles and help to the elderly: Attitudes of women in the United States and Japan. *The Gerontologist, 25*, 584–592.
Elliott, K.S., and Campbell, R. (1993). From shared household to "separate togetherness": Variations in the family living arrangements of Japanese elders. Paper presented at the annual meeting of the Gerontological Society of America, New Orleans, LA.
Hashimoto, A. (1996). *The gift of generations: Japanese and American perspectives on aging and the social contract*. Cambridge: Cambridge University Press.
Ikegami, N., and Yamada T. (1996). Comparison of long-term care for the elderly between Japan and the United States. In N. Ikegami and J.C. Campbell (Eds.), *Containing health care costs in Japan* (pp. 155–171). Ann Arbor: University of Michigan Press.

Ingersoll-Dayton, B., Campbell, R., Kurokawa, Y., and Saito, M. (1996). Separateness and togetherness: Interdependence over the life course in Japanese and American marriages. *Journal of Social and Personal Relationships, 13*, 387–400.

Ingersoll-Dayton, B., Campbell, R., and Mattson, J. (1998). Forms of communication: A cross-cultural comparison of older married couples in the United States and Japan. *Journal of Cross-Cultural Gerontology, 13*, 1, 63–80.

Kobrin, F.E. (1976). The fall in household size and the rise of the primary individual in the United States. *Demography, 13*, 127–138.

Kōseishō (Ministry of Health and Welfare). (1997). *Kokumin Eisei no Dōkō* (Trends in Public Health), *44*, 9. Tokyo: Kōsei Tōkei Kyōkai.

Long, S.O. (1996). Nurturing and femininity: The ideal of caregiving in post-war Japan. In A.E. Imamura (Ed.), *Re-imaging Japanese women* (pp. 156–176). Berkeley: University of California Press.

Maeda, D., and Nakatani, Y. (1992). Family care of the elderly in Japan. In J.I. Kosberg (Ed.), *Family care of the elderly: Social and cultural changes* (pp. 196–209). Newbury Park, CA: Sage.

Moen, P.H., and Forest, K.B. (1995). Family policy for an aging society: Moving to the twenty-first century. *Gerontologist, 35*, 825–830.

Morgan, S.P., and Hirosima, K. (1983). The persistence of extended family residence in Japan: Anachronism or alternative strategy? *American Sociological Review, 48*, 269–281.

Ogawa, N., and Retherford, R.D. (1996). Shifting costs of caring for the elderly back to families in Japan: Will it work? *Population and Development Review, 23*, 59–64.

Policy Office for the Aged. (1991). The international study on living and consciousness of elderly people: An outline of the results. Tokyo: Management and Coordination Agency.

Sodei, T. (1998). Role of the family in long-term care. Paper presented at the Keio University International Symposium for Life Science and Medicine: Long-term care for frail older people – Reaching for the ideal system.

US Bureau of the Census. *Statistical abstract of the United States.* (1992). Washington, DC: US Department of Commerce.

12 Recognizing the need for gender-responsive family caregiving policy

Lessons from male caregivers

Phyllis Braudy Harris and Susan Orpett Long

> It was just like they [particularly women professionals] were humoring me. I don't know how else to characterize it, but they questioned that you would even be in the least bit involved or concerned or interested in all of this.
>
> Forty-two-year-old son caring for his mother with Alzheimer's disease, United States

> I think this study of male caregivers is important. I wonder why Americans are here looking at this issue when our own government and service providers aren't. The problem of elder care will only get greater.
>
> Sixty-eight-year-old son caring for his frail 95-year-old mother, Japan

In recent years, Japanese and American policies for providing for the needs of their growing elderly population have come to diverge significantly, in part because of differing political ideologies about the appropriate role of government in providing social welfare services. Many Japanese scholars, social critics, and ordinary citizens have looked to the government for leadership in assuming responsibility for creating an egalitarian system which offers older members of society opportunities for work, reasonably priced medical services, and means of financial and physical support if they become impaired. (See, for example, Hashimoto, 1996.) The dominant American political ideology of the past two decades has, in contrast, emphasized government fiscal restraint, and thus the need for developing private methods of post-retirement income, medical care, and social services. Despite these philosophical differences, policies are alike in their expectation that the majority of care of impaired elderly will be provided by families. Our study of male family caregivers points to the conscious and unconscious assumptions relating gender and nurturance that lie behind and within caregiving policy in both countries.

Focusing on caregiving in cross-cultural comparison allows us to see more clearly how caregivers in different countries may experience similar demographic and social changes. The way people experience their roles is shaped in part by cultural factors that define the meaning of what they do in a particular context. Since historically people in Japan and the United States have interpreted their activities and their lives in the context of quite different world views – for example, Christian ideas of love versus Confucian notions of filial piety – we wished to explore the similarities and differences in the ways in which contemporary male caregivers in the two countries describe their experiences. This small-scale exploratory study begins to investigate whether the meanings caregiving men take from these experiences vary within and across societies.

In Japan and the United States, families are providing more complex care to their elderly family members for more extended periods of time than ever before, and it has placed unprecedented stress on families (Aneshensel *et al.* 1995; Brody, 1990; Harris and Long, 1993; Lock, 1993; Pearlin *et al.*, 1990). However, the majority of Japanese as well as Americans continue to express preference for being cared for in their homes and by family members if they become ill (Martin, 1989). Institutionalization is the choice of last resort for the majority of families in both countries (Ikegami and Yamada, 1996).

Family caregiving policy in both countries has been implemented without acknowledging cultural assumptions that caring for an elderly family member is a gendered experience. In Japan and in the United States, women have constituted the majority of caregivers of the elderly, reinforcing cultural assumptions that caregiving is "naturally" women's work. These assumptions have made men who have taken on the caregiving role "non-normative." Policy makers have incorporated these assumptions about gender into work, family, and long-term care policy, thus creating policy in which there has been little recognition that men too care for elderly family members. We believe that by recognizing the role of men in elder care and acknowledging the cultural assumptions behind seemingly gender-neutral policy, we can develop better policies and programs that are gender-responsive. Gender-responsive policies can better support caregivers by adapting programs to the needs and responsibilities experienced by men and women, so that the burden that often comes with caregiving will be lessened for all who care for elderly spouses or parents.

Both Japan and the United States have experienced the demographic changes of increased life expectancy and decreased fertility. There is a positive correlation between increased age and chronic disability, leading to increased need for family caregiving at the same time that family size is declining (see Harris and Long, 1999 and Long and Harris, 1997 for fuller discussion). The majority of caregivers in both countries are women. Wives, daughters, and in Japan, daughters-in-law have borne most of the responsibility. However, in both countries, men are also involved in caregiving: 28 percent in the United States (Stone, Cafferata and Sangl, 1987; National Alliance for Caregiving, 1997) and 15 percent in Japan (Kōseishō, 1997, p. 111). Yet because of cultural norms and stereotypes about male caregivers, we know little about who they are, what tasks they perform, how they cope with the difficulties of caregiving, how their lives are affected, and how they interpret their experiences as caregivers. Studies in Japan are beginning to recognize the need to examine male caregiving (Harris, Long, and Fujii, 1998; Odahara and Nakayama, 1992; Okuyama, 1996 and 1997; Takenaga, 1998).

A small number of American studies have focused mainly on husbands, who make up approximately half of the male caregivers. These studies have concluded that husbands are committed to caring for their wives, are comfortable taking control of the situation, and fare better emotionally than women caregivers. There is inconsistency in their findings regarding coping ability and strategies, total number of hours involved in caregiving, and use of formal and informal help. Little information is available about the meaning of the caregiving experience for these men (Harris and Bichler, 1997; Horowitz, 1985; Kramer, 1997; Miller, 1990; Miller and Cafasso, 1992; Mui, 1995; Stoller, 1992). The data available on son caregiving is even more sparse, though sons constitute 11 percent of all primary caregivers and 52 percent of all secondary caregivers in the United States (Stone, Cafferata and Sangl, 1987). For the most part, these studies have compared sons to daughters and have found them lacking as caregivers in terms of commitment, tasks provided, and overall involvement (Horowitz, 1985; Montgomery and Kamo, 1987; Stoller, 1992), but these conclusions are based mainly on small quantitative samples. There has been no previous in-depth research that focuses on understanding their motivation for caregiving or the meaning they derive from the experience.

In this chapter we argue that we need to listen more closely to the caregiving experience of men, the non-normative caregivers, because their personal experiences as caregivers reflect the gendered assumptions found in caregiving policy in both societies. Gender has been the subject of research studies and policy concern regarding the frail elderly themselves, especially in the United States, where the poverty of many older women has been taken up as a women's issue (Hooyman and Gonyea, 1995). In Japan, feminists have seen caregiving as a women's issue because of the recognition of the heavy responsibilities that have fallen to them (Sodei, 1997).

Yet focusing on gender is to do more than identify women's issues; caregiving as a gendered activity cannot be fully understood without consideration of both women's *and* men's lives. The complex relationships among men and women, their ideas and their opportunities, create and reinforce a *gender system* which is the context for any social activity or cultural interpretation of caregiving. A gender system is grounded in both recognition of difference and valuation of that difference. This chapter points to widespread assumptions about the existence of differential abilities to nurture others based on gender, and relates these differences to unequal opportunities provided by government and workplace policies under a veil of gender-neutrality.

We begin this chapter by providing an account of male caregiving experiences as described to us during interviews of men in both countries. They related the tasks they perform, their motivations for taking on the role, the impact of caregiving on their lives, and the responses of others to their activities. We then point out the ways that their male gender has impacted on the meaning they derive from this role. Their experiences challenge cultural assumptions that lie behind elder care policy and point to issues that need to be considered in the development of gender-responsive policy and programs.

Male caregiving

Three separate purposive non-random samples were collected for this study. From 1991–1996, we conducted exploratory studies of men caring for an elderly family member in a large metropolitan area of the American Midwest and in the Kansai area of Japan, to begin to answer these questions about the nature of male caregiving in two societies historically different in family relationships, attitudes toward disability, and ideals of caregiving.

Believing that in this new area of research listening to the men's experiences would aid our understanding, we conducted open-ended personal interviews lasting one to two hours utilizing an interview guide which allowed the men to take the discussion in their own directions while focusing on the key questions of the research. The topics included in the interview schedules were broken into four major categories and then were broken down into more specific areas, with minor changes depending if the interviewee was a husband or son. The four major topics were:

- the role of caregiver: tasks, new roles, definitions of the roles, changes over time, difficulties, losses, disappointments, accomplishments, satisfactions, impact of the role on work and family, and life style changes
- stress and coping: types of stresses, coping strategies, social support, financial impact of illness, service usage, and role of health care professionals
- marital and family relationships: impact of caregiving on relationship with wife, children, and siblings; role and expectations of wife, children, and siblings, and impact on relationship with ill parent
- meaning and motivation: reason for taking on caregiving role, meaning of the experience, sense of purpose, personal growth, and societal reaction.

The interview guide was pre-tested on an American sample of four husbands and sons. Before being translated for the Japanese sample, the interview guide was discussed at length with a Japanese social worker/researcher to assess the guide's cultural relevance. Then the guide was translated by the Japanese researcher and back translated by a Japanese-speaking American researcher to ensure that the choice of the Japanese words captured the meaning that was intended. All the interviews were taped and then transcribed and compared with field notes for accuracy.

In the United States, fifteen husbands and fifteen sons of demented elderly persons volunteered to participate in the study through the local Alzheimer's Association. The samples were collected through newspaper ads in an

Alzheimer's Association newsletter, from a review of calls made to a local Alzheimer's help line, and from referrals from the staff of a local Alzheimer's Association. The sample included men with a broad range of demographic characteristics such as socioeconomic class, race, urban/rural residence, number of years of caregiving, and employment status. The primary diagnosis of the impaired family member was dementia. The majority of the care recipients were living in the community either with their spouse or children. In Japan, eleven husbands and five sons of demented and/or physically frail elderly patients who were referred by local physicians, a senior center, or a dementia assessment center agreed to be interviewed. Because contact with these men was made through health care providers, additional information about the men's caregiving situations was obtained through conversations with these health care professionals. (See Harris and Long, 1999 for fuller description of methodology and sample.)

There were no major demographic differences in the age and social class of the samples of American and Japanese caregivers. The average age of the impaired parents, 77 for the American sons and 87 for the Japanese sons, did differ significantly. Other important differences between the samples are in the parents' diagnoses and in living arrangements. In the American sample the major diagnosis was cognitive impairment, but the Japanese sample also included a portion of people who had severe physical impairments due to stroke or arthritis which rendered them bedridden. In Japan, 1.2 million elderly are classified as bedridden (Kōseishō 1996), a category not used in the United States due to a strong emphasis on rehabilitation. Researchers disagree about the significance of the type of impairment for the caregiving experience (Montgomery, Kosloski, and Borgatta, 1990).

There were also more multigenerational households in Japan, and in the United States more nursing home placements by sons. In the United States nursing homes are more available than in Japan, and placement is more acceptable. Although nationally the proportion of elderly-only households has risen in Japan from less than 5 percent of all households in 1975 to over 13 percent in 1994 (Kōseishō, 1996, p. 328), more parents in our American than Japanese sample were living alone, reflecting the national difference that 40 percent of the elderly in the United States live in elderly-only households (US Bureau of the Census, 1996). A brief summary of the findings is presented below.

Motivations

The men in our study expressed that they had taken on the caregiving role because of love, a sense of duty, or some combination of these motives. Interesting cross-cultural differences emerged in the differences in motivation between husbands and sons. American husbands frequently referred to their wedding vows and expressed the expectation that they would care for a spouse "in sickness and in health." They appreciated any support they received from their children, but saw caregiving as their own responsibility. American sons provided care out of love, duty, and a sense of wishing to repay the parent, but for the most part were able to set boundaries and time limits on their caregiving. In contrast, Japanese sons (who were caregivers) expected that the obligation to care for an ailing, elderly parent was theirs, whether viewed as traditional Confucian filial piety or a "modern" sense of responsibility to repay their parent for their care. They provided extensive care, setting few limits to what they would do. Japanese husbands, not expecting to have caregiving responsibilities in old age, often expressed their assumption of the caregiving role as a result of default: a son had not married, the children had all moved away, or the general sense that society had changed and "now old people must take care of each other." They accepted their new burdens, sometimes out of love, but more often they chose to reinterpret the situation as an opportunity to repay their wives for their many years of care for them.

Tasks

The men in both countries provided a broad range of services, from hands-on care to physical presence to emotional support. They performed nursing tasks such as giving medication and intravenous feeding, turning, and exercising the patient. They assisted with or took over housekeeping tasks of cooking, cleaning, and laundry. Other tasks frequently reported by the men included bathing, feeding, dressing, and toileting the elderly relative. They took them to doctors' appointments and out for walks. Which of these various tasks were performed by which men depended upon the relative's impairment, and on factors such as the caregiver's personal predilections, work status, and the availability, in economic terms in the United States and in programmatic terms in Japan, of home services such as visiting nurses and home helpers. In general, husbands did more hands-on care than sons, who were more often employed and more likely to make use of social services to assist in caregiving tasks. An important task for the American sons was providing emotional support.

Impact on the men's family lives

The need to provide care and the burdens of doing so created conflict in some families and brought others closer together. The extent of conflict (whether open or internalized) appeared to depend on cultural expectations of who should provide care. American husbands were grateful for the assistance of siblings or children, but expected little from them. A few of the American sons whose fathers were not involved in caring for their wives were resentful and angry at their father's "abdication of his responsibility." Japanese husband caregivers expressed varying degrees of resignation to their unexpected role, but some also expressed a great deal of disappointment and frustration when children, particularly those living nearby, refused to help, or ignored their mother's situation entirely. (See, for example, the discussion of the Suzuki family in Campbell and Ingersoll-Dayton, Chapter 11 this volume.) In the families in which children (or daughters-in-law) brought meals and/or visited regularly, family relations appeared to be a great source of support and happiness for the husband caregiver. In both countries, some of the son caregivers experienced disagreements with siblings if there was an expectation that siblings would help out more than they did. However, the Japanese sons were all the eldest son in their family, and the expectation that they would be the sole or primary caregiver was strong. Most of these sons, however, experienced role conflict and sometimes openly argued with their wives concerning their responsibilities for caring for their parent. The American sons reported that their wives were supportive of their activities and sometimes assisted them in caring for their parent, though the sons sometimes experienced conflicts between responsibilities toward their parent and toward their own nuclear family due to time limitations.

Conflict between caregiving and work

Generational differences in this area were pronounced in both countries. Most of the American husbands were already retired when they began taking care of their wives. Many Japanese husbands had retired from their career jobs and although some were working in post-retirement jobs when their wives became ill, they expressed little conflict over leaving that job to provide care. They missed their more social experiences of work as well as the spending money it provided, but their pensions made it possible to make caregiving their priority. On the other hand, most sons in both countries were employed and their caregiving forced them to make sacrifices in their careers by giving up promotions, changing jobs, or moving to be closer to their parent.

Impact on the men's personal lives

Caregiving impacted on the personal lives of all of the men in both positive and negative ways. One of the greatest and most consistently reported problems faced by all caregivers is the lack of time for themselves, time to pursue friendships and hobbies. This seemed particularly acute in Japan, where the continuous physical presence of the caregiver is experienced as a form of reassurance and thus seen as an important aspect of the caregiving role (Long, 1996; Long, 1997). Being a caregiver was, for most of the men, a lonely experience.

Many of the men in both countries, however, indicated that their sad and unpleasant situation was also a source of personal growth for them. They took pride in learning new roles and in gaining knowledge about their relatives' disease, negotiating service systems, and developing greater awareness of social problems related to the elderly. A few noted that they had developed closer relationships with their impaired relatives or with other family members, had learned to communicate more openly, or had come to understand the satisfactions of nurturing.

The impact of gender on men's caregiving experiences

Many of the tasks, burdens, and variation in experience described by the men we interviewed are similar to those described for female caregivers of the elderly. In both countries, cultural expectations influence the style and expectations of caregiving for both men and women. Yet one of the strongest cultural assumptions in both Japan and the US is that women are the natural nurturers, and therefore that it is women who should and do care for the elderly. Does this assumption make a difference in the experience of men who take on this responsibility in spite of cultural norms about appropriate gender roles? Our data suggest that gender role socialization and gendered societal expectations *do* make a difference in the ways that men experience and interpret their caregiving activities.

Skills for caregiving

When a woman becomes a caregiver of an elderly relative, in many ways it is a continuation of other roles she has performed over her life course. Despite more flexibility in gender roles in recent years, particularly in the United States, most women continue to perform the majority of household tasks and are the primary caretakers of children. They are more likely than their husbands to have cared for ill children or other relatives, and are more likely to have a job that involves these skills. Furthermore, society expects women to have such skills either through nature (their female genes), or nurture (their life experiences) (Anderson, 1997; Bonvillain, 1998; Hochschild and Machung, 1989; O'Connell, 1993; Renzetti and Curran, 1995).

In contrast, caregiving for men most often means moving into uncharted territory for them. Particularly for the husbands in our study, they were challenged to learn new skills in their later years, a source of both stress and pride. The American husbands talked about learning to cook and to plan nutritionally balanced meals. They were concerned with learning about female hygiene, with toileting, grooming, bathing, and dressing another person. For some, their wives' illnesses caused them for the first time to be responsible for household financial matters such as paying bills and balancing checkbooks. Japanese husbands stressed that they had needed to learn housekeeping tasks, cooking, shopping, and laundry activities, which previously their wives had performed, although in some cases nearby daughters or daughters-in-law now assisted with these tasks. Despite the physical hardship of getting the impaired elderly person in and out of the deep tubs, the Japanese men seemed more comfortable than the Americans with bathing another person, perhaps due to a lifetime of experiences bathing with others, including assisting children (Clark, 1994). Men in both countries said that they learned these skills informally, through trial and error, practice, and advice from health professionals, female relatives, and home helpers. Some of the American men participated in support groups for male caregivers which provided a source of suggestions and advice from other men in similar situations. A few local governments in Japan have begun to offer adult education classes for men in homemaking (Jenike, 1997, p. 334), but none of the men in our study had participated in these programs. Several had joined support groups for families of the demented elderly, which offered a forum to discuss problems in a sympathetic group.

Acquisition of another set of skills was more subtle. Older men in both countries generally have less developed friendship networks outside of the workplace, and relationships with neighbors and relatives are often maintained through the efforts of their wives. Communication styles in both countries are also gendered. In Japanese, differences in vocabulary and levels of politeness between masculine and feminine speech clearly and continuously indicate men's superior social status, so that, for example, men may commonly refer to their wives as *gusai* ("foolish wife") or *kanai* ("[the one] in the house"), while women refer to their husbands with the term for household head or master. Japanese women may not be encouraged to express their emotions, but they are expected to take the responsibility for anticipating the physical and emotional needs of others in a way that men are not (Iwao, 1993; Lebra, 1984). American women are often encouraged to be more expressive, to talk more about emotions and social relationships, than are men (Tannen, 1990; Wood, 1997).

These social and communication skills are related to obtaining information, assistance and support, to providing comfort and companionship to the elderly relative, and sometimes to coping with the difficulties of caregiving. Some of the men in our study responded to their lack of skills in this area by bringing a different set of "masculine" skills to the job. American sons, in particular, attempted to assert control over the situation, relentlessly searching out information, and being assertive in obtaining the medical and social services their parents needed. Some of the men brought skills from the workplace to the job of caregiving, such as planning and coordinating the schedules and activities of numerous service providers, organizing the household, and utilizing a problem-solving approach to difficulties that arose in the course of caregiving. Yet some men in both countries also spoke of learning new ways to communicate, and of becoming closer to their wives or parents through nurturing.

Gender also mattered in the men's descriptions of their means of coping with caregiver burden, though cultural differences are also important. American women cope by talking with a confidante, utilizing their social networks, and sometimes by using psychotropic drugs (George, 1984). Japanese women caregivers seem more reluctant to ask for assistance in caregiving and express that they must bear the burden, but they do complain of physical pain and illness for which it is acceptable to obtain treatment. (See Ohnuki-Tierney, 1984 and Lock, 1987 regarding somatization in Japanese society.) Some of the literature on caregiver burden in the United States has reported that men experience less of a burden, suggesting that men either do not do as much or do not experience what they do as so stressful (Fitting *et al.*, 1986; Miller and Cafasso, 1992). However, it is also possible that they are less willing to use complaining as a coping method. The men in our study described a strong sense of burden when given the opportunity to talk about their experiences. But their methods of coping seemed different from those of women caregivers. Whereas women in both countries use respite care to fulfill other responsibilities such as housekeeping or childcare, some of the men, particularly American husbands, saw respite as a chance to reconnect with their former lives. It was assumed that this break to pursue their own hobbies or to get out to socialize would be temporary and that they would come back to their caregiving duties refreshed and better prepared to continue their caregiving. In contrast to the somatization of stress among Japanese women, several of the Japanese husbands emphasized the need to maintain their own health in order to continue to provide care. They believed this could be accomplished by eating properly and by going for walks when they had time. Other methods of coping were less effective. The men rarely spoke of turning to friends or other confidantes. Although not gender-specific, we did hear over the course of our research that some of the men used alcohol as an escape from problems, took psychoactive drugs for depression, or occasionally lashed out in physical abuse of the elderly family member. (See also Ono, 1998.)

Identity issues: masculinity and nurturing activity

As women perform caregiving tasks, they are acting consistently with gender role expectations in both Japan and the United States. However, as men take on caregiving, they may experience it as a discontinuity in their lives, one that implicitly challenges the masculine self-identity they have constructed over the years. In our study, this seemed less of an issue for sons than for husbands. Sons continued working and thus maintained active participation in some elements of their "normal life." Being younger, some of the sons may have more androgynous role expectations than did their parents' generation.

Consequently, husband caregivers give up more of their previous lifestyles than sons when they assume responsibility for caregiving. One husband's account reflects the feelings of others in the study when he spoke of his need to go out to the garage now and then to work on his projects in order to get back in touch with his masculine self. Other American husbands spoke of issues of sexuality, not wanting to "take advantage" of their demented wives but experiencing loss of their masculinity. Japanese husbands seemed more resigned to the change in gendered activity, but nonetheless spoke regretfully of a loss of the sociability and autonomy characteristic of the world of adult men. They, like many of the American husbands, coped with this sense of loss by reinterpreting caregiving as an opportunity for *kaeshi*, repaying their wives for years of care, rather than focusing on issues of gender identity.

Societal responses to men providing elder care

Since, in both societies, women are expected to be the family caregivers, men who take on this role are in some sense deviant. Their non-normative gender behavior evokes two types of responses that differ from responses to women caregivers. First, the men are sometimes praised or given special recognition for caregiving that women doing the same activities would not receive because it is expected of women, but not of men. People may offer assistance; for example, many American husbands were aided by their own sisters. Daughters and daughters-in-law may cook and do other "feminine" tasks to help a father who is caregiving that they would not do for a caregiving mother. Female neighbors may offer advice. Men are told that they are doing a difficult job well, as one Japanese husband reported: "I have a good reputation in the community."

Yet the more common response is disbelief that men are actually doing all that women family caregivers do. American men complained in interviews that people treated them as though they were incompetent, although they themselves felt comfortable with their role. Health care providers failed to include American husbands and sons in planning meetings about the patient. Some employers, even when personally understanding of the strains on Japanese and American sons, officially ignored the family situation or treated these sons as anomalies in the work force rather than assisting them in getting through a difficult period in their lives. In short, male caregivers were not expected to be able to provide comparable care to that provided by women, and thus at times were not taken seriously. Their crossing gender roles rendered them less capable or invisible in the eyes of others.

Men's caregiving experiences: challenges to public assumptions about caregiving

We have described the activities and ideas of the male caregivers we interviewed, and have found that although they share many experiences with women caregivers, gender does make a difference in the way they experience other aspects of their role. These gender-specific issues challenge general public assumptions about the caregiving role and the policies based upon them. In this section, we delineate some of these areas.

Who is providing the care?

In both the United States and Japan, it has been assumed that women are not only the normative caregivers, but are the most competent. The men we interviewed, despite limited caregiving experiences, showed that men are able to provide a wide range of hands-on instrumental and emotional support for an extended period of time for a spouse or parent. Although we are not aware of policies specifying that caregivers must be female, directly and indirectly, the two governments have supported workplace policy that has encouraged a continued subordinate role of women in the labor force (Anderson, 1997; Boling, 1998; Bonvillain, 1998; Brinton, 1993; Renzetti and Curran, 1995; Sugimoto, 1997), which in turn makes it more likely that a woman will remain outside of the labor force or be more likely than her husband to leave the labor force to take on family responsibilities. The main economic resources of society are in the hands of men, leaving women to define their most significant roles in other directions such as nurturing. Mandatory retirement ages in Japan differ for men and women, making middle-aged women more available for caregiving. But if men can be competent caregivers, should not family caregiving policy encourage them to take on that role and to be seen as competent by others?

Motivations for caregiving

In Japan, caregiving is often portrayed as an onerous burden, done by wives, daughters, and daughters-in-law out of a sense of duty and with great resentment. Together with the realities of demographics and the genuine difficulties of caregiving, these portrayals have pushed the Japanese government toward increasing funding for services and to accept increased responsibility for the welfare of the elderly with the Gold Plan (Ten Year Strategy to Promote Health Care and Welfare Services for the Elderly) and the Long-Term Care Insurance (*Kaigo Hoken*) program. In the United States, there has been a cultural assumption that men will provide care only when there is no available female relative to do so, a phenomenon labeled by sociologists as the "hierarchy of family substitution" (Cantor, 1983). The men in our study indicate that there is a much broader range of motivations for caregiving. Although many did express a sense of duty, their commitment to carry through was often also motivated by other factors such as love, keeping promises, and repaying past nurturing. The significance of recognizing varying motivations is that the individual's reasons for taking on this role, in the case of men, colors the ways in which they assign meaning to the tasks they perform. For some of the men, this made their caregiving a different kind of experience from the common assumptions of it as a burden to be avoided, despite the fact that they were performing the same onerous tasks.

Relation between work and caregiving

Husband caregivers clearly point to the need for financial security in later years. Japanese husbands often gave up post-retirement jobs when they became caregivers, and were able to do so financially only because of pension benefits. American husbands were usually retired, but as fear of the breakdown of the social security system leads to increased privatization of pensions and medical benefits, more men will be pressured to work to pay for these, impacting on their availability and energy for caregiving.

In both countries, sons were faced with tremendous stress as they tried to juggle work and caregiving responsibilities in workplaces which assume that workers have wives at home to be nurturers for the family. Women have either remained out of the work force or in subordinate positions with lower pay, both reflecting and reinforcing their movement in and out of the labor force to take on caregiving responsibilities for children and elderly relatives. Policies in both countries have maintained a separation between the work and family lives of their employees, rendering family caregiving needs invisible or secondary. Labor laws have protected individual workers by regulating such things as hours, conditions, and child labor, but have not protected family needs. Son caregivers in both countries challenge the assumptions that work and family can be kept separate.

Service utilization

The men in our study challenge several assumptions about service utilization, though these assumptions have been different in the two countries. In Japan, there is a myth that caregivers are reluctant to utilize services because of the stigma (people afraid they will be criticized for not doing a good job) and the reluctance to have strangers come into the home. Most of the Japanese husbands did make grateful use of home help. For sons, the availability of help was critical to their ability to continue working. Both sons and husbands wished for greater availability of services.

The American assumption is labeled the Hydra-headed myth of gerontology. Policy makers have believed that Americans do not take care of their family members, and that providing more services will only promote that tendency. The male caregivers we interviewed, like their female counterparts, challenged that myth with their commitment even while utilizing formal services. When they used respite services, it was done as a means of coping with stress, not to abandon their caregiving responsibilities. For American sons, like Japanese sons, the availability of high quality services was critical to their ability to continue working.

Thus, men *are* providing care, and doing so with a variety of motivations. They have shown commitment to taking on this role despite their society's stereotypes about their competence and their lack of experience in nurturing roles. However, they need policies to support their efforts in the areas of financial security, the workplace, and service provision.

Policy and program implications

Thus, listening to the experiences of caregiving men has led us to question some of the gendered assumptions behind policies and programs in Japan and the United States. Policies and programs will need to be rethought and restructured if we are to meet the specific gendered needs of this developing new group of caregivers. Both countries would benefit from program development that implements gender-responsive, rather than gender-neutral, policy. These are policies that recognize the need for financial security for caregivers and care recipients, encourage more responsive, family-oriented workplaces, and in the public arena provide economic incentives and increased funding for innovative long-term, community-based care services that empower men as well as women caregivers.

Financial security

Meeting basic financial needs was a problem for some of the men in our study. In the United States, there was great variability among the husbands in their financial security. For men who had retired from professional and managerial positions, their private pensions, social security benefits, savings, and other investment income provided them with a comfortable retirement income. However, for less affluent men in the study, their limited retirement incomes were based mainly on their social security benefits. This often meant having to make a choice between needed medications, proper nutrition, or respite care. This was particularly true of the African Americans in our study, consistent with national data showing that older African-American men are five times more likely to be poor than older white men (Gonyea, 1995).

In Japan, we were impressed with the changes that have occurred in the pension system that allow elderly couples to maintain economic independence from their children (see Campbell, 1992 for history of the pension system in Japan). In the recent past, social security pensions were so small that they were considered little more than "spending money." By the mid-1990s, a two-tier national pension system provided at least a minimal level of universal coverage for those over 65, including non-wage-earning housewives (Hoshino, 1996). About the same time, however, the system was reformed to encourage continued participation of older workers in the labor force by allowing for partial working pensions and creating wage subsidies for older workers (Koshiro, 1996; see also Roberts, 1996 on Silver Human Resource Centers). This system seems to take into account the need for pensions for those who are impaired and unable to continue working; however, it does not recognize that an older person caring for an impaired spouse will also be unable to continue to participate in the labor force. Thus the system still seems to be based on the assumption that wives and daughters-in-law, who are not in the labor force, will be the primary caregivers. The husbands we interviewed in Japan did not complain of economic difficulties. However, as more of the costs previously covered by Medical Care for the Elderly (*Rōjin Hoken*) are shifted to the family, particularly limitations of stay in hospitals and higher out-of-pocket copayments for medical care and drugs, the loss of the husband's wages will be more strongly felt. Financial security is the backbone of good family caregiving policy.

Workplace

For caregiving sons and some husbands, there is no option but to remain in the labor force. We believe that a number of changes in workplace policy would encourage men to take on caregiving responsibilities, and be able to offer more assistance to other family caregivers. Many of the company policies that have been developed to make workplaces more family-friendly regarding child care can be extended and adapted for elder care. Although some companies have taken the lead in this regard, it is often public policy that encourages such programs through laws and incentives.

The first step in a family-oriented workplace is the recognition that men too are involved in family care, both elder and child care. Recognition of the need for better balance between work and family responsibilities, and promotion of such an underlying philosophy, form the cornerstone of progressive workplace policies. For men as well as for women, employers might provide flextime opportunities, opportunities for job sharing, more opportunities for home-based work, expanded family care leave, employee assistance programs with counselors that are knowledgeable about elder care issues, and a cafeteria-type benefit plan that includes elder care options. Some American companies such as Stride Rite and Campbell's Soup were innovators a decade ago by offering on-site intergenerational day care programs for employees' family members.

American policies such as The Federal Family and Medical Leave Act of 1993 are written in gender-neutral language. The extent to which men take advantage of such policies will depend not only on their personal commitment, but on wider economic policies which determine men's and women's employment options, and on cultural attitudes about men's relative involvement in work and family. It will also depend on the opportunities available to women.

Japan has moved rapidly in the past decade to develop family-friendly policy regarding children, offering tax deductions and an extensive network of publicly subsidized day care centers. A child care leave law gives either parent up to a year's leave of absence following childbirth, and subsidies are provided to employers for compliance; however compliance remains voluntary. Over 99 percent of employees who take such leave are women (Rōdōshō, 1996; Boling, 1998). As in the US, there is no national-level policy supporting *paid* leave for elder care. Despite this, a larger proportion of those who take elder care leave than those who take child care leave are men, about 19 percent (Rōdōshō, 1996). Yet generally workers who can no longer juggle work and caregiving responsibilities leave their jobs permanently; these are most often low-paid women (see Brinton, 1993) whose departure leaves employers little sense of responsibility for developing policy and programs. Only two of the five sons we interviewed in Japan had corporate jobs (two others were self-employed and one was unemployed). Although they believed that their supervisors were "understanding," there was no attempt to institutionalize such understanding in workplace policy regarding work hours, qualifications for promotions, or referral services. Rather, they were relieved of some individual work responsibilities, but with, they believed, significant consequences for their future careers. The Japanese government has the opportunity to take a leadership role in promoting family-oriented workplaces in ways similar to what it has done for child care, but as in the United States, significant cultural change will need to accompany policy before most men are likely to feel comfortable taking advantage of such programs.

Long-term care

Policy that provides economic incentives and funding for family care is a critical factor to encourage male caregiving. In Japan, programs and policy for the elderly have been divided between those for medical care and those considered social services. There was little attempt to coordinate policy across this divide, with results such as the use of hospitals as long-term residential facilities. While the Medical Care for the Elderly program has been well funded through a combination of premiums, tax money, and government-sponsored redistribution among insurance programs, social services have had to rely largely on local government funding, resulting in great variation in the type and amount of services provided from one municipality to another, even with the 1994 revision of the Gold Plan. This lack of coordination has meant lack of integration of services to support not only the impaired elderly person, but also his or her caregivers. The passing of the Long-Term Care Insurance Act in 1997 will create a system intended to coordinate medical and social services in individualized care plans (Kimura, 1996). As programs are developed, government welfare workers at all levels should consider options for care plans involving husbands and sons, and work to provide all caregivers with the support that they need to fulfill those responsibilities.

In contrast, the United States has not had an overall long-term care policy, but has relied only on Medicare and Medicaid to assist older adults who have become ill. These programs have focused little on supporting family caregiving. The economic incentives in the United States for elder care, though changing, still promote institutional care. In the United States, it has been estimated that out-of-pocket long-term care costs for families are as much as $54 billion annually (McConnell and Riggs, 1994). A higher percentage of family caregivers compared to the overall elderly population have incomes below the poverty line (Hooyman and Gonyea, 1995). Only 25 percent of non-institutional care is publicly subsidized (Leutz et al., 1992). Medicare, the major health program for the elderly, is structured to pay primarily for acute hospital care, and only 3 percent of its expenditures pay for home health care (Binstock, 1990).

American policy can be made more supportive of both male and female family caregivers by expanding dependent care tax credits, with fewer restrictions on whom and how the funds should be spent, and more recognition given to the impact of the level of the care recipient's impairment. This would give the family more options to purchase services or to provide the care themselves. More funding needs to be made available for innovative community-based care that would promote male caregiving. The always present fear in the minds of American policy makers that if funding for elder care is made available, families will abdicate their responsibility has to finally be abandoned. More funding to aid families in elder care will only promote more family care, not discourage families, as shown by the men in our study.

Social support programs

To varying degrees, husband and son caregivers in both countries experienced social isolation and had limited support networks. This can be addressed through a number of approaches. One approach is support groups, gender mixed or gender specific. Support groups for caregivers organized around specific diseases have become popular in the United States and are increasing in Japan as well. These types of self-help groups provide emotional support, a chance to expand social networks, and accurate up-to-date information about a disease with concrete helpful advice for handling the daily struggles of caregiving (Montgomery, 1995). Another approach would be a time-limited educational-based group with a format like a workshop. This more formal presentation of material, with emphasis on education rather than support, may appeal to men more than a traditional support group (Harris, 1993; Harris and Bichler, 1997). In Japan, support groups sometimes function as interest groups which lobby for particular policies or legislation, often at the local or prefectural level. We would expect cultural differences in the way such groups are organized and conducted (see, for example, Smith, 1998 on alcoholics' groups). The educational format might appeal more to Japanese caregivers given the social value of life-long learning (Vogel, 1979). One problem, however, is the reluctance of Japanese husbands to leave their wives for a period of time, especially if it is not absolutely necessary (see Harris and Long, 1999; Long, 1997). Sons, on the other hand, may not feel that they have time to attend even an educational session because of work commitments.

A more accessible method of support for many men, both in Japan and the United States, might be the use of computer support networks, such as is available through the internet (Smyth and Harris, 1993). This support has features unique to this medium that are congruent with the needs of the male caregivers we described. A computer support group is available twenty-four hours a day with up-to-date helpful concrete suggestions about the "how-to" of caregiving. The system allows the participants to remain anonymous, if they choose, so men who have difficulty expressing their thoughts and feelings to others do not have to reveal their identities. Governmental funding can promote the development of such networks through hospitals and social service agencies that could also reach rural districts, which may have more limited availability of services.

Social networking opportunities can be promoted through male friendship clubs at senior centers and golden age clubs in either country. As mentioned earlier, male caregivers frequently lack confidants. For older employees, companies could develop "hobby clubs" or drop-in centers where men with similar interests could meet and establish some bonds of friendship that would extend beyond their work-related ties. These clubs on the companies' grounds could continue into the post-retirement years.

Educational/skill enhancement programs

Male caregivers needed skill development and education, as well as information about the medical problems of their family member and the services available for them.

Caregiver education includes a broad array of topics. Besides covering general information such as disease and behavior management, men need classes and workshops that specifically address issues of personal care skills, cooking, household and financial management, and (in the United States) hiring and supervising home help. Personal care classes that particularly emphasize female hygiene, grooming, clothes shopping, toileting and bathroom safety, and bathing, can be held in local senior and adult day care centers (see reference to such a program sponsored by local government in Jenike, 1997). Cooking was a big hurdle for many men to overcome in both countries, and courses that focus on the fundamentals of nutrition and cooking need to be developed. Some husbands in both the American and Japanese samples had turned over their paychecks to their wives who managed the finances of the house. These husbands had no experience in paying the bills or personal banking. The American husbands were further burdened with handling the overwhelming number of health care statements and bills from Medicare and Medigap insurance policies.

In the United States, where home help is not available through governmental sources as it is in Japan, sons and husbands expressed a great need for a class that would teach them how to screen, hire, and supervise home help aides. The American son caregivers felt frustrated and bewildered by the maze of services and programs available, which often had different eligibility and financing requirements. They wanted individually tailored professional advice in the care and management of their parents. Sons wanted case management services available from a centrally located social service agency. They expected and demanded more service options and availability than husbands. If this type of information were also available through company employment assistance programs, the information would be even more accessible for son caregivers. Although services in Japan are similarly scattered across a number of institutions and offices, the Long-Term Care Insurance program in Japan is being designed to centralize services in that country, which will relieve some of the coordinating and assessment functions now daunting family caregivers (Bungei Shunjū, 1996).

Respite care and related services

The American samples, both sons and husbands, made more use of respite care than the Japanese sample, since this service was congruent with the American model of good care. Time away was seen as being beneficial to caregivers so they could rejuvenate themselves and return refreshed to resume their caregiving responsibilities. It was the service most sought after by these caregivers. Both Americans and Japanese complained of very limited availability of respite programs and of their restrictive hours. There were few weekend and evening respite care programs available. In the United States there also was the compounded problem of affordability. Most American respite programs were paid out of pocket by caregivers since there is little government funding to cover these services. In Japan, despite the expansion of services under the 1989 Gold Plan and its 1994 revision, Japanese caregivers, especially the working sons, had to supplement government services with private ones. This is an area where funds are sorely needed, and where the decision of what services would be most useful and who should provide these services should be left to the families' discretion, or worked out together with service providers.

Conclusion

Neither Japan nor America has sufficiently recognized that a significant number of men are caring for elderly relatives who need assistance. Without this awareness, there is little research that explores the significance of gender in caregiving, and programs that address special needs of male caregivers remain underdeveloped. Policy that on the surface is gender-neutral continues to be based on models of female nurturance. Thus, the men in our study often felt they were facing a monumental task alone and unprepared. This chapter has exposed some of the underlying assumptions that have left gaps in the policies and service-delivery systems in both countries, and serves as a challenge to policy makers and service providers to recognize and meet the growing needs of male caregivers. In both countries, a paradigm shift is needed that redefines caregiving not as a woman's role, but as an experience shaped in part by gender. This opens the way for recognizing men's roles and responsibilities in elder care and leads to better understanding of the experiences of *all* family caregivers.

Implications for caregivers

Clearly, in both societies, men can no longer be considered exceptional or temporary caregivers. They represent an important option for families for providing consistent and competent care for older family members. Men may experience the caregiver role differently than women because they come to it with different life experiences. When families, friends, and neighbors recognize that men's experiences can be integrated into the caregiving role, they will be more accepting of alternative ways to provide care beyond the stereotype of female nurturing. Thus they will be more accepting and more supportive of men who do care for elderly relatives.

By viewing caregiving as a gendered experience, social service and health care providers will be better able to discern the role that men play in elder care, and the strengths and weaknesses they bring to these tasks. For example, many men come to caregiving with limited nursing and housekeeping skills and with minimal social support networks, yet they broaden the role with their problem-solving and coping strategies.

Recognizing the gendered nature of caregiving will benefit daughters and wives as well as sons and husbands. Increasingly, in both countries women remain in the labor market as full-time workers. Like the husbands and sons in our study, many women are committed to caring for elderly parents, and face struggles of time and income, incongruities of necessary caregiving skills with past experiences, and issues of personal identity. Thus it is not the *sex* of the caregiver that is the crux of our argument, but rather the changing *gendered* experiences that men and women bring to caregiving that need to be recognized.

Implications for policy and programs

The words of the men we interviewed cause us to rethink assumptions that are often incorporated into policy: Who provides the care for impaired elderly relatives? What are their motivations? How do caregivers balance work and caregiving responsibilities? What types of services are desired and needed? Their responses point to the impact of numerous areas of policy that can be reformulated to better meet the needs of these caregivers and of society at large.

- In the area of financial security, policy should recognize the need for pensions not only for those who are impaired, but also on the part of caregivers who must retire or take unpaid leave to provide care for an elderly relative, regardless of the age or gender of the caregiver.
- Labor policy must encourage greater gender equity in the workplace, family-oriented workplace policies, and an environment in which workers are not penalized for taking on caregiver responsibilities.
- Long-term care policy needs to incorporate specific programs which meet the needs of men for social support, skill development, and respite care rather than assume women will be available for caregiving.

Policies in these areas that encourage men to be caregivers will simultaneously ease the burden on women caregivers as well. Gender-responsive caregiver policy and programs will enable more elderly people to receive family care by relatives who are better prepared, are financially able to take on the burdens, experience less conflict with other roles, and have more support in dealing with the anxieties and strains of their responsibilities.

Comparative, qualitative research and policy analysis

The findings of this study illustrate that a comparative research approach can clearly expose the cultural assumptions upon which caregiving is based. Through comparison, we can identifying how cultural and personal factors help shape the way men experience their roles. Qualitative studies such as this one can identify changing social roles and provide policy makers and service providers with guidance as they move toward the future. These studies broaden perspectives, leading people to ask new questions and look for new options. By their immediacy, they also serve as a reminder that humans are first of all social and cultural beings who are not only shaped by policy, but should have a strong voice in its creation.

Policy makers must be concerned with a variety of issues, ranging from practical political considerations to satisfying the broadest possible range of constituents. They must be concerned wtih financial cost and feasibility. However, by beginning to understand the day-to-day experience of caregivers and the meanings they assign to that experience, policy makers can move toward designing better policy and programs to support *all* family caregivers.

Acknowledgments

The authors are grateful to Miwa Fujii for research assistance, to Michiko Naoi and Takako Sodei for assistance in locating Japanese literature and statistics, to John Traphagan for helpful comments on an earlier draft, and to the participants in the Abe colloquium for their insights and suggestions.

References

Anderson, M.L. (1997). *Thinking about women: Sociological perspectives on sex and gender*. Boston: Allyn and Bacon.

Aneshensel, C.S., Pearlin, L.I., Mullan, T.J., and Witlatch, C.J. (1995). *Profiles in caregiving: The unexpected career*. San Diego: Academic Press.

Binstock, R. (1990). The politics and economics of aging and diversity. In S. Bass, E. Kutea, and F.M. Torres-Gel (Eds.), *Diversity in aging* (pp. 73–98). Glenview, IL: Scott Foresman.

Boling, P. (1998). Family policy in Japan. *Journal of Social Policy, 27*, 2, 173–190.

Bonvillain, N. (1998). *Women and men: Cultural constructs of gender* (2nd ed.). Upper Saddle River, NJ: Prentice Hall.

Brinton, M.C. (1993). *Women and the economic miracle: Gender and work in postwar Japan*. Berkeley: University of California Press.

Brody, E.M. (1990). *Women in the middle*. New York: Springer.

Bungei Shunjū (Ed.). (1996). *Nihon no ronten '97*, Chapter 13 (pp. 476–507). Tokyo: Bungei Shunjū.

Campbell, J.C. (1992). *How policies change: The Japanese government and the aging society*. Princeton, NJ: Princeton University Press.

Cantor, M.H. (1983). Strain among caregivers: A study of experience in the United States. *The Gerontologist, 23*, 597–604.

Clark, S. (1994). *Japan: A view from the bath*. Honolulu: University of Hawaii Press.

Fitting, M., Ragins, P., Lucas, M.J., and Eastham, J. (1986). Caregivers of demented patients: A comparison of husbands and wives. *The Gerontologist, 26*, 248–252.

George, L.K. (1984). The burden of caregiving: How much? What kinds? For what? *Advances in Research, 8*, 2. Durham, North Carolina: Duke University Center for the Study of Aging and Human Development.

Gonyea, J. (1995). Making gender visible in public policy. In E. Thompson (Ed.), *Older men* (pp. 237–255). Thousand Oaks, CA: Sage.

Harris, P.B. (1993). The misunderstood caregiver? A qualitative study of the male caregiver of Alzheimer's disease victims. *The Gerontologist, 33*, 4, 551–556.

Harris, P.B., and Bichler, J. (1997). *Men giving care: Reflections of husbands and sons.* New York: Garland Publishing.

Harris, P.B., and Long, S.O. (1993). Daughter-in-law's burden: An exploratory study of caregiving in Japan. *Journal of Cross-Cultural Gerontology, 8*, 97–118.

Harris, P.B., and Long, S.O. (1999). Male caregivers in the United States and Japan: Does culture matter? *Journal of Aging Studies, 13*, 3, 241–268.

Harris, P.B., Long, S.O., and Fujii, M. (1998). Men and elder care in Japan: A ripple of change? *Journal of Cross-Cultural Gerontology, 13*, 177–198.

Hashimoto, A. (1996). *The gift of generations: Japanese and American perspectives of aging and the social contract.* Cambridge: Cambridge University Press.

Hochschild, A., and Machung, A. (1989). *The second shift.* New York: Viking Penguin.

Hooyman, N., and Gonyea, J. (1995). *Feminist perspectives on family care.* Thousand Oaks, CA: Sage.

Horowitz, A. (1985). Family caregiving to the frail elderly. *Annual Review of Gerontology and Geriatrics, 5*, 194–246.

Hoshino, S. (1996). Paying for the health and social care of the elderly. In S.A. Bass, R. Morris, and M. Oka (Eds.), *Public policy and the old age revolution in Japan* (pp. 37–56). Binghamton, NY: Haworth Press.

Ikegami, N., and Yamada, T. (1996). Comparison of long-term care for the elderly between Japan and the United States. In N. Ikegami and J.C. Campbell (Eds.), *Containing health care costs in Japan* (pp. 155–171). Ann Arbor: University of Michigan Press.

Iwao, S. (1993). *The Japanese woman: Traditional image and changing reality.* New York: The Free Press.

Jenike, B.R. (1997). Home-based health care for the elderly in Japan: A silent system of gender and duty. In S. Formanek and S. Linhardt (Eds.), *Aging: Asian concepts and experiences, past and present* (pp. 329–346). Wien: Der Österreichischen Akademie der Wissenschaften.

Kimura, T. (1996). From transfer to social services: A new emphasis on social policies for the aged in Japan. In S.A. Bass, R. Morris, and M. Oka (Eds.), *Public policy and the old age revolution in Japan* (pp. 177–190). Binghamton, NY: Haworth Press.

Kōseishō (Ministry of Health and Welfare). (1996). *Kōsei hakusho, Heisei 8 nenpan (1996 Health and Welfare White Paper).* Tokyo: Kōseishō.

Kōseishō (Ministry of Health and Welfare). (1997). *Kōsei hakusho, Heisei 9 nenpan (1997 Health and Welfare White Paper).* Tokyo: Kōseishō.

Koshiro, K. (1996). Policies for a smoother transition from work to retirement. In S.A. Bass, R. Morris, and M. Oka (Eds.), *Public policy and the old age revolution in Japan* (pp. 97–114). Binghamton, NY: Haworth Press.

Kramer, B.J. (1997). Differential predictors of strain and gain among husbands caring for wives with dementia. *The Gerontologist, 37*, 2, 239–249.

Lebra, T.S. (1984). *Japanese women: Constraint and fulfillment.* Honolulu: University of Hawaii Press.

Leutz, W.N., Capitman, J.A., MacAdam, M., and Abrahams, R. (1992). *Care for frail elders: Developing community solutions.* Westport, CT: Auburn House.

Lock, M.M. (1987). Protests of a good wife and wise mother: The medicalization of distress in Japan. In E. Norbeck and M. Lock (Eds.), *Health, illness, and medical care in Japan: Cultural and social dimensions* (pp. 130–157). Honolulu: University of Hawaii Press.

Lock, M.M. (1993). *Encounters with aging: Mythologies of menopause in Japan and North America.* Berkeley: University of California Press.

Long, S.O. (1996). Nurturing and femininity: The ideal of caregiving in postwar Japan. In A. Imamura (Ed.), *Re-imaging Japanese women* (pp. 156–176). Berkeley: University of California Press.

Long, S.O. (1997). Risōteki na kaigo to wa? Amerika kara mita Nihon no rinen to genjitsu (What is ideal caregiving? Japanese ideals and reality from an American's perspective). *Hospisu Kea to Zaitaku Kea, 5*, 1, 37–43.

Long, S.O., and Harris, P.B. (1997). Caring for bedridden elderly: Ideals, realities, and social change in Japan. In S. Formanek and S. Linhardt (Eds.), *Aging: Asian concepts and experiences, past and present* (pp. 347–368). Wien: Der Österreichischen Akademie der Wissenschaften.

Martin, L.G. (1989). The graying of Japan. *Population Bulletin, 44*, 2, 1–41.

McConnell, S., and Riggs, J. (1994). A public policy agenda: Supporting family caregiving. In M. Cantor (Ed.), *Family caregiving: An agenda for the future* (pp. 25–34). San Francisco: American Society on Aging.

Miller, B. (1990). Gender differences in spouse management of the caregiver role. In *Circles of care: Work and identity in women's lives* (pp. 92–104). Albany: State University of New York Press.

Miller, B., and Cafasso, L. (1992). Gender differences in caregiving: Fact or artifact? *The Gerontologist, 32*, 498–507.

Montgomery, R. (1995). Molding interventions to the caregivers mosaic. Paper presented at the Center for Practice Innovations Conference, Case Western Reserve University, Cleveland.

Montgomery, R., and Kamo, Y. (1987). Differences between sons and daughters in parental caregiving. Paper presented at the 36th Annual Scientific Meeting of the Gerontological Society of America, Washington, D.C.

Montgomery, R., Kosloski, K., and Borgatta, E. (1990). Service use and the caregiving experience: Does Alzheimer's disease make a difference? In D.E. Biegel and A. Blum (Eds.), *Aging and caregiving: Theory, research, and policy* (pp. 139–159). Newbury Park, CA: Sage.

Mui, A.C. (1995). Caring for frail elderly parents: A comparison of adult sons and daughters. *The Gerontologist, 35*, 86–93.

National Alliance for Caregiving, and The American Association of Retired Persons. (1997). *Family caregiving in the United States: Findings from a national study*. Washington, DC: National Alliance for Caregiving and the American Association of Retired Persons.

O'Connell, M. (1993). *Where's papa? Father's role in child care*. Washington, DC: Population Reference Bureau.

Odahara, H., and Nakayama, T. (1992). *Chihōsei rōjin kanja no zaitaku kango ni oyobasu eikyō no kentō: Dansei kaigosha no ishiki to jittai chōsa* (Factors affecting home care for the elderly with dementia: Survey of awareness and actual situation of male caregivers). *Rōnen Shakai Kagaku, 14 Suppl.*, 84–89.

Ohnuki-Tierney, E. (1984). *Illness and culture in contemporary Japan*. Cambridge: Cambridge University Press.

Okuyama, N. (1996). *Seibetsu yakuwari kara mita kōrei dansei kaigosha no kaigo* (A study on gender role and male elderly caregivers). *Shakaigaku Kenkyūka Ronshū, 3*, 27–38.

Okuyama, N. (1997). *Bunken kara mita zaitaku de no dansei kaigosha no kaigo* (A study on the literature concerning male caregivers). *Tōkyō Toritsu Iryō Gijutsu Tanki Daigaku Kiyō, 10*, 267–272.

Ono, S. (1998). Taking care of ill wives pushes elderly men over the edge. *AERA*. July 14, 1998. Asahi English Language Edition, at http://www.asahi.com/english/english.html.

Pearlin, L.I., Mullan, J., Semple, J.T., and Skaff, M.M. (1990). Caregiving and the stress process: An overview of concepts and their measures. *The Gerontologist, 30,* 583–594.
Renzetti, C.M., and Curran, D.J. (1995). *Women, men, and society* (3rd ed.). Boston: Allyn & Bacon.
Roberts, G.S. (1996). Between policy and practice: Japan's Silver Human Resource Centers as viewed from the inside. In S.A. Bass, R. Morris, and M. Oka (Eds.), *Public policy and the old age revolution in Japan* (pp. 115–132). Binghamton, NY: Haworth Press.
Rōdōshō. (Ministry of Labor). (1996). *Joshi koyō kanri chōsa* (Survey on the management of working women). Tokyo: Rōdōshō.
Smith, S. (1998). Good old boy into alcoholic: *Danshukai* and learning a new drinking role in Japan. In J. Singleton (Ed.), *Learning in likely places: Varieties of apprenticeship in Japan.* Cambridge: Cambridge University Press.
Smyth, K.A., and Harris, P.B. (1993). Using telecomputing to provide information and support to caregivers of persons with dementia. *The Gerontologist, 33,* 123–127.
Sodei, T. (1997). Women's two roles and gender equity. *Journal of Home Economics of Japan, 48,* 1, 91–98.
Stone, R., Cafferata, G., and Sangl, J. (1987). Caregivers of the frail elderly: A national profile. *The Gerontologist, 29,* 677–683.
Stoller, E.P. (1992). Gender differences in the experiences of caregiving spouses. In J.W. Dwyer and R.T. Coward (Eds.), *Gender, families, and elder care* (pp. 49–64). Newbury Park, CA: Sage.
Sugimoto, Y. (1997). *An introduction to Japanese society.* Cambridge: Cambridge University Press.
Takenaga, M. (1998). *Otoko no kaigo* (Male caregiving). Tokyo: Hoken.
Tannen, D. (1990). *You just don't understand: Women and men in conversation.* New York: Ballantine.
US Bureau of the Census. (1996). *Current population reports, Special studies, P23–190, 65+ in the United States.* Washington, DC: US Government Printing Office.
Vogel, E. (1979). *Japan as number one.* Cambridge: Harvard University Press.
Wood, J.T. (1997). *Gendered lives: Communication, gender, and culture* (2nd ed.). Belmont, CA: Wadsworth Publishing Co.

Part V
Facilitating care of self

13 The creativity of the demented elderly

The use of psychological approaches in a Japanese outpatient clinic

Yukiko Kurokawa

The creativity of the demented elderly

In Japan as well as in other countries, professionals spend a lot of time discussing solutions for the negative aspects of dementia. Much effort has been devoted to improving the quality of their physical care, including the development of new wheelchairs and all sorts of diapers. As for mental care, the focus of research and practice has been put on the management of problematic situations due to cognitive dysfunction, such as wandering and agitation. This kind of approach aims to minimize problems and primarily serves to benefit caregivers. Yet each person with dementia has a long history of living as an individual and does not wish to be treated merely as a "problem" for caregivers to manage. Rather, caring for people with dementia means assisting them to continue to live as individuals and recognizing their continuity of self despite cognitive impairments.

Professionals have come to a common understanding that they should watch and listen to people with dementia as whole persons, paying attention to their past history, how they lived, what they liked or disliked, and so on. This is made difficult in cases of people with dementia due to their cognitive impairment. Nonetheless, the core of one's personhood remains beyond cognitive impairment. With this understanding in mind, a number of attempts such as reality orientation (Holden and Woods, 1995), reminiscence and life review (Butler, 1963), validation therapy (Feil, 1989) and positive integrated approach (Holden and Woods, 1995) were developed to treat and care for people with dementia. These have proven to be effective, at least to some extent, for the psychological well-being of people with dementia.

Both in Japan and the United States, creativity is believed to be one of the most precious treasures of a human being. Thus professionals have tried to both be creative and to encourage the creativity of people with dementia. Campbell (1997) has pointed out the importance of finding solutions to problems associated with aging in a creative manner by considering the older person's strengths, emotions, experiences, and existing supports to fuel creative client-centered interventions. Have professionals tried hard enough to approach and appreciate the creativity of people with dementia? If professionals want clients to be creative, they need a strong desire for being creative themselves, encouraging people with dementia to express themselves in acceptable ways, not only creating problems, but expressing themselves through those problems.

The British poet, J. Killick (1994: 12) has scrupulously edited the written and verbal communications of people with dementia into written poetry. A person in a nursing home said to the poet,

> Are we all kidnapped?
> I'm not at all sure
> what kidnapping is, but
> I know I'm very frightened.
>
> I could go out there
> and sit on that swing
> and I would enjoy it.
> I want my freedom.
>
> But we none of us have our freedom.
> I don't understand so much
> that I'll just do without it,
> chuck the whole lot in the air.

These people with dementia appreciated the poet for coming and sitting down beside them, listening to them wholeheartedly, and trying to assist them to express themselves creatively without any practical purpose such as to feed, bathe, or dress them. This led many of them to really open up, although often the words needed to be edited to make sense. It is important to realize that a person with dementia, especially in its early stage, has great possibility for expressing him- or herself in extremely creative ways with appropriate assistance and on appropriate occasions. Moreover, the process of self-expression seems to be "interesting" and meaningful for them.

Little attention has been paid to the creativity of demented elderly. This chapter describes the present situation concerning activities for people with dementia in Japan. I then present two cases of people with dementia, focusing on their creativity and the methods we have developed to aid their self-expression. The quality of life of the demented elderly may be considerably improved by professional assistance in maintaining continuity of self, which suggests the need for policy which goes beyond custodial care.

Activities: the present situation in Japan

Current activities for people with dementia

There are a number of activities for people with dementia in Japan. Typical activities include creative work without large body movement; artwork such as *shodō*, calligraphy, flower arranging, pottery, sewing, knitting, and carving;

creative work with physical movement such as dance, singing, and drama; birthday parties; cooking; hiking; enjoying nature; tea time; outings; travel; music therapy; and reminiscence (Kurokawa, 1994, 1995).

Evaluation of activities by professionals

In 1996, the Foundation for the Prevention of Dementia conducted a survey concerning professional evaluation of these activities for demented people (Boke Yobō Kyōkai, 1996). Results showed that enjoying hobbies with physical movement and group rehabilitation were the two activities evaluated most highly by professionals as contributing to the physical well-being of people with dementia. The third most highly regarded were role-enhancing activities such as cooking, washing, and gardening. As for psychological well-being, reminiscence was the most highly evaluated program. Hiking and observing nature as well as role-enhancing activities were seen as valuable, whereas birthday parties and cooking activities were the least highly regarded. While birthday parties and cooking activities seem to be lively and popular everywhere, reminiscence is a more personalized, individualized approach. This survey suggests that professionals tend to prefer a personal, individualized approach, and gain less professional satisfaction through what they call the "stereotyped approach" utilized in many institutions both in Japan and the United States.

One of the reasons that health care professionals specializing in the care and treatment of people with dementia prefer personalized, individualized activities may be that they enrich the quality of life for the professionals themselves. Many professionals aim toward the psychological well-being of the person with dementia, but this is most often indirectly through physical care. Few attempts in Japan aim directly at psychological well-being, such as counseling or group approaches, or to enhancing the creativity of people with dementia.

Regardless of disciplinary background, some amount of training in psychological approaches is necessary for understanding and creating a rich personal relationship that will be meaningful for both the professional and the person with dementia, and will encourage their creativity.

Skills required for communicating with people with dementia

In this section, I will discuss issues concerning skills that facilitate communication with demented elderly people and can be used to approach their creativity.

Knowledge of the aging process

Dementia is a disease related to the aging process, although it is not caused by it. Thus knowledge of the aging process is crucial in understanding people with dementia. Most people with dementia experience both the process of aging and the course of their disease. Imagine if we did not have knowledge of the simple facts we know. How can we make care plans without knowing that the average length of life is around 70 or 80 years? Dealing with dementia without knowledge of the aging process is as if one was making a care plan for someone up to 300 years old. The areas to be covered may be extremely wide, from physical to mental, social or spiritual areas. Elderly people are the best teachers in the area of psychological understanding. We should listen carefully to what elderly people wish to say and observe what elderly people do.

Knowledge of dementia

It is harmful and unethical to care for people with dementia without adequate knowledge of it. Several areas to be covered in a training course would be: diagnostic assessment, natural courses of dementia, types and characteristics of dementia, stages of dementia, management of problem behaviors, social resources and services, activities for dementia, family care, terminal care, and ethical issues. The areas of brain damage and its effects should be understood, as well as remaining abilities, interests, and skills.

Knowledge and experience of working in a team

No single discipline can provide a comprehensive approach for people with dementia. Collaboration of a team is essential in meeting the needs of people with dementia. It is not as easy to work in a team as might be expected. The reason the team approach is difficult is the reason it is essential, that is, the diversity of backgrounds and points of view (Campbell, 1997). Each discipline has its own specialities and skills which overlap in practice. Presently, the psychological approach in a narrow sense is provided by psychiatrists, psychologists, and social workers in most countries. The psychological approach in a broader sense can be provided by people from any discipline.

Different disciplines often compete with each other for funds in a limited budget. Since the governments of most countries are increasingly cutting budgets, it appears much more productive to work together to insist on the importance of using more funds for improving the quality of psychological care for the demented elderly. This would enable more training which enriches the quality of life of the professionals by allowing them to enter into the lives of people with dementia beyond the provision of custodial care.

Many institutions and hospital professionals in Japan point to two major problems which must be addressed in order to improve the care of the elderly with dementia: first, a shortage of staff, and second, inadequate knowledge and skill of the staff (Boke Yobō Kyōkai, 1996). Most institutions for dementia care in Japan provide opportunities for staff training. On the other hand, the majority of these training programs are fragmented and nonsystematic. Moreover, due to insufficient numbers, the staff are fully occupied with the tremendous job of daily care for people with dementia. Thus, although the staff are quite well-motivated for training, there is little time left for continuous systematic education. Adequate numbers of staff as well as continuous training and education, including opportunities for supervision, should be systematized.

Counseling skills

Basic counseling skills are useful in relating to people with dementia. Such skills as listening, acceptance, empathy, nonjudgmental approaches, and genuine and unconditional positive regard are not easy to achieve. Learning these requires an ongoing continuous process, which includes practice and care supervision. Difficulty lies within these concepts, as was pointed out by Randall and Downie (1996) in the context of palliative care ethics. They claim that these concepts which lie at the heart of counseling are problematic, unrealistic, and even contrary to human relationships. That is, "genuineness" must be sacrificed to some extent while exhibiting a "nonjudgmental" attitude in order to be "empathetic." Elderly people have much experience in terms of human relationships, and they are sensitive to these contradictory aspects of professional skills. Most knowledge and skills of counseling and psychotherapy are based on experiences from the perspective of the younger generation, but there are many areas to be investigated from experiences of elderly people.

Case presentation

A psychological approach emphasizing creativity with two patients with dementia, one man and one woman, at a university hospital in Japan will be briefly discussed. In both cases, care was provided by a team of a doctor and a psychologist collaborating with a certified caseworker, a social worker, a nurse, and an occupational therapist from community agencies. Limitations on the services that can be provided at a university hospital guide us to work in a team in almost all cases. Here my focus will be on the psychological approach which was applied at the outpatient clinic of the university hospital, trying to stimulate and enhance the creativity of patients with dementia.

Mrs K: age 67, female, Alzheimer's disease

Mrs K, a 67-year-old woman, was accompanied by her husband to the psychiatric clinic of the university hospital. She looked much older than her age, with long, messy hair and an anxious expression on her face. She appeared extremely defensive, insisting that nothing was wrong with her and there was no reason to come to the hospital, especially to the neuropsychiatry division. Her husband, a businessman, seemed to be overwhelmed by his wife's inability to calculate numbers properly, her forgetfulness, and her ineptness in cooking, making dishes either too salty or without any salt. While her husband went out to work, she was left alone in the house and became very anxious, especially in the evenings. This is not an unusual case and after she had been through several examinations, including an EEG, a CAT scan, and neuropsychological tests, she was diagnosed as having Alzheimer's disease.

There were not many services to provide medical treatment for her. When the neuropsychiatrist asked me to interview her for an hour each month using reminiscence, Mrs K started reviewing her life with me. Because Mrs K was not able to come to the hospital on her own, her husband, Mr K, accompanied her each time. We referred them to a certified caseworker who later accompanied Mrs K to the hospital when her husband was not available.

I tried to explain to Mrs K the purpose of our session in a way that she could understand:

Kurokawa: I understand that you feel you are quite alright.
Mrs K: Oh, yes, I don't worry about things. I am an easy-going person.
Kurokawa: That's good. It is so nice that you seem to be spending your days pleasantly. You don't like coming to a hospital, do you?
Mrs K: Well … (looks at her husband)
Kurokawa: Normally nobody likes to come to hospitals. It's unnatural to love coming to hospitals.
Mrs K: (laughs)
Kurokawa: As a person grows older, compared to when they are younger, it is not a big surprise to have some new problems.
Mrs K: Oh yes, I am okay, but umm … I forget things.
Kurokawa: Do you?
Mrs K: Not very often, but … you know.
Kurokawa: You seem to be okay, but are you spending your days without talking with anybody?
Mrs K: Well …
Kurokawa: We can talk and deal with any issues, if you have any in the future. A kind of prevention. How does that sound to you?
Mrs K: I have many friends, umm … Mrs O, we are good friends. We went to Europe together. Mrs O likes poetry. I haven't done much of it.
Kurokawa: That's good. You have many friends. It must be your warm personality that you have so many friends. I suppose you would not want to come here anymore?
Mrs K: (silence) I saw many people in the waiting room. It was so interesting to see them. Watching people, I learn a lot. All sorts of different people. I'm enjoying it.

She seemed not to understand what was going to happen, but showed a slightly positive change in her attitude about coming to the hospital.

Kurokawa: I think it would be good for you to come here once in a while and stimulate your brain. You must have so many precious experiences that I have never had.

Mrs K:	Just that I have lived long. I have come through so many events.
Kurokawa:	Would you like to use this opportunity for reviewing your life? I am so curious to learn from your experiences.
Mrs K:	(smiles)
Kurokawa:	Would you like to talk about your past?
Mrs K:	Past stories. I can talk about that. So many things happened in my life.
Kurokawa:	What about your days when you were a child?

As the interview proceeded she seemed to start to enjoy it greatly, though her memory was not very well organized. She told me how beautiful the sea was in Tokyo when she was a child, how excited she had been when she got in a taxi for the first time, how her parents cherished her so much as their only daughter.

Mrs K:	Oh, you cannot imagine, the beautiful sea of Tokyo then.
Kurokawa:	It's not so beautiful these days, filled with factories and buildings and cars. Was it so beautiful?
Mrs K:	Yes, yes. I must tell you. We went to the sea and collected shells. Up in the sky, the balloon, what did we call it … umm … an airship was floating. That was amazing.
Kurokawa:	An airship?
Mrs K:	Yes, the name was … umm … I forget it … I can't remember.
Kurokawa:	It had a name, how interesting.
Mrs K:	Yes, it had a name … I can't remember.

When Mrs K could not remember the name of the airship, Mr K helped her.

Mr K:	Was it "Akron," and … "Zeppelin"?
Mrs K:	Oh yes, "Akron" and "Zeppelin," that was it.

When she had finished reminiscing about her days before marriage, I suggested that she and her husband should reminisce together about their married life. Her husband was bringing her to the hospital each time, and was there, ready to join the session. They both thought it would be a good chance to recall their marital life, since they never had such an opportunity to sit down and review their life.

Mr K:	We went to England and Scotland in 1990. Didn't we?
Mrs K:	Yes, we went recently. The beautiful rose garden, I remember.
Mr K:	You liked the gardens so much.
Mrs K:	I would love to visit once again.

At one point, Mr K told his wife that he recognized, in reviewing their life, that she had taken the major responsibilities in raising their children. Mrs K smiled, looking very content.

Mr K: I was so busy, you were the key person in raising the children.

Mrs K: I really enjoyed it. We were the type not to take things too seriously. Sometimes thieves came to steal our flowers, and the thief would come back to drop them off later, do you remember?

Mr K: Well ... yes, but I should thank you.

Mrs K: (with a big smile) It's not such a big deal. I enjoyed it so much. There were those women, working so hard with their small babies on their back. Oh, no. I was not the type. I said goodbye and good luck to them, you see.

Kurokawa: So you are saying you quit your job when you had your baby?

Mrs K: Yes, I didn't want to continue with my baby on my back. So I said, "Excuse me, excuse me," and quit my work.

Kurokawa: You were a very responsible mother.

Mrs K: I enjoyed raising children.

As the process of their life review went on, the demented wife started accepting what her life had been, and gradually came to accept her present situation, her forgetfulness and her condition of dependency on others.

Kurokawa: Are you going to have lunch at the restaurant in the hospital?

Mrs K: (whispers) Yes, somehow it was revealed that the food at the restaurant is better than my cooking. I am sorry about that, but I feel sorry for my husband if I feel too sorry, so I think I'll take it okay.

Kurokawa: Oh, you must have prepared wonderful dishes every day for your husband and you would also enjoy the food at the restaurant with your husband.

Mrs K: Yes. It's not good to work too hard. It's important to take it easy. I shall follow my husband. It's sometimes tough to remember everything. I'm in an easy situation, quite lucky.

During one session, I asked Mrs K whether she would like to draw a picture. She did not, but Mr K spontaneously took the crayon and drew a landscape. We were amazed that three weeks later Mrs K made a collage of a landscape which was exactly the same shape as her husband's drawing that she did not even remember at all.

The experience of couple reminiscence turned out to be very fruitful, as if the non-demented husband supported not only the wife's memory but also her life itself. The form of reminiscence in this case started as an individual reminiscence and changed to couple reminiscence. As the interviews went on, the content of reminiscence altered from defensive reminiscence to story-telling reminiscence and finally to integrative reminiscence.

When either member of a couple develops dementia, it becomes a very important issue to support the non-demented spouse who is facing aging issues him/herself, and thus may have tremendous difficulty accepting her or his spouse's situation. In a recent study of family caregivers in Japan, it was reported that more problems occur when the caregiver is the spouse compared to the caregiver being the child or other younger relatives. Of course it is important to reduce their physical burden, but we should never forget the psychological burden. The psychological burden of the spouse may be different from the burden of the children. In the case of Mrs and Mr K, couple reminiscence worked as a useful method for the psychological support of the demented wife, but also a meaningful way to support the spouse as well.

Reviewing their life together, couples get a chance to share their memory of their experiences, meeting each other for the first time, getting married, raising children, surviving difficult times during the war, and traveling to many places together. Clinicians and researchers point out that concrete cues are useful in this process (Burnside, 1984; Campbell, 1997). Through psychological approaches such as reminiscence work, memories long kept in storage can emerge to give insight and deep emotional interaction between the couple involved. In the case of Mr and Mrs K, couple reminiscence and nonverbal art methods such as collages or drawings allowed them opportunities to share their being as whole persons and dramatically synchronize in creative expression.

Mr M: age 79, male, Alzheimer's disease, early stage

Mr M was born the second son of a farmer in a village in the Tokyo area. He helped his father raise vegetables and rice as did many other Japanese boys of those days. He graduated from elementary school and without further education helped his father. Later he married and worked for an electric company. He currently lives with his wife and his unmarried daughter.

His wife, Mrs M, noticed his recent memory loss and anticipating that it might be dementia, brought Mr M to the hospital. After several examinations he was diagnosed as having Alzheimer's disease. Mr M was encouraged to participate in an early-stage support group for people with dementia, and he said he would like to try. This is a weekly support group at the outpatient clinic of a university hospital in Tokyo, run by a team of psychologists, a doctor, and a nurse. An average of eight patients with mild to moderate dementia participated in the program which uses methods such as reminiscence, reality orientation, collage, and present problem focusing. Topics chosen for the support group are shown in Table 13.1. Table 13.2 provides information on the content of the program. At one point we asked the patients what they themselves wanted to discuss in the support group. One of the patients raised the issue of her memory loss. The 77-year-old woman explained, "I have a terrible, terrible memory problem. I wonder how other people deal with memory loss," and other patients nodded their heads. Patients made the staff recognize the importance of taking up their major concerns, especially in the early stages when they feel a tremendous loss and anxiety. Following the need and the request of the group members we decided to focus on current topics such as memory

Table 13.1 Examples of themes of the support group

Reminiscence
    Childhood
    What we learned from our parents
    New Year's Day
    War
    Girl's Festival
Current topics
    Memory loss
    My concerns
    My joys
    What we want to tell the young
    How to maintain our health
Collage

Table 13.2 Support Group Program

Introduction
Reality orientation
Relaxation
Theme of the day
Tea with Japanese cakes

loss, fear, and anxiety. This was the point at which patients really started to support each other.

Early in the first few sessions, Mr M seemed to be quite aggressive towards other patients, accusing them of poor memory and pointing out trivial mistakes in a harsh manner. He preferred not to talk about his upbringing as the second son of a farmer, saying to another participant who was a former teacher:

> You were special. You have led a wealthy life. We were so poor we could not wear new kimonos even on New Year's Day. I always had to wear my brother's old clothing. It was not good to be born as the second son of a farmer.

He seemed to be expressing his anger. Mr M also told us repeatedly that he was sorry he could not climb mountains any more. He made a series of collages in the group which contained the following elements:

Collage 1: Australia, Egypt, mountain, *tatami* room, coconut.
Collage 2: Mountain.
Collage 3: Religious: "Can any religion answer my question?"
Collage 4: Man with a radish: "What is your question? A new life starts from one's turning point."
Collage 5: Trees, fruit, nature in fall, *haiku*: "As the fall advances, appreciating the harvest."
Collage 6: Mountains, *haiku*: "Nature is a gift from our God."

The first collage consisted of four pictures. He explained,

> This is Australia. It was my dream to travel there. This is Egypt. I have traveled there once with my wife. I wanted to live in a house like this but it was too expensive. I renovated one room of my house, not as fancy as this picture, but I loved being there. This is a coconut. It reminds me of the days I went to Southeast Asia during the war and coconuts were just like this. I am terribly sorry that I cannot climb mountains any more. My wife won't let me go.

On a small piece of paper, Mr M was able to express his accomplishments, his memory of an enjoyable trip with his wife, his dreams of the past, the harsh experience of war, and his discouragement in a sophisticated, creative way. His struggle to negotiate between his dream and his reality seemed to be expressed symbolically through the process of renovating his house, which given the limitations of the real world was not ideally accomplished. Nevertheless, Mr M was capable enough to come to terms with his given situation, which brought him great satisfaction.

In the collages which Mr M made over time, he repeatedly chose pictures of mountains, saying he was so sorry he was no longer able to climb mountains. He expressed strong feelings of anger and sorrow at his loss. While Mr M was struggling to accept his situation, he made a collage with a man trying to climb a high mountain carrying a big load on his back.

As the sessions went on, Mr M gradually started to share life stories from his childhood to those present in the support group. Several months after his initial collage, Mr M picked up a picture of a man, holding a large white radish at his harvest. Mr M had seemed ashamed of "just being the son of a farmer," as mentioned before. Yet after participating in the group for several months, sharing his life histories and experiences with the staff and other participants, he gradually recovered his psychological strength and appeared to come to terms with his past, his memory loss, and his aging process. He became proud of his past, which was unique and different from that of the other participants.

Mr M used several phrases cut from magazines which reflected his feelings and thoughts. The following verses put into his work of collage reflect part of his struggle to come to terms with his own situation:

> "Where do men come from, and where do men go, can religion provide the answer to this question?"

> "New life starts from one's turning point. Why do you feel you are bewildered?"

> "The road to peace is long away, but I will never give up."

Mr M. said to the participants, "Is there any cure for our memory loss? No. Then I would rather like to enjoy the rest of my days peacefully. There is no point in worrying." To our surprise, during the process Mr M started writing *haiku*, short poems of 17 syllables. In these creative works the maturity of his integrated personality and deep thoughts of life emerged.

> The fall advancing, appreciating the harvest with life.
> The fall advancing, mountains robed in honorable colors.
> Appreciating great Nature as the gift of our God.

Mr M commented along with his work, "We are all responsible for maintaining this beautiful nature, and we should pass it down to our descendants."

Discussion

We expect that professionals will increasingly recognize the importance of providing psychosocial care for people with dementia, including the encouragement of their creativity. It is not reasonable to expect people to express their creativity by handing them paper and crayon and letting them go. Time as well as professional skill is required to enable people with dementia to express their creativity. Balancing subjective involvement and objective observation, knowledge of negative responses in the psychological approach, knowing the limits to what professionals can or may do, and knowledge and experience of teamwork are all necessary for a successful psychosocial approach. Different techniques and psychosocial approaches need to be applied according to each individual and his or her family, the stage of dementia, and current cognitive abilities. Despite the fact that training and the process of improving one's skills in psychosocial clinical work takes time, the psychological approach offers great potential for enhancing the quality of life of people with dementia and their families.

The psychosocial approach should be considered a preventive intervention, not the prevention of dementia, but the prevention of problem behaviors or psychiatric symptoms which accompany dementia. Many people, professionals and caregivers, have discussed the management of problem behaviors, sometimes referred to as "challenging behaviors." However, many of these behaviors can be prevented by using a psychosocial approach. Fewer resources and less manpower are required if we can prevent these behaviors through psychosocial approaches, rather than spending a huge amount of time and energy struggling to manage them.

The ethical issue of informing people of the disease at the early stages of dementia is strongly related to the extent to which professionals are able to provide psychosocial support. There is no treatment, biological or psychosocial, that will cure the disease, but there are ways to support the well-being of the demented person through psychosocial approaches. That is the reason it is so important to support a person who faces a tremendous amount of fear, loss, and anxiety. Through psychosocial approaches at the early stage of dementia, and encouraging creativity in particular, people with dementia may be able to maintain their self-esteem. As they share their precious life experiences and express "themselves" as independent mature human beings with determination, families and professionals will be better able to understand each as a whole person and thus provide better care in the future course of their disease. Psychological intervention with Mrs K enabled the professional to understand what she would want to say when she had lost her ability of verbal communication. Otherwise, her words might have meant nothing more than series of fragmented disorganized words. It also helped her husband to accept his wife's disease by reviewing their marital life, trying to come to terms with their unfinished business while Mrs K was still able to share the task.

Due to their cognitive impairment it is often difficult for people with dementia to create something from nothing. Our professional role is to encourage their creativity by using skills and techniques based on an assessment of what the person *can* do. Most of the current activities for and approaches to dementia underestimate the possibility that people with dementia can achieve integration of their personality. Facing one's overwhelming situation and struggle to come to terms with the disease enables people with dementia to confront the vulnerability of human beings, as we see in the case of Mr M.

This process will not happen naturally among people with dementia. Psychological approaches can help maximize the strength of people with dementia and highlight the creativity and wisdom cultivated over years of various experiences. To determine the best approach for a particular person, correct assessments of his or her cognitive function and other related abilities are necessary. Stimulating the procedural memory (memory learned through physical exercise, such as riding a bicycle or knitting) of the person is known to be effective for those who have lost their verbal function. Procedural memory is strongly related to the process of creative work. The question is, what kind of procedural memory can be stimulated for each person? It depends on the person's past history, what he or she liked, what attracted them, what is available, and the present level and type of the disease.

The cultural heritage of both Japan and the United States can contribute to our understanding of the relationship between creativity, life experiences, and dementia. Currently, artistic activities such as *ikebana* (flower arranging), *haiku*, tea ceremonies, music, and dance are popular in Japanese day service centers and nursing homes, but these are mostly applied in a group for recreation and enjoyment. Through the investigation and methods for adapting these activities for people with dementia in an individualized manner, other populations will be able to enjoy their fruits. Cultural exchange between the two countries can contribute to our ability to care for people with dementia offering more diverse and better understood avenues for personal expression.

Offering a psychological approach for dementia requires time and money. Funding for approaches such as reminiscence and reality orientation has been supported for up to six months by the Japanese government for patients with dementia admitted to hospitals for the elderly where enrichment is stressed over aggressive treatment. However, the importance of psychological support at early stages of dementia, when people generally live at home and receive only outpatient treatment, is not yet well recognized.

The cognitive function and the memory of a person with dementia declines as time goes by. Today is the best time to implement psychosocial approaches for people with dementia. When needed, professionals can help them to cherish their special memories and share the gift of their creativity with others. The meaning of dementia is well expressed in the creative work they produce. Although their products are not always joyful and beautiful, neither are they always miserable and desperate. They can inspire and affect our sensibility in searching for and appreciating meaning in our own lives.

References

Boke Yobō Kyōkai. (1996). *Chihō kōreisha kea no zenkoku jittai chōsa* (Survey of dementia care in Japan). Tokyo: Mainichi Shinbunsha.

Burnside, I. et al. (1994). *Working with elder adults* (3rd ed.). Boston: Jones and Barlett.

Butler, R.N. (1963). The life review: An interpretation of reminiscence in the aged. *Psychiatry*, 26, 65–76.

Campbell, R. (1997). Creativity in diverse populations: Giving voice to the unexpressed. Program abstracts of the 50th Annual Scientific Meeting of the Gerontological Society of America. *The Gerontologist*, 37, Special issue 1, 235–236.

Feil, N. (1989). Validation: An empathetic approach to the care of dementia. *Clinical Gerontologist*, 8, 89–94.

Holden, U., and Woods, R.T. (1995). *Positive approach to dementia* (3rd ed.). Edinburgh: Churchill Livingston.

Killick, J. (1994). *Please give me back my personality*. Stirling, Scotland: University of Stirling, Dementia Services Development Centre.

Kurokawa, Y. (1994). *Chihō rōjin ni taisuru kaisōhō gurūpu* (Reminiscence group approach for the cognitively impaired elderly). *Japanese Journal of Geriatric Psychiatry*, 5, 1, 73–81.

Kurokawa, Y. (1995). *Chihō rōjin ni taisuru shinriteki apurōchi* (Reminiscence groups with Japanese dementia patients). *Journal of Japanese Clinical Psychology*, 13, 2, 169–179.

Kurokawa, Y. (1996). *Chihōsei shikkan o yūsuru kanja ni taisuru shinri ryōhō to shite no kaisōhō no yūkōsei* (Reminiscence groups with the elderly with dementia). Dissertation, University of Tokyo.

Randall, F., and Downie, R.S. (1996). *Palliative care ethics*. Oxford: Oxford Medical Publications.

14 Visible lives

Life stories and ritual in American nursing homes[1]

Thu Tram T. Nguyen, Joal M. Hill and Thomas R. Cole

Elderly people who enter American nursing homes experience a great deal of anxiety, stress, and depression – especially during the first six months after admission (Oleson and Shadick, 1993; Schneewind, 1990). In the nursing home, routines and tasks precede individual residents' needs (Hepburn *et al.*, 1997; Gubrium, 1975; Williams, 1990), impoverishing already uneasy relationships between residents and care providers. Emphasis on routine physical tasks contributes to residents' dependency (Brandriet, 1995) and learned helplessness (Seligman, 1975). Therefore, care providers view residents through old-age stereotypes (Pietrukowicz and Johnson, 1991) that exacerbate residents' feelings of low self-worth and uselessness. In this typical nursing home environment, residents, families, and care providers become convinced that elders have little to offer and experience – that they cannot reciprocate care, are unable to participate in pleasurable or communal activities, and are incapable of growth. Thus, new nursing home residents often feel invisible – to themselves as well as to others.

This chapter describes the Visible Lives project, undertaken in several Texas nursing homes. Our work is inspired by a broader movement for nursing home culture change in the United States which aims to place individuals ahead of tasks, to address the needs of the spirit as well as the body, to accept risk-taking as a normal part of life, to begin decision-making with the resident, and to respect and enjoy residents and staff as unique and valuable individuals (Fagan *et al.*, 1997). The Visible Lives project has three primary goals:

- to render residents' life histories and identities visible and accessible to the nursing home community – care providers, staff, volunteers, residents, families, and friends
- to facilitate individualized care planning
- to ease the transition from independent or assisted living to a nursing home.

Following a brief overview of the project, we describe the clinical background of Visible Lives, define individualized care, elucidate the three stages of the project (life story interview, storyboard construction, and "definitional ceremonies"), describe our experience creating storyboard prototypes with two nursing home residents, and offer concluding remarks.

Visible Lives, still in a formative stage, helps a resident represent who he or she is, has been, and wants to be. As a resident reviews and "re-members" his or her life story with an interviewer, visual material (such as family photographs, personal documents, certificates, and cards) and textual material (for example audiotaped life story experiences, personal letters, religious passages, poems, adages, and favorite recipes) are collected. These artifacts are then collaboratively crafted onto a 20 × 30-inch colored poster board subsequently referred to as a "storyboard." Such a collage of lived experiences allows a resident to communicate his or her life story as he or she would like to tell and share it. Thus, we take what is not visible – an elder's memories and interpretation of his or her past – and render it palpably present. In the future, we plan to develop a series of storyboard communal presentations and to study the effects of this intervention on residents and staff.

Until the early 1960s, the tendency of old people to talk about the past was viewed as either an understandable preoccupation with happier times or a form of pathology. In a seminal article published in 1963, Robert Butler argued that the tendency among elderly to review their lives was a universal and potentially therapeutic process stimulated by proximity to death. Butler's work stimulated new forms of practice and research in gerontological social work (Kaminsky, 1984), nursing (Chubon, 1980; Ebersole, 1976), medicine (Butler, 1974; Harris and Harris, 1980), and psychiatry (Lesser et al., 1981; Lewis, 1973). In the 1980s, scholars in the interpretive social sciences (Bruner, 1986; Cohler, 1982; Gergen, 1981; Myerhoff, 1992; Polkinghorne, 1988) and the humanities (Manheimer, 1992; Ricouer, 1971) began to articulate narrative as the central concept underlying various forms of remembering – life review, reminiscence, memoir, autobiography, and life story. Narrative, defined as an organized discourse, is presented in an ordered and coherent manner to a potential listener or reader. Today, scholars and researchers accept narrative as a means of maintaining a sense of personal integrity or coherence, making sense of life changes, and therefore an essential way of maintaining morale and positive well-being (McAdams, 1993; McAdams and Ochberg, 1988; Polkinghorne, 1983, 1988; Schafer, 1980, 1981).

Preserving a satisfactory self-image and maintaining a sense of competence and mastery have been identified as important adaptive tools for positive transition to nursing home living (Moos and Schaefer, 1986). Reminiscence and life review have become common interventions for honing these adaptive skills. Cohler and Cole (1996) noted that one element missing from previous research is an awareness that all narrative takes place in a specific, reciprocal process of telling and listening. In other words, each life story is a joint construction, the product of a dialogue or collaboration between storyteller (in this case the nursing home resident) and listener (researcher, care provider, family, and other residents). This insight has been central to the development of the Visible Lives project, which focuses on the possibilities that may result from collaboration, rather than upon the effects of a reminiscing elder individually.

Our project has also grown out of collaborative experiences in clinical ethics consultation (Cole, Thompson, and Rounds, 1995); research and writing about what it means to grow old in American culture (Cole, 1992; Cole and Gadow, 1986); readings in the anthropology of aging (Kertzer and Keith, 1984; Myerhoff, 1992); readings in clinical nursing and social work with nursing home residents (Bramlett and Gueldner, 1993; Haight and Olson, 1989; Murphy, 1990; Oleson and Shadick, 1993; Schneewind, 1990); field work gathering personal narratives in nursing homes; and interest in the use of visual images for memory, identity, and understanding. Visible Lives is also guided by the emerging theory and practice of individualized care.

Individualized care is "an interdisciplinary approach which acknowledges elders as unique persons and is practiced through caring, consistent relationships. Personal knowledge is used to create ways of living that are congruent with past patterns and individual preferences" (Happ *et al.*, 1996, p. 7). We believe that delivery of individualized care is possible within institutions such as nursing homes, and that it can be facilitated by using elders' life stories to build and strengthen meaningful relationships among care providers, nursing home residents and their families. Defined in this manner, care involves three fundamental principles best articulated by one of the pioneers of nursing home culture change, Dr William H. Thomas:

> First, we must recognize, appreciate and promote each resident's capacity for growth ... It is much harder to accept as true for the severely demented and disabled ...
>
> Second, when we dedicate ourselves to helping other people grow, our work must be defined by their needs and capacities, not ours ... Treatment is selfish ... Care is selfless. It must be guided by the capacities and needs of the person being cared for.
>
> Third, while treatment can be intermittent and brief, care must be continuous and long lasting. In this light, the words "long-term care" are redundant ... All real care is long term.
>
> (Thomas, 1994, pp. 21–22)

Each of these principles requires knowledge of the nursing home resident, not merely knowledge about him or her. Biographical narrative and images alone are subject to the same limitations we find in the medical chart – if we do not collaborate with elderly residents. We gather data about the person and still fail to know him or her as a person. Where decision-making opportunities are few, life story interview and collaborative storyboard construction assist residents to focus on significant life events, while also allowing for creativity and control.

Having no past life history to explain a resident's behavior, most care providers misunderstand their elderly charges. Care providers can only interpret and imagine what they now see before their eyes: wrinkled skin, white hair, impaired memories, frail bodies, demanding attitudes. It is true, but not often made explicit, that "the way we see things is affected by what we know or what we believe" (Berger et al., 1977, p. 8). Unless care providers have spent time with older people, such as grandparents or family friends, they may have only old-age stereotypes and myths to identify and connect with their everyday experience in the nursing home.

However, Pietrukowicz and Johnson (1991) found that nurse aides who received a resident's life history prior to interacting with that elder demonstrated improved attitudes about that resident's capacity. Imparting knowledge of an individual's life provides a fuller picture as well as possible explanations for current behavior and preferences. For example, a resident may not venture out of his or her room. If a preference for privacy is elicited from the life story, care providers can avoid stereotyping the resident as antisocial, maladaptive, or depressed. Perhaps the resident has always been accustomed to quiet and solitude. His or her behavior is not necessarily a failure to adapt to the new environment. Creative alternatives to institutional structure may then be explored, such as opportunities for the resident to eat in his or her room or in a quiet place in the nursing home.

Life stories impart knowledge and understanding of residents as individuals with unique experiences and with particular values, needs, strengths, and preferences. Such knowledge and information, while necessary for individualizing care, are largely unavailable in nursing home records. In fact, the important medical information comprising a resident's medical chart can overshadow the knowledge and personal understanding required for care. People enter nursing homes because they are frail or sick. The nursing home resident may thus be reduced to an assortment of physiological diagnoses rather than viewed as a unique individual who experiences illness and treatment in a particular way.

Life story interviews, storyboard construction, and "definitional ceremonies"

The full Visible Lives project enables a resident to re-cover and re-work his or her unique life experiences in three phases: life story interviews, storyboard construction, and definitional ceremonies. These phases provide three successive occasions for residents to "re-member" and re-present themselves. The terms "re-membering" and "definitional ceremony" are taken from the work of Barbara Myerhoff, who developed them while studying elderly Jewish immigrants at a senior center in Venice, California in the 1970s. Myerhoff observed that these Holocaust survivors felt unseen. They competed fiercely for opportunities to stage appearances that would make their individual and communal existence continuous and palpable to themselves and to others. Myerhoff also noticed that her listening presence gave people an opportunity to "become visible ... [and to] exercise power over their images ... Sometimes the image is the only part of their lives subject to control," wrote Myerhoff. "But this is not a small thing to control" (1992, p. 232). As Myerhoff gathered collective and individual life histories of these Eastern European Jews, she coined the word "re-membering" which nicely captures the active, creative process of selecting, arranging, and connecting that characterizes life history work.

The Aliyah Center in Venice also offered Myerhoff a poignant setting in which to observe the creative work of ritual. Since these people had moved to California later in life, they were cut off from their children and from their culture of origin. At the Aliyah Center they carried on various celebrations, festivals, religious services, and other communal events which allowed them to re-member themselves, to stake "claims regarding their vanished past and proof of their continuing existence and honor" (Myerhoff, 1984, p. 320). Myerhoff called these public occasions "definitional ceremonies," which she defined as ritualized performance "for enacting and displaying one's own interpretation of oneself, against the play of accident, chaos, and negative interpretations that may be offered up by history and outsiders" (Myerhoff, 1984, p. 320).

Although we use ethnographic methods and Myerhoff's concepts of "re-membering" and "definitional ceremonies," Visible Lives does not primarily aim to reproduce a detailed biography of residents' lives or of nursing home culture. Instead, we collaborate with residents to visually depict what they consider significant aspects of their lives. Visible Lives provides an opportunity for the elderly nursing home resident to articulate how they wish to be viewed by others, gives them narrative and perceptual control over that image, and offers the nursing home community a new way of seeing the resident.

Life story interviews

Life story interviews investigate what is meaningful to the aged individual. Interviewers pose the same questions to each participant, but the questions are open-ended, allowing for individual, idiosyncratic responses. Patterned after other interview methodologies, our ethnographic inquiries explore social and cultural features of the elder's life, help construct a narrative of personal identity and history, and finally, encourage expressing problems and concerns about nursing home adjustment. The respondent can then come to terms with particular realities (for example, that one will not return to independent living), and achieve a sense of enhanced morale or meaning (Cohler and Cole, 1996).

Several recorded in-depth interviews elicit the main themes, interests, turning points, problems, and accomplishments of a resident's life. During life story interviews, we probe for details, clarification and connections, helping residents organize their memories. Open-ended questions and probes include: "Tell me about your childhood ... Describe your most vivid memories of your parents ... Tell me about your adolescent years ... What is most memorable about your adult life? ... Tell me about being old ... If you could relive your life, tell me what you would change ... What do you want people to know about you and your life?" The interview quickly becomes more like a conversation than a formal interview, since it is emotionally engaging and follow-up questions depend upon previous answers rather than a prescribed set of questions.

During the course of the interviews, the resident and family (if available and with the resident's consent) are asked to share family photographs, memorabilia, pieces of art, or family heirlooms collected over a lifetime. A professional photographer captures animated contemporary images of the resident to place on the storyboard, alongside duplicates or reproductions of old photographs or documents. Clip art or other images relevant to the resident's life are brought in or downloaded from the Internet. The recorded interviews are transcribed and read by (or to) the resident, who chooses the main themes for the storyboard.

Storyboard construction

We begin storyboard construction once all narrative and visual images have been assembled (including phrases or vignettes from interviews that have been enlarged for easier viewing); we work collaboratively with the resident, arranging the images on the storyboard. Since the layout frequently reflects the symbolic importance of a resident's significant memories, we encourage him or her to lead in arranging images. For example, our preference might be to center the resident's current portrait on the storyboard, but actually a resident is more likely to place his or her own image peripheral to a wedding portrait or photographs of grandchildren.

Arranging visual and narrative images on the storyboard is a physical "re-membering" and visual placing of which "members" belong where in the story. Most interventions involving reminiscence and life review depend on memory, creating several limitations, even for the cognitively intact resident. We provide written accounts of interview sessions to participating residents. Therefore, the resident directly benefits from written or visual reinforcement of his or her recollections. We have also noted that visual material elicits memories that may not have been communicated during the interview sessions.

Definitional ceremonies

In the future, we plan to develop the third stage of the project: communal storyboard presentation. This "definitional ceremony" hopefully will be witnessed by care providers, other nursing home residents, family and friends. Although juxtaposed texts – visual and narrative, present and past – afford an opportunity for the elder to be seen beyond the current confines of time and place, they are likely to be undervalued by the nursing home community. Therefore after a storyboard is complete, we plan to implement a series of ritual ceremonies to publicly communicate and affirm an elder's life story. First, each storyboard is presented to care providers, staff, volunteers, other residents, family, and friends; then it is displayed on the resident's door or in some prominent place in the nursing home. According to the preference of each participating resident, a storyboard is periodically modified to depict changes in the individual's life story (such as the birth or adoption of a grandchild, remembrance of a close friend recently deceased, or involvement in a nursing home activity). Finally, after a resident's death, the storyboard is re-presented to the nursing home community as a memorial and public acknowledgment of loss. The storyboard will then be given to a family member or friend previously designated by the elder.

Life stories recall the reality of life before nursing home placement and old-age frailties – a reality not clearly seen by those charged with the care of elders. The routines of nursing home care only make apparent the difficulties of aging. They do not tell us what it is like to experience those difficulties or attempt to live with them. Furthermore, they do not tell us about the individual and his or her preferences, values, and strengths. "Definitional ceremonies" in the nursing home serve to connect human beings through stories to those places between what is believed and what is seen about old age. Without this understanding, we are ill-equipped to provide individualized care, and to reflect on what it means to grow old.

We conceive the creation and presentation of each visual and textual storyboard as a collaborative recreation of the self, a narrative bridge helping to span the ambiguous time between a former, independent self and a new identity as nursing home resident. In creating a storyboard, we are not so much participant-observers as participant-collaborators. Thus our project is collaborative at three levels: listening and responding to the life story, the collaborative process of constructing the storyboard, and the presentation or "definitional ceremony" of the shaped life story. We are providing the repetition necessary for ritual in the symbolic form of life story – a "re-membered" re-presentation of the elder. For this reason, we emphasize the collaborative and ritual aspects of Visible Lives, which, at its core, consists of repeated reciprocal acts of listening and telling.

Two visible lives: Sarita Johnson and Lily Matthews[2]

Kitwood and Bredin (1992) articulate a theory of dementia care which we believe has wider applicability to non-demented nursing home residents. They suggest that self-esteem (a sense of worth or one's self); sense of agency (the ability to make a mark on others and the world); social confidence (the ability to move toward others, be at ease with them and offer advice and comfort); and hope (a sense that the future will be good even with loss and change) contribute to a state of well-being. We have found these characteristics of well-being feature prominently in a good transition to nursing home life regardless of cognitive impairment, as illustrated by Sarita Johnson's participation in Visible Lives. Not only her storyboard, but each stage of the project in itself, enhanced Mrs Johnson's well-being in demonstrable ways.

Mrs Sarita Johnson

Thu Tram Nguyen met the 79-year-old woman in the summer of 1996. Mrs Johnson was then living on the third floor of the nursing home with her husband Roy, who was paralyzed from a stroke he had suffered the previous winter.

When Ms Nguyen began visiting, Mrs Johnson would ask, "Do you have any advice for me?" She responded softly to questions with only, "Yes, ma'am," or "No, ma'am." In late August, Roy died. Mrs Johnson stopped sleeping in her bed, wouldn't eat much, and rarely ventured out of her room. In September, Mrs Johnson began to tell stories about her husband:

> He wasn't just a man. He was a provider, he was a husband ... Roy was very religious, very dutiful to the usher board. Not a Sunday came that he didn't go to church. He was always at his post at Jerusalem Baptist Church ... I sat next to Roy in my recliner after he got sick and held his hand. That was all that I could do. It was very hard after he died. But as I sit and talk it eases my mind quite a bit. Sometimes I talk to his picture. And I ask God to let me be with my husband forever in Heaven, and I believe He will do that.

Gradually, Mrs Johnson began to reminisce about her own life, which began on a farm in Arcadia, Louisiana in 1917. During the process of "re-membering" Mrs Johnson recaptured a sense of self-worth that was greatly diminished by nursing home placement and her husband's death. As care providers, family and other residents became interested in both the story-telling process and the collaborative storyboard, Mrs Johnson's self-esteem, sense of agency and social confidence grew. Mrs Johnson "re-membered" her life and as her life experiences became visible, she emerged from the depths of her grief. Joking and sharing her advice and experience of marriage, she communicated more with care providers and staff. She found that her life makes an impact on others, and began leaving her room more frequently to interact with other nursing home residents. Eventually she acquired a beau.

We believe that "re-membering" her life story helped facilitate Mrs Johnson's grieving process – for husband, home and independence. Allowed to grieve, it then became possible for her to hope – to believe that in spite of irretrievable losses, her future in the nursing home could be good. At the outset of our interviews, for example, Mrs Johnson frequently expressed her desire to go home, even though she acknowledged that home was an unsafe environment for her. By the close of our collaboration, she said more than once, "I miss my home, but I know this is the best place for me to be."

Visible Lives presented Mrs Johnson's life as she described it. She was not just an old woman who talked to a picture on the wall. At present Mrs Johnson is a grieving widow, self-conscious about her missing teeth, but proud of her still-thick hair, which an attendant braids and arranges in different styles. She suffers from arthritis and poor vision. But she is also a little girl in Arcadia, Louisiana, picking cotton alongside her four brothers, a young woman working at her first job in a meat-packing plant in Galveston, Texas, and a young bride. She is a mother, grandmother and great-grandmother, who finds comfort and continuity in remembering her husband and her large extended family.

Mrs Johnson's participation in Visible Lives not only helped her explore new opportunities for herself, it also helped caregivers see and re-interpret her personality and demeanor. When we first met Mrs Johnson, she was considered to have some dementia, in part because she had the habit of talking to her husband's picture. Care providers not acquainted with Mrs Johnson did not know that she spoke to Roy even as he lay bedridden and aphasic. They therefore interpreted her behavior as delusional or as evidence of senility. But Mrs Johnson told us, "As I sit and talk it eases my mind quite a bit. Sometimes I talk to his picture. And I ask God to let me be with my husband forever in Heaven, and I believe He will do that." Placed in the context of her 50-year marriage and strong spiritual beliefs, Mrs Johnson's behavior can be re-interpreted not as organic or psychic disintegration, but as a productive means of coping which allowed her to integrate the loss of her husband into her present life. After placing her husband's memory into her life story, she befriended staff and residents. Mrs Johnson still lives in the nursing home, where her Visible Lives photographer Marilyn Brodwick recently found her napping in the lobby with her gentleman friend.

Mrs Lily Matthews

Our experience with a second participant demonstrates how visual depiction of a life can modify stereotypes or negative impressions of a nursing home resident. Born in the early 1920s on Long Island, Lily Matthews traveled with her best girlfriend Helen to Galveston to study nursing. Enjoying the warm climate, she and eventually her family established permanent residence.

Mrs Matthews had been acquainted with her husband John only a couple of days before he eventually proposed marriage, "But we had to wait until he got back from the ship in August. We married on August 11, 1957." Mrs Matthews recounted that before her marriage to John she would pray to St Jude to bring her an honest man, "And he answered my prayers. My husband was so honest and so good. We didn't have too many years together, but it was enough to remember. We were married 31 years."

Mrs Matthews remembers her life was not exciting like other people's, but it was stable with work and weekend family get-togethers: "We had a nice time. But when the babies came they made all the difference in the world." Later she shared with Ms Nguyen and Ms Hill that she could not have children of her own, but eventually adopted her babies Sally and Johnny.

Lily Matthews came to Galveston to become a nurse, and, although retired for fifteen years, this identity remains of central importance to her. She vividly remembers living through numerous natural disasters, an industrial disaster in Texas, and the polio epidemic in America. She remembers these times explicitly through her nursing career. Not a woman of many words nor descriptive of events, Mrs Matthews recalls:

> The Texas City disaster happened April 16, 1947. I was on duty that night and we all went to Texas City. Shifts were eight hours. I worked from 11 p.m. to 7 a.m., but during the disaster I helped where I could during the

day. I didn't care about sleeping. It was hard work, but I felt sorry for the patients. A lot of them had gangrene so we had to separate them from the rest. From 1947 to 1948 there was a polio epidemic in America. I was so happy when they found the Salk vaccine. The vaccine came in 1964, I think. I was so thankful. I used to have to wrap the babies. I was one of the nurses who could operate the iron lung. I was not afraid of contracting polio. I was never afraid. I guess that was why God was good to me.

Mrs Matthews is a difficult person to know even though she is more cognitively competent than most residents, care providers, and staff in her nursing home. She offers little information and description unless explicitly asked. Even when she talks easily, she provides sparse details that do not reveal her interests or needs: "I don't like growing old. I don't like it. But I have to accept it. It's my turn now to be old." Care providers are misled into thinking that she has adjusted fully to nursing home living. When asked about nursing home living, Mrs Matthews, who is wheelchair bound, replied:

> I miss doing things for myself. I miss driving. I miss shopping. I miss those things that we take for granted. I miss those things. I try to be independent. I try to help the staff. I hope I can just do a little bit for somebody.

Mrs Matthews, proud-spirited and disciplined, lonely without her family and friends, is unable to discuss her situation with care providers because she appears less needy than other residents and asserts her independence. Although Mrs Matthews has a sense of self-worth and knows she has made an impact on others, she is unable to engage others.

Mrs Matthews' life story narrative provided Ms Nguyen and Ms Hill with a better perspective on her personality. They understood Mrs Matthews' need to maintain her independence. She survived natural and chemical disasters, cared for the sick, and outlived her husband. However, after Mrs Matthews constructed her storyboard, Ms Nguyen and Ms Hill learned from the visual placement of images what Mrs Matthews had not explicitly conveyed in her narrative. Another story was revealed when storyboard construction was completed.

On the storyboard, she centered pictures of her "grandbabies," placed an image of a nurse with the Texas City disaster in the upper right-hand corner, an image of the movie poster *Now, Voyager* in the upper left-hand corner, underneath which she placed an Impressionist reproduction of a dancing couple, and she placed an image of three sisters near her contemporary portrait in the lower left-hand corner. Mrs Matthews lost most of her photographs in floods and fires. The *Now, Voyager* image was chosen because the star Paul Henreid reminded Mrs Matthews of her husband John. Ms Nguyen and Ms Hill were unaware of Mrs Matthews' love of Impressionist art, dancing, entertaining, and animals until she selected images for her storyboard.

Individual narrative made visible disrupts preconceived stereotypes or shadowy impressions, and opens up opportunities to pause – to question and rework "odd" connections and assumptions about an individual and to understand at another level what is not revealed or uncovered during the life story interviews. Lily Matthews, more aggressive and mentally competent than other nursing home residents, is more likely to voice her requests rather than wait for her needs to be anticipated. Knowing that she was a nurse, care providers have created an "institutional myth" about Lily Matthews: "She's a mean woman. She was a mean nurse too. And she is trying to be nice now because she is approaching death." A story circulates that the "mean nurse" is getting what she deserves in the nursing home.

Care providers may have a different way of seeing Mrs Matthews when they see on her storyboard elements of her untold life story. Looking at images allows residents to revisit, recover, and "re-member" their life story in ways not possible through textual construction. It also affords care providers opportunity to see and know more about their residents, and perhaps re-interpret and rethink previous judgments. Care providers may have a different way of seeing Mrs Matthews when they become aware of the disasters lived through, her commitment to nursing, her love of family, the adoption of her two children, and her loving marriage. Behaviors interpreted as "demands," "meanness," or "bossiness" may be reinterpreted as awkward but sincere efforts to be independent and help others. Ms Nguyen and Ms Hill received a different story because they listened to the story Lily Matthews wanted told – and they saw Lily the way Lily wanted others to see her.

Conclusion

Using ritual, we want to build a culture in the nursing home in which lives are linked – where the storytellers are heard and seen, and where the listeners receive stories and see reflections of themselves in their charges' lives. There is then a communion of participants and witnesses, and a better understanding of individuals and the role each member has in the lives of nursing home residents. Whether care providers, residents, family, or friends, we are all listeners, and re-memberers. We can never presume to completely know another person, which is both the mystery and delight of human companionship. However, by listening, seeing, and responding to stories, we can illuminate what would otherwise remain unexplored. As Berger and colleagues state, "The relation between what we see and what we know is never settled ... We only see what we look at. To look at is an act of choice. As a result of this act, what we see is brought within our reach – though not necessarily within arms reach" (Berger *et al.*, 1977, p. 8)

For Mrs Johnson, Visible Lives helped articulate and find new possibilities for life in a nursing home which we believe can occur for others, not only on an individual basis, but corporately as well. Instead of structuring group activities according to tradition and/or the convenience and interests of staff, nursing homes can shape activities based on knowledge gained in life story work and individualized care. Eliciting residents' past interests, values, and strengths may result in positive and achievable group activities, such as groups for Bible study, poetry writing and reading, a "festival" of favorite movies, or demonstrations and presentations from community members about historical events, local flora and fauna, or other topics.

In *Writing Lives*, a book on the principles of biography, Leon Edel writes, "lives are composed in most instances as if they were mosaics. Mosaics before they are composed are not fiction; they are an accumulation of little pieces of reality, shaped into an image" (Edel, 1984, p. 16). The Visible Lives project shapes little narrative and visual pieces of reality into a composite image which visibly symbolizes the resident to herself, her family and the nursing home community.

Notes

1 Research for this chapter was supported in part by a Pre-Doctoral Fellowship from the Sealy Center on Aging, University of Texas Medical Branch, Galveston.
2 Although the two nursing home residents referred to in this chapter consented to use of their stories, we have changed names to guard their privacy.

References

Berger, J., Blomberg, S., Fox, C., Dibb, M., and Hollis, R. (1977). *Ways of seeing*. New York: Penguin Books.

Bramlett, M.H., and Gueldner, S.H. (1993). Reminiscence: A viable option to enhance power in elders. *Clinical Nurse Specialist*, 7, 2, 68–74.

Brandriet, L.M. (1995). Changing nurse aide behavior to decrease learned helplessness in nursing home elders. *Gerontology and Geriatrics Education*, 6, 3–19.

Bruner, J. (1986). *Actual minds, possible worlds*. Cambridge, MA: Harvard University Press.

Butler, R. (1963). The life review: An interpretation of reminiscence in the aged. *Psychiatry*, 26, 65–76.

Butler, R. (1974). Successful aging and the role of life review. *Journal of the American Geriatric Society*, 22, 529–535.

Chubon, S. (1980). A novel approach to the process of life review. *Journal of Gerontological Nursing*, 6, 543–546.

Cohler, B. (1982). Personal narrative and the life-course. In P. Baltes and O.G. Brim, Jr. (Eds.), *Life span development and behavior* (Vol. 4, pp. 205–241). New York: Academic Press.

Cohler, B., and Cole, T. (1996). Studying older lives: Reciprocal acts of telling and listening. In J.E. Birren, G.M. Kenyon, J.E. Ruth, J.J.F. Schroots, and T. Svensson (Eds.), *Aging and biography* (pp. 61–76). New York: Springer.

Cole, T. (1992). *The journey of life: A cultural history of aging in America*. New York: Cambridge University Press.

Cole, T., and Gadow, S. (Eds.). (1986). *What does it mean to grow old: Reflections from the humanities*. Durham: Duke University Press.

Cole, T., Thompson, B., and Rounds, L. (1995). In whose voice? Composing an ethics case as a song of life. *Journal of Long Term Home Health Care*, 14, 4, 23–31.

Ebersole, P.P. (1976). Reminiscing. *American Journal of Nursing*, 79, 1304–1305.

Edel, L. (1984). *Writing lives: Principia biographica*. New York: Norton.

Fagan, R.M., Williams, C.C., Strumpf, N.E., and Burger, S.G. (1997). *Final report of a meeting of pioneers in nursing home culture change*. Rochester, New York.

Gergen, K. (1981). The functions and foibles of negotiating self-conceptions. In M. Lynch, A. Norem-Hebeisen, and K. George (Eds.), *Self-concept: Advances in theory and research* (pp. 59–76). Cambridge, MA: Ballinger.

Gubrium, J. (1975). *Living and dying at Murray Manor*. New York: St Martin's Press.

Haight, B., and Olson, M. (1989). Teaching home health aides the use of life review. *Journal of Nursing Staff Development*, 5, 1, 11–16.

Happ, M.B., Williams, C.C., Strumpf, N.E., and Burger, S.G. (1996). Individualized care for frail elders: theory and practice. *Journal of Gerontological Nursing*, 22, 3, 7–13.

Harris, R., and Harris, S. (1980). Therapeutic uses of oral history techniques in medicine. *International Journal of Aging and Human Development*, 12, 1, 27–34.

Hepburn, K.W., Caron, W., Luptak, M., Ostwald, S.K., Grant, L., and Keenan, J.M. (1997). The family stories workshop: Stories for those who cannot remember. *The Gerontologist*, 37, 6, 827–832.

Kaminsky, M. (Ed.). (1984). *Uses of reminiscence: New ways of working with older adults*. New York: Haworth Press.

Kertzer, D.I., and Keith, J. (Eds.) (1984). *Age and anthropological theory*. Ithaca: Cornell University Press.

Kitwood, T., and Bredin, K. (1992). Towards a theory of dementia care: Personhood and well-being. *Aging and Society*, 12, 269–287.

Lesser, J., Lazarus, L.W., Frankel, R., and Havasy, S. (1981). Reminiscence group therapy with psychotic geriatric inpatients. *The Gerontologist*, 21, 3, 291–296.

Lewis, C.N. (1973). The adaptive value of reminiscing in old age. *Journal of Geriatric Psychiatry*, 6, 1, 117–121.

Manheimer, R. (1992). Remember to remember. In M. Kaminsky (Ed.), *All that our lives have witnessed*. New York: Horizon Press.

McAdams, D.P. (1993). *The stories we live by: Personal myths and the making of the self*. New York: Morrow.

McAdams, D.P., and Ochberg, R.L. (Eds.). (1988). Psychobiography and life narratives (special issue). *Journal of Personality*, 56, 1.

Moos, R.H., and Schaefer, J.A. (Eds.). (1986). *Coping with life crises: An integrated approach*. New York: Plenum Press.

Murphy, S.A. (1990). Human responses to transitions: A holistic nursing perspective. *Holistic Nurse Practitioner*, 4, 3, 1–7.

Myerhoff, B.G. (1984). Rites and signs of ripening: The intertwining of ritual, time and growing older. In D.I. Kertzer and J. Keith (Eds.), *Age and anthropological theory* (pp.305–330). Ithaca: Cornell University Press.

Myerhoff, B.G. (1992). Life history among the elderly: Performance, visibility, and remembering. In M. Kaminsky (Ed.), *Remembered lives: The work of ritual, storytelling, and growing older*. Ann Arbor: University of Michigan Press.

Oleson, M., and Shadick, K.M. (1993). Application of Moos and Schaefer's (1986) model to nursing care of elderly persons relocating to a nursing home. *Journal of Advanced Nursing*, 18, 3, 479–485.

Pietrukowicz, M.A., and Johnson, M.M.S. (1991). Using life histories to individualize nursing home staff attitudes toward residents. *The Gerontologist*, 31, 1, 102–106.

Polkinghorne, D. (1983). *Methodology for the human sciences: Systems of inquiry*. Albany: State University of New York Press.

Polkinghorne, D. (1988). *Narrative knowing and the human sciences*. Albany: State University of New York Press.

Ricoeur, P. (1971). The model of the text: meaningful action considered as text. *Social Research*, 38, 529–562.

Schafer, R. (1980). Narration in the psychoanalytic dialogue. *Critical Inquiry, 7*, 29–53.
Schafer, R. (1981). *Narrative actions in psychoanalysis.* Worcester, MA: Clark University Press.
Schneewind, E.H. (1990). The reaction of the family to the institutionalization of an elderly member: Factors influencing adjustment and suggestions for easing the transition to a new life phase. *Journal of Gerontological Social Work, 15,* 1/2, 121–135.
Seligman, M.E.P. (1975). *Helplessness: On depression, development, and death.* San Francisco: W.H. Freeman.
Thomas, W.H. (1994). *The Eden Alternative: Nature, hope and nursing homes.* Sherburne, New York: The Eden Alternative Foundation.
Williams, C.C. (1990). Long-term care and the human spirit. *Generations, 14,* 25–28.

15 Disclosure, decisions, and dementia in Japan

Maximizing the continuity of self

Masahiko Saito

Except in very unusual circumstances, Japanese patients are not told a diagnosis of dementia. In the past it was assumed that family members would care for elderly relatives and that there was thus no need to concern the person with unhappy details over which they had no control. So both doctors and family members have been hesitant to tell patients the truth. It is not only because of the character of the disease itself or the age of the patients. In other fatal or difficult-to-treat disease like cancer or schizophrenia, the same tendency exists. The Japanese government reports that only 18.2 percent of cancer patients who died in March and April, 1992 were informed of their true diagnosis (Kōseishō Kenko Seisaku Kyoku Sōmuka, 1994). About 30 percent of them were informed of their diagnoses not by their doctors but by family members. In some cases, the will of the family has been more important than the will of the individual family members in Japanese society. Edwards (1989) pointed out that the Japanese view the individual as incomplete and unable to function in society alone, needing the structure of the family unit to be complete. Once a person gets ill and needs to be cared for by family members, such a tendency becomes more apparent.

Yet a variety of social, economic, and cultural changes have led to more elderly people living separately from their children, and family caregiving can no longer be assumed. Moreover, there are legal means to deal with the management of the property of people who are retarded or otherwise unable to make good decisions, and as we have increasing numbers of elderly people experiencing dementia, these laws are sometimes applied to them. However, these legal steps are inappropriate for their cases because they do not recognize that these elderly people are often capable, especially in the early stages of their diseases, of making decisions about how they will live their lives and the kind of medical and social care they will receive. But their participation in these decisions depends on their being informed of their disease and educated about it in detail. This in turn necessitates providing psychological support for the elderly and their families. In this chapter I will present four scenarios drawn from my clinical experiences which represent different approaches to decision-making in cases of demented elderly patients, illustrating the complex relationships among family, health care professionals, the law and the patients' care. I conclude that we need changes in both the medical and legal systems to provide the best care for demented people by encouraging continuity of selfhood through involvement in decisions about their care to the extent they are capable.

Demographic change in Japanese society

In recent decades, Japan's social structure has been changing rapidly. The population of Japan was 125.57 million in 1995 and 14.54 percent of those were 65 years old or older (Eigingu Sōgō Kenkyū Sentā, 1998). Figure 15.1 shows the types of households with elderly people in Japan from 1975 to 1995. In 1975, Japan had 6.9 million households with people aged 65 or older. Among these, there were 1.53 million single or couple households in 1975, 4.57 in 1995, and it is estimated that there will be 9.05 million in 2200. Figure 15.2 shows the breakdown of household types in Yamagata, a prefecture in northern Japan, Kagoshima Prefecture on the southern island of Kyushu, and Tokyo. In Yamagata, 77 percent of the elderly live with their children, in contrast to 48 percent in Tokyo and 35 percent in Kagoshima. Generally speaking, the ratio of the elderly living with their children is small in large cities such as Tokyo, and in the southwestern part of Japan such as Kyushu. The rapid increase of the number of elderly people living by themselves has resulted in the decline of traditional family functions in Japan.

Who cares for the elderly in Japan?

Figure 15.3 indicates where the elderly with dementia receive care. It shows that 74.5 percent of them are cared for in their homes in which caregiving family members also reside (Ōtsuka *et al.*, 1992). Figure 15.4 shows who provides home care (Miura, 1997). In general, nearly half of them are cared for by their daughters-in-law. The daughter-in-law, most often the wife of the eldest son, has been the main caregiver in traditional Japanese society, and this remains true in rural areas today. But in Tokyo, elderly spouses (mainly wives) are the most common caregivers (37.7 percent), daughters-in-law constitute 30.0 percent, and daughters 21.1 percent of caregivers. Some of the daughters are married and some are single. In any case, most of the caregivers at home are women who live with the elderly in the same household.

The number of residents of special nursing homes for the elderly (*tokubetsu yōgo rōjin hōmu*) are presented in Figure 15.5 (Miura, 1997). In 1975, there were 41,606 residents in these homes, and in 1995 there were 220,916. However, the number of elderly who want or have to live in such facilities has been increasing much more rapidly, so that in Tokyo, there is long waiting list of two to three years to be admitted to these nursing homes.

The hospital is another option for where the elderly "live" in Japan. Because of the health insurance system and social welfare law of Japan, for some elderly people who have higher incomes, staying in a hospital is a cheaper option than living in a public nursing home due to the sliding fee scale of these homes. In rural areas, caregiving of elderly relatives is still considered to be an obligation

Disclosure, decisions, and dementia in Japan   305

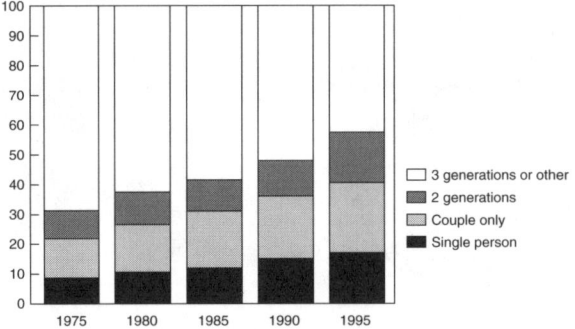

Figure 15.1 Households with people aged over 65 in Japan
Source: Ministry of Health and Welfare Japan, 1992.

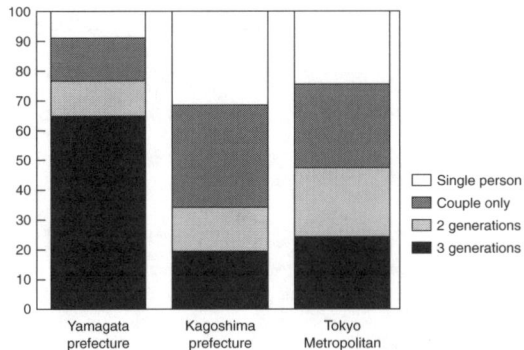

Figure 15.2 Households with people aged over 65 in Yamagata, Kagoshima and Tokyo (1995)
Source: Statisitcs Bureau, General affairs Agency, Natinal Census, 1995

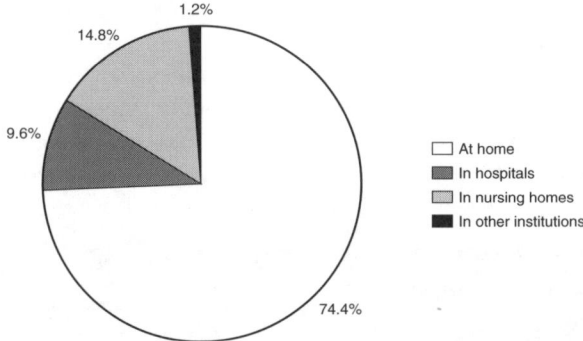

Figure 15.3 Where patients with dementia receive care in Japan
Source: Ōtsuka *et al*, 1992.

306 Facilitating care of self

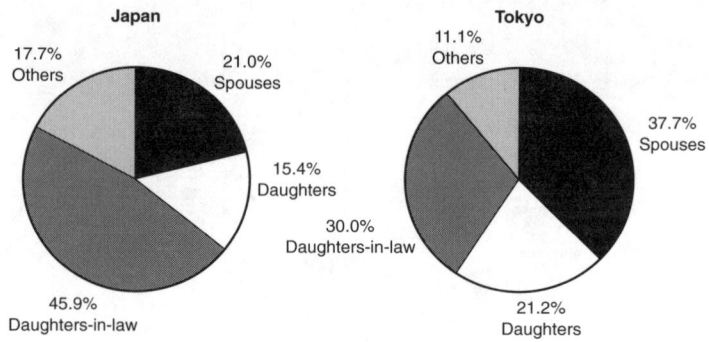

Figure 15.4 Care providers of patients with dementia

Source: Tokyo Metropolitan Government, *Survey on the Status of National Livelihood*, 1995.

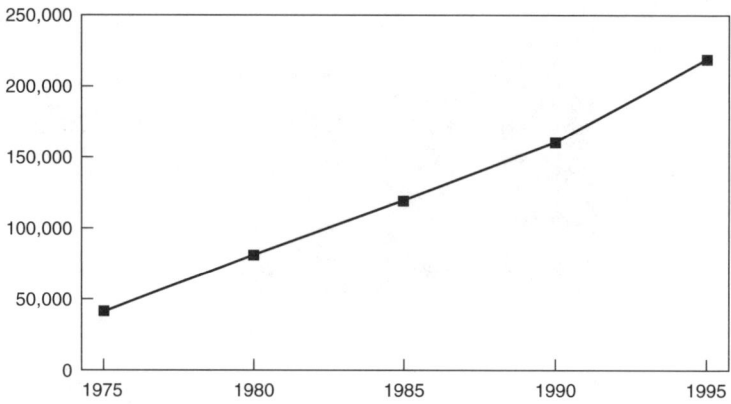

Figure 15.5 Number of residents of nursing homes in Japan 1975–1995

Source: Ministry of Health and Welfare, *Social Welfare Facility Survey*, 1995.

of the eldest son's wife. In such areas, nursing home placement is thought to be shameful behavior for the daughters-in-law. Hospitalization due to some kind of disease (most elderly people have one or two "diseases") is a good excuse for family caregivers to turn the care of their relative over to someone else.

Case studies of decision-making regarding demented family members

Case 1

K.A. was a 55-year-old man. He came to the University Hospital because of his slight language problem. He had been a jet pilot of the Japanese Defense

Force. When he retired from the service, he got a job as a professor of a technical college. When he came to the hospital for the first time, he himself did not feel any problems at all. His younger sister was the first person who recognized his problem. When she spoke with K.A. on the telephone, she found that he sometimes echoed her words. The Japanese language distinguishes words of respect used when addressing others and words of modesty used when talking about oneself. Thus, when someone asks something about you in words of respect, you should answer in words of modesty. When K.A.'s sister asked about his condition in words of respect, he responded using words of respect speaking of himself. This made her feel strange, so afterwards she asked K.A.'s wife whether there was anything wrong with him. When K.A. came to see us at the University Hospital, his wife told us that she had felt some change in him over the years, but she could not identify what it was. When K.A.'s sister pointed out his inappropriate speech, she at last could make up her mind to take him to a hospital to clarify what had happened.

After the initial interview, we arranged a number of medical and psychological examinations. His verbal intelligence and memory had apparently declined more than his nonverbal intelligence and memory. Magnetic resonance imaging (MRI) showed moderate atrophy of his temporal lobe, especially in the left hemisphere. We arranged for a second visit to explain the diagnosis. For the second visit, his wife came to the hospital with her son and daughter, but without K.A. She told us that they would like to decide whether they should tell him the truth or not after we inform them of the diagnosis. We explained his diagnosis, his present condition, and his prognosis. When leaving us, his wife asked us not to inform him of the diagnosis or prognosis. At that time, he was still able to teach at the college. Probably because of the effect of his character change due to his disease, this intelligent man did not recognize the decline of his ability. But if we had explained his medical condition and prognosis at that time, he might have been able to understand what was happening to him.

It was one year after the initial visit that he and his wife again came to see us at the University Hospital. His dementia had progressed severely and he had already completely withdrawn from social activity. He needed assistance in daily activities such as dressing and bathing. He had already lost any insight about his condition. When I asked him if there was anything wrong with his mental or physical condition, he just smiled and said no. When I asked him the reason he retired from his career at the college, he replied that it was just because his wife had told him to do so.

His wife told me that it had been a terrible year. When she was informed of the diagnosis and prognosis, she could not believe it. She did not want to know any more about the disease. But after a few weeks of confusion, she made up her mind to do anything she could for him and her family. First, she told her mother-in-law the facts. This stouthearted old woman said that she would support anything that her daughter-in-law decided. These two women decided at the beginning that he should resign from his work before his colleagues recognized his problem, because they thought if people outside of the family became aware of his disease, his son and daughter might be disadvantaged in getting a job or in marriage. So he resigned without knowing the reasons, but he did not appear seriously concerned about it, she said.

After this visit, which was one year after the initial one, he started coming to the hospital every two months. Two years after the initial visit, he came to see us in a wheelchair. He was almost mutistic. His wife continued to care for him in their home, but she had already abandoned her attempts to cover up his disease, because her son and daughter insisted that they needed social services to take care of him at home.

Three years have passed since his first visit. He is now bedridden, and completely mutistic but is still living at home. His son got married and lives apart from his parents. The son's wife has a full-time job, but the son and his wife come to see the parents on holidays and help take care of him. The daughter has graduated from the university and is employed in a company. She lives with her parents and also helps her mother on holidays. But most of the care is given by the wife with some support from home helpers and public health nurses.

Case 2

Y.T. died just before her 80th birthday. She was a widow with two sons and two daughters. The two sons and elder daughter were married and the youngest daughter was single. When her eldest son got married, she and her husband had expected the young couple to live with them, but her daughter-in-law refused to do so. Her husband died nine years ago, leaving her alone. Y.T. did not want to live with any of her married children at that time, so she asked her youngest daughter to come back home and live with her. At that time, no sign of dementia was apparent. She enjoyed her life, teaching tea ceremony for several years. It was also convenient for her youngest daughter to live with her mother because she could devote herself to her work without worrying about housekeeping which was done by Y.T. When Y.T. was 70 years old, the youngest daughter recognized that Y.T.'s memory loss was somewhat extraordinary. She was surprised to find that Y.T. forgot the fact that she had forgotten something. She wanted Y.T. to see a doctor, but her brothers and sister, especially the eldest brother, was strongly against the idea of going to the hospital. When the son visited Y.T., he did not see anything wrong with her. If he had stayed to live with her for a week or so, he would have discovered his mother's problems. Two years later Y.T. got lost in the neighborhood and was rescued by a police officer. After such an accident, Y.T.'s sons and daughter finally agreed to have Y.T. see a doctor. She came to the hospital with her youngest daughter, and was diagnosed as having moderate to severe Alzheimer's disease. When we told the youngest daughter about the diagnosis and prognosis, she wanted to register Y.T. on the nursing home waiting list, which was three years long at that point. But again, her eldest brother opposed it, insisting that their mother be taken care of at home by one of her children. The second son lived in Osaka, the married daughter was taking care of her parents-in-law, and the eldest son's wife refused to live with Y.T. Thus there was no one but the youngest daughter who could take the responsibility. The eldest son suggested that if the youngest sister would resign from her job and devote herself to caregiving, he and the younger brother would support them financially. However, she refused her brother's offer. She had been working in a publishing company as an editor for nearly 20 years, and she loved her job. She decided to continue working and also take care of her mother at home without help from her brothers, obtaining the assistance of social services, volunteers' services, and support from her company.

When Y.T. was 78 years old, a cancer was found in her breast. The surgeon suggested an operation, but the youngest daughter hesitated to agree to radical therapy. Y.T.'s dementia was so progressed that she needed assistance in daily activities such as eating, dressing and excreting. The daughter was afraid that Y.T. might be unable to cooperate with the doctor concerning the intensive treatment following the operation and this threatened her life seriously. Moreover, at that time, Y.T. had shown no symptoms of the cancer. On this occasion, a conflict again arose with her elder brothers and sister, who insisted that Y.T. have the operation if there was any possibility it would prolong her life. Finally, the youngest daughter carried her point, and this time, her brothers and sister left decisions about their mother's care to her. Y.T. lived two more years, cared for by the youngest daughter at home, and died of pneumonia.

Case 3

T.Y. was a 76-year-old woman who came to see us because of progressive memory loss. She had lived by herself since her husband died 20 years ago. She was born in Tokyo as her parents' first child. Her mother died when she was 2 years old. Her father later remarried, and she had two younger half brothers. However she had not had any contact with them for 20 years. She married a merchant when she was 18. Her husband worked very hard and left her a large inheritance. Since his death, she had devoted herself to supporting young artists such as dancers, singers, and painters, enjoying herself very much in these years.

When she came to our hospital for the first time, she was accompanied by a 50-year-old man who was a dance master of Japanese traditional dancing. He said that she had supported him for a long time, so he would like to take care of her for the rest of her life. He was the person who first recognized her memory problems and persuaded her to see a doctor. She was an intelligent charming old woman, but her memory deficit was apparent at the initial interview. We arranged several examinations for her. Her brain CT and MRI indicated Alzheimer's disease.

When all the examinations were over, T.Y. came to see us with the dance master. T.Y. told us that she was afraid of not being able to understand the doctor's explanation so she wanted him to hear the results with her. So, we explained her disease to them, and also advised them to think about how to manage her properties in the future because she might lose her ability to do so by herself in a year or so. But I never mentioned the diagnosis and they did not ask. I just told her that her memory loss and brain atrophy were not the kind due to the ordinary aging process and that I was afraid her psychological function might decline further. I was worried about the man who came with her. Although T.Y. seemed to trust him very much, he was just a neighborhood friend, not her relative. So I advised them to discuss her future care with her half-brothers.

A week later, T.Y. came to see us again. This time, she was accompanied by her two half-brothers, their wives and the dance master. T.Y. told me that she had asked the dance master to call her half brothers to tell them what happened, and they wanted to see the doctor to hear the explanation directly. T.Y. wanted me to tell her half-brothers exactly the same story we had told her a week before, so we did.

Another week had passed, and T.Y. and the dance master came again. She asked me whether she had Alzheimer's disease. She said that after the last visit, her half-brothers told her that she might have Alzheimer's disease, and that either of them would be willing to serve as her guardian. I verified that she did have Alzheimer's disease, my first experience of disclosing a diagnosis of Alzheimer's disease to the patient herself. She did not look very upset, but only asked me what would happen to her in the future. She said that she did not want to be cared for by her half brothers. She wanted to give part of her property to the dance master and entrust the rest to him for her own care. Although her memory function at that point was insufficient, she was still able to make such a judgment. I advised her to consult a lawyer to go through the necessary formalities. She subsequently met with a lawyer and made arrangements to give a part of her property to the dance master and entrust the rest to the lawyer for her care.

Case 4

M.S. is a 72-year-old widow. She was born in Hokkaido, but moved to Manchuria with her husband in the 1930s. He died in the war, and she came back to Japan alone. Since then, she has been living in Tokyo by herself. When she turned 70 she retired from her work. She lived in a small apartment, with no friends or relatives in Tokyo.

The person living next door had gone to the Social Welfare Office claiming that the office should pay more attention to this isolated old woman. What frightened the residents of the apartment was the potential for an accidental fire because she sometimes left her room forgetting that she was cooking. She also could not abide by the rules among the residents of the apartment, although she had previously been a very precise woman. The residents of the apartment believed she was no longer able to live by herself and that the Social Welfare Department should place her in a special nursing home for the aged.

When the case worker of the Social Welfare Office visited her, her clothes looked dirty and her small room was full of smelling rubbish. It was almost impossible for him to find even a small space to sit in the room. It looked like it was very difficult for her to live by herself. The social worker tried to persuade her to move in to a nursing home, but she wanted to continue living there and refused to sign the application form for the nursing home. Her memory disturbance was apparent but she could speak rather reasonably. She said that she had been living by herself for more than fifty years, and that she was afraid she might not be able to adapt to living in the nursing home. She did agree reluctantly to a home helper's visit three times a week.

After the initial visit, the social worker looked for a relative who would make an application for the nursing home care on her behalf, and finally found a niece living in a small town in the Tohoku district far from Tokyo. He asked if she could take care of M.S., but she had never met her, and did not want to be involved in the case. The social worker asked the niece to place her seal on the application for the nursing home, and so she did.

M.S. continued to live by herself with home helpers' assistance for two more years, before she was admitted to a nursing home from the waiting list. By that time, her physical ability had declined so much that she no longer refused to move to the nursing home. Her mental function had declined so much that she never asked who had registered her name on the waiting list, but even at that point she wanted to continue to live by herself.

Discussion

The process of decision-making seen in case 1 was previously the most common in dementia care in Japan. Most Japanese doctors do not tell the patient the diagnosis or the prognosis of dementia, and most family members do not want doctors to tell the patient the truth. In case 1, the patient's wife was the key person in the decision-making. She took the patient to the hospital. When the doctors explained the results of the medical and psychological examinations, she came to the hospital without her husband, although he might have been able to understand what had happened. After that, the wife immediately consulted with her mother-in-law about what they should do. This was a holdover from the traditional structure of Japanese society. In this case, the patient's wife took the initiative in decision-making because her mother-in-law was too old to do so. They were anxious about the impact of societal responses to the disease on their children's job and marriage opportunities. The burden of caregiving could be a hazard for the marriage of children, especially a son, because the son's wife might be expected to take part in the caregiving. This was another remnant of traditional society. But the burden of caregiving in this case was too much for the wife. It was the younger generation who broke through the bottleneck by consulting the Social Welfare Office and introducing social resources which could provide support to their mother.

K.A. is now in the final stage of Pick's disease. He has been getting good mental and physical care from his family members, but his own will has been excluded from the decision-making about his life from the beginning of the disease.

Case 2 represents a recent trend in Japan. The number of elderly people who are cared for not by the daughter-in-law, but by the daughter (married or unmarried), has been increasing rapidly in large cities.

The first reaction of the eldest son to his mother's dementia, resistance to facing the facts, is a common reaction of patients' children, especially sons. Although such a reaction is also common in western countries, in Japan, such an attitude may be more apparent. Dore (1978) found that the mother–son relationship was a particularly strong tie in Japanese families. The son in this case did not want to acknowledge the situation, so until his mother's dementia became severe, he would never agree to have her seen at the hospital, nor did he come to see the medical staff to hear her diagnosis and prognosis. At the first stage of care, the son refused to consider the idea of his mother's admission into a nursing home. Although he took no responsibility for his mother's care, his youngest sister, who lived with her and looked after their mother, always consulted him. In the traditional family structure, the eldest son had been the leader of the whole family.

Once the youngest daughter decided to take care of her mother at home and also continue working, she took advantage of all the social resources available to her. Her mother had long experience working as a volunteer in the community nursing home when she was in good health, and thus her old friends were willing to help. The publishing company in which the youngest daughter was working offered ways to support her in her caregiving of her mother. In the process of the care, the youngest daughter consulted with her elder brothers and sister at important phases of decision-making. They did not fully understand their mother's situation or the hard work of the youngest sister, and this often made her irritable. Fortunately, she had a supportive social network. Her friends looked after her and her mother and offered their opinions occasionally. It helped her to view her own situation objectively and to make the right decisions. By the time her mother's cancer came to light, she was confident enough in her own decision-making concerning her mother's care. The mother could not decide anything so the youngest daughter decided to avoid radical treatment for her mother. Her elder brothers and sister, who had initially wanted their mother to have the operation, finally agreed with her. At first, she had left every decision about her mother's care to her eldest brother, which may have been the most comfortable way to proceed. However, in the process of caring for her mother, the youngest daughter became more and more independent from expectations derived from family structure. She used her own social network as much as possible, and finally came to take on the responsibility for managing her mother's end stage care.

Case 3 was the only patient described in this chapter who came to the hospital of her own will, and also the only one who wanted to know her own diagnosis. It is very exceptional in Japan for the doctor to tell a patient about the diagnosis of a disease such as Alzheimer's. In most cases, doctors tell the family members, as illustrated in case 1. The decision as to whether the doctor should tell the truth to patients or not is often left to family members, and almost all families do not want the patient to be told the exact diagnosis and prognosis. The attitude of dementia patients and family members in Japan may not be very different from that of the United States. Maguire *et al.* (1996) reported that although 83 percent of relatives of people with Alzheimer's disease in the United States did not want the patients to be told their diagnosis, 71 percent would want to be told if they had the disorder themselves. High (1994) reviewed fifty-three papers and concluded that elderly patients in western countries almost always prefer that family members serve in the role of surrogate decision makers. Rice and Warner (1994) surveyed attitudes of geriatric psychiatrists in the United States about the disclosure of the diagnosis of dementia to patients. They found that severely demented patients were rarely told their diagnosis, while caregivers were almost always told. The moderately demented were more often informed, while the mildly demented tended to be told the diagnosis without the prognosis. Numerous articles discuss disclosure of a dementia diagnosis in the United States and United Kingdom (for example, Cutcliffe and Milton, 1996; Dickamer and Lachs, 1992; Meyers, 1997; Rohde *et al.*, 1995). In Japan, however, there seems to be even less disclosure, regardless of the severity of the dementia. (See Chapter 7 by Long and Chihara, this volume, concerning disclosure of a cancer diagnosis.) Family caregivers are almost always told, and they make all the decisions for the patients. But the present rapid increase of elderly people living alone makes it impossible for such family relationships to continue. Yet disclosure of the diagnosis to dementia patients is still an extraordinary circumstance.

In case 3, the patient was very wealthy, so many people around her wanted to be her guardian. No one knew who was the most appropriate person to support her. If she had been in a rural district in Japan, a half brother would have become her guardian and looked after her. In such a district, not only the complex kinship network but also the community bond would function as a safeguard for a person such as T.Y. If ever the half-brother were to do something not to her benefit, he would have to risk facing the criticism of his community. But in a large city like Tokyo, such kinship and community bonds no longer exist. It seemed to be risky to leave her life and fortune to the half brothers with whom she had no contact for a long time. Neither was there a way to guarantee that the dance master would support her after she lost her ability to manage her property and daily living. But she declared that she would like to rely on him, so we arranged for them to see a lawyer to prevent expected troubles with her relatives and also to have the lawyer function as a guardian for her. In this way she was able to decide her own way of living and arrange matters according to her own wishes.

Case 4 describes the situation of a single person without property. She had many difficulties living in an apartment by herself, so the claims made by other residents that she should move into a special nursing home for the aged were reasonable. But on the other hand, it is also important that her right to live on her own in her own way be respected as much as possible. When a social worker visited her, she told him that a safe life might not necessarily be a happy life. The social worker gave up trying to persuade her, but he had to respond to the complaints of the neighbors. He arranged all possible resources to help her manage in the apartment, but this was apparently insufficient. At present, the social welfare system for the demented elderly is mainly aimed at supporting coresiding caregivers, not elderly people living alone. There is little effect for those with moderate to severe mental dysfunction. At the same time, the social worker arranged for a relative to sign an application form for a special nursing home for the aged. When a resident applies for admission, the admissions committee in the Social Welfare Office examines the situation and decides whether he or she can be admitted. There is no due process of law for the application of a person without reasonable will, such as a demented older person, or of a person who refuses to apply even though living alone is apparently dangerous for himself and his neighbors. Case 4 is not an exception in Tokyo. In such cases, social workers usually look for a relative and persuade him or her to apply for the nursing home, but in many cases, these relatives are indifferent to the elderly person. Lieberman and Kramer (1991) and Cohen *et al.* (1993) found that not the characteristics of the dementia itself, but the social and psychological variables around the patients, predicted the decision to institutionalize the demented elderly. The same is true in Japan.

As described through these four cases, the legal, medical and social welfare system in Japan is not catching up with the rapid changes of Japanese society. In the medical system, hospital staff are not accustomed to informing patients of a diagnosis like Alzheimer's disease or other dementias in the early stage, or to supporting the psychological reaction of the patient and the family. Whether or not we can inform patients of the diagnosis of dementia depends on the ability of medical professionals to support and respond to the anxiety and depression of patients after the disclosure. In this sense, training doctors, psychologists, nurses and social workers in this field is crucial. At the Department of Neuropsychiatry in Tokyo University Hospital, we have offered psychological support to these early dementia patients in groups, couples, and as individuals. (These are described by Y. Kurokawa in Chapter 13, this volume.) These programs seem to be effective for relieving the anxiety not only of the patients, but also of family members, especially spouses. They also seem to help prevent behavioral disturbances of patients. Novack *et al.* (1979) noted that American physicians moved quickly from believing it inappropriate to tell patients a cancer diagnosis to considering it a duty to inform them. Although disclosure of cancer in Japan remains less widespread than in the United States, the number of people in Japan who want to know their own diagnosis has been increasing rapidly. I expect that the same kind of change concerning the disclosure of the diagnosis of dementia will take place in the near future.

In the Japanese social welfare system, most special nursing homes for the aged now accept dementia patients. However, the laws concerning the operation of special nursing homes for the aged are still based on the assumption that applications from residents are voluntary. The Welfare Law for the Aged (Rōjin Fukushi Hō) does not recognize that there may be many old people whose wishes are not reasonable or are unexpressed because of their dementia. For dementia care in institutions like nursing homes, locked wards or other methods which restrict the freedom of residents are sometimes necessary. Yet there are no legal standards for operating such locked wards. At the end of 1997, the Long-Term Care Insurance Act (*Kaigo Hoken Hō*) was passed. The private sector is expected to launch into the field of providing social welfare services to the elderly. Thus quality control of dementia care, including issues of involuntary admission and restrictions of freedom, has become increasingly important.

In Japanese civil law, the interdiction order and the quasi-incompetence order are the procedures for guardianship of people without the ability to manage their property. However, in such procedures, the people who need guardianship must relinquish other rights which they might still be able to enjoy. These systems were established to assist the mentally retarded or severely psychotic patients. But it is the elderly who now need such assistance. Those with mild dementia have impairments in some areas but remain intact in others. They show rather high IQs and it is difficult to determine the presence or the level of dementia by the standards of mental retardation. Yet Japanese psychiatrists continue to provide evidence for guardianship of elderly people according to these standards. Even in western countries, a medical standard of competency for dementia patients has not yet been established (Fornsworth, 1989; Kaplan *et al.*, 1988; Marson *et al.*, 1997). In Japan, research in this field is urgently needed.

The use of the interdiction order and the quasi-incompetence order of Japanese civil law is far behind the present situation in both legal and medical aspects. Moreover, the thoughts of the general public in Japan are far behind the current reality. Even in Tokyo, more than 50 percent of family caregivers think that there is no need to establish any legal procedure for family members to manage the property of the demented person, such as selling real estate (Saito, 1997). When most elderly people lived with their eldest son's family, this was convenient, but it is no longer realistic when most of the elderly live alone. The Japanese government announced in 1997 that they were preparing a bill concerning guardianship for adults in which they will propose establishing a new form of guardianship that is less restrictive than the interdiction and quasi-incompetence orders. Meanwhile, some local authorities in Tokyo, Osaka, Kanagawa, and other large cities are experimenting with new systems to assist in the management of the property of elderly people. Most of these are systems of private guardianship under voluntary contract, modeled after the British Enduring Powers of Attorney Act. These private or voluntary systems may be more appropriate for elderly people who live alone.

These programs, however, have been limited to concern for the management of property. Decision-making about medical care or other matters of daily living of the demented elderly have not become a topic of discussion in Japan. When the elderly person is living with his or her family, as in case 1 and case 2, a family member's decisions are automatically assumed to be the patient's decision. As the numbers of elderly living alone increase, problems like case 3 and case 4 are becoming more common. Systems such as the American durable power of attorney for health care would be helpful in some of these situations.

Conclusion

In the past, decisions about health care, social welfare, and daily living affairs of elderly people with dementia were left to family members. But the rapid aging of the Japanese population has been accompanied by a dramatic increase in the number of households in which an elderly person lives alone or only with an elderly spouse, making family-based decision-making more difficult.

To catch up with these demographic changes, we need to shift from the traditional decision-making process to more individualized and more autonomous ways to make decisions. For such a shift to occur, medical professionals need more systematic training on how to inform their patients of the truth about their illness and how to support them psychologically to establish more individually oriented medical services and to encourage the patient to make their own decisions for as long as possible. Laws relevant to the decision-making process urgently need to be established. More flexible and less restrictive guardianship systems such as the enduring powers of attorney system of Great Britain and the durable power of attorney for health care of the Untied States should be welcomed. Yet even with such laws in place, new legal standards for the judgment of competency need to be established. Today, medical opinion about the competency of elderly people in Japan is still based on the standards for mentally retarded or psychotic patients. We need clear standards for judging a demented patient's capacity for conducting legal affairs such as testament, marriage, divorce, adoption, private contracts, and other activities.

The function of the family as decision-maker and caregiver of the demented elderly has been on the decline in Japan, while the role of the individual and the autonomy of the elderly have become more important. It is difficult to say whether such a change represents progress or regression for the Japanese. As professional caregivers we must recognize the different experiences and expectations that different age cohorts bring to decision-making. While demographic changes force us to deal with a new reality, we need both to be sensitive to these differences and to recognize that we cannot return to the past.

References

Cohen, C.A., Gold, D.P., Shulman, K.I., Wortley, J.T., McDonald, G., and Wargon, M. (1993). Factors determining the decision to institutionalize dementing individuals: A prospective study. *The Gerontologist, 33*, 714–720.

Cutcliffe, J., and Milton, J. (1996). In defense of telling lies to cognitively impaired patients. *International Journal of Psychiatry, 11*, 1117–1118.

Dickamer, M.A., and Lachs, M.S. (1992). Should patients with Alzheimer's disease be told their diagnosis? *New England Journal of Medicine, 326*, 947–951.

Dore, R.P. (1978). *Shinohata : A portrait of Japanese village*. New York: Pantheon Books.

Edwards, W.E. (1989). *Modern Japan through its weddings*. Stanford: Stanford University Press.

Eigingu Sōgō Kenkyū Sentā (Japan Aging Center) (1998). Kōrei Shakai Kisō Shiryō Nenkan 1998–1999 (Basic Statistics of the Aging Society, 1998–1999). Tokyo: Chūō Hōki.

Fornsworth, M.G. (1989). Evaluation of mental competency. *American Family Physician, 39*, 182–190.

High, D.M. (1994). Surrogate decision-making: Who will make decisions for me when I can't? *Clinics in Geriatric Medicine, 10*, 445–462.

Kaplan, K.H., Strang, J.P., and Ahmed, I. (1988). Dementia, mental retardation, and competency to make decisions. *General Hospital Psychiatry, 10*, 385–388.

Kōseishō Kenko Seisaku Kyoku Sōmuka (General Affairs Division, Health Policy Section, Ministry of Health and Welfare). (1994). Makki iryō o kangaeru (Consideration of Terminal Medical Care). Tokyo: Daiichi Hōki Shuppan.

Lieberman, M.A., and Kramer, J.H. (1991). Factors affecting decisions to institutionalize demented elderly. *The Gerontologist, 31*, 371–374.

Maguire, C.P., Kirby, M., Coen, R., Coakly, D., Lawlor, B.A., and O'Neill, D. (1996). Family members' attitudes toward telling the patient with Alzheimer's disease their diagnosis. *British Medical Journal, 313*, 529–560.

Marson, D.C., McInturff, B., Hawkins, L., Bartolucci, A., and Harrell, L.E.. (1997). Consistency of physician judgments of capacity to consent in mild Alzheimer's disease. *Journal of the American Geriatric Society, 45*, 453–457.

Meyers, B.S. (1997). Telling patients they have Alzheimer's disease. *British Medical Journal, 314*, 321–322.

Miura, F. (1997). *Zusetsu Kōreisha Hakusho* (White Paper on Aging in Japan 1997). Tokyo: Japanese Council of Social Welfare.

Novack, D.H., Plumer, R., Smith, R.L., Ochtihill, H., Morrow, G.R., and Bennet, J.M. (1979). Change in physicians' attitude towards telling the cancer patient. *Journal of the American Medical Association, 241*, 897–900.

Ōtsuka, T., Karasawa, A., and Matsushita, M. (1992). Wagakuni no chihō rōjin no shutsu genritsu (The prevalence of dementia in Japan). *Japanese Journal of Geriatric Psychiatry, 3*, 435–439.

Rice, K., and Warner, N. (1994). Breaking the bad news: What do psychiatrists tell patients with dementia about their illness. *International Journal of Geriatric Psychiatry, 9*, 467–472.

Rohde, K., Peskind, E.R., and Raskind, M.A. (1995). Suicide in two patients with Alzheimer's disease. *Journal of the American Geriatric Society, 43*, 187–189.

Saito, M. (1997). Chihō seishikkan o yūsuru kōreisha no zaisan kanri (Financial affairs of the elderly people with dementia). *Rinshō Seishin Igaku* (Japanese Journal of Clinical Psychiatry), *26*, 1399–1405.

16 Concepts of personhood in Alzheimer's disease

Considering Japanese notions of a relational self

William E. Deal and Peter J. Whitehouse[1]

Recent discussions of Alzheimer's disease – and other diseases of which dementia is an integral symptom – often focus on the perspective of the person experiencing the disease. Alzheimer's disease patients are frequently described in terms of the status of their "self."[2] In some cases, persons affected by Alzheimer's disease have been characterized as selves in various stages of deterioration or dissolution. They are seen as having become incomplete persons, or, in the extreme, as having lost their selves altogether – Alzheimer's disease has been called the "death of self" (Cohen and Eisdorfer, 1986, p. 259). By extension, these perceptions of the effects of Alzheimer's disease have shaped the care regimens advocated and developed by researchers and caregivers.

Conceptions of self, then, are critical to our understanding and treatment of persons affected by Alzheimer's disease. In this chapter, we discuss and revise an emerging model of self in dementia and/or Alzheimer's disease advanced in recent literature.[3] The vast majority of studies on the deterioration of self in Alzheimer's disease have been written by western researchers focusing on western – mostly British and American – Alzheimer's disease patients and treatment regimens (Sabat and Harré, 1992; Kitwood, 1990; Kitwood and Bredin, 1992; Herskovits, 1995; Gubrium, 1986; Fontana and Smith, 1989; Cohen and Eisdorfer, 1986). Some scholars have questioned the prevalent paradigm which casts Alzheimer's disease as a condition in which the self is eventually "lost." However, even researchers who have maintained that the patient's self is not entirely absent have contended that in Alzheimer's disease, the self becomes "shattered" (Kitwood and Bredin, 1992, p. 277) or the self is in the process of "unbecoming" (Fontana and Smith, 1989, p. 35).

The problem of self has been particularly important to health care professionals involved with Alzheimer's disease because of the radical changes in personality, mood, and cognitive function that are typical of the disease. Of course, the struggle to better pinpoint the nature of the self has not been the sole domain of those working with Alzheimer's disease – it has long been a preoccupation for people working in various fields. We do not propose to resolve this debate in this chapter, but we do wish to move toward an understanding of self that can better accommodate the extensive changes, across many aspects of human experience, that Alzheimer's disease patients encounter during the disease. We recognize that this notion of self may seem at first rather imprecise, but as we will discuss further below, we believe that the self *is* characteristically elusive, and thus the best way to endeavor to comprehend it is through comparison. In order to reconceive a concept of self, and the nature of the self in Alzheimer's disease, we will contrast views of self in the United States with Japanese perceptions.

For most caregivers, restoring a sense of self, or preventing any further slippage, has been the goal of Alzheimer's disease care philosophies. Recent studies have attempted to change the caregiver view of the patient's self, thereby aiming to reinstate the caregiver's sense of the "personhood" of Alzheimer's disease patients. This type of study takes as one of its assumptions that personhood is socially constructed. For this reason, the caregiver must participate in establishing a sense of personhood in the caregiving relationship (Sabat and Harré, 1992, pp. 445–446; Kitwood and Bredin, 1992, p. 275). In this kind of approach, once the existence of self – understood to be divided into individual and social components – has been recognized, caregiving efforts are aimed at restoring or maintaining the social self, thereby validating personhood. From this perspective, personhood is not possible, at least in any meaningful way, without self.

The language of "personhood" and "self" employed in these theories is crucial to an understanding of issues of self in Alzheimer's disease. As we have seen in the research cited above, personhood is usually defined in part by a construct of self. The self inscribed in personhood runs along a continuum that has at its opposite ends notions of individual self and relational (or social) self, with different cultures locating the self at different points along this

high emphasis	US view of personhood	low emphasis
individual self		relational self

low emphasis	Japanese view of personhood	high emphasis
individual self		relational self

continuum.[4] US and Japanese views are often said to differ in the following way:

The "individual self" and the "relational self" ends of the continuum demonstrate the direct correlation between status of self and personhood. Thus, in a worldview in which there is high emphasis placed upon the relational self – as is the case in Japan – personhood will be primarily defined socially or relationally. By contrast, in worldviews that emphasize the individual self, personhood is principally conceptualized in terms of the autonomous self. When the latter association is made – as it often is in the western views of self discussed in this chapter – the idea that Alzheimer's disease results in a loss or death of self is consequently extended to include a loss of personhood as well.

In cultural conceptions that tend to view self as relational – for instance in the Japanese views discussed below – the self altered by Alzheimer's does not result in a loss of personhood. Rather, personhood is defined in part as a relationship between people that remains intact. Family and caregivers still perceive the Alzheimer's patient as having personhood insofar as the fundamental relationship between them is still conceived to exist. For example, consider the relationship between a woman who has Alzheimer's, no longer able to talk or care for herself, and her son. She continues to exist in the minds of others as a self, even if she is unable to maintain her sense of her own identity. From the son's perspective, she is still his mother even if she cannot think of herself as his mother. The act of ascribing a self thus shifts to others and social interaction becomes the primary means through which the mother's identity is maintained. We can define personhood, therefore, as the status accorded in social interactions to persons recognized as selves. As Kitwood and Bredin argue, "[p]ersonhood is not, at first, a property of the individual; rather, it is provided or guaranteed by the presence of others" (Kitwood and Bredin, 1992, p. 275).[5]

In the studies cited above, the aim of restoring personhood is laudably compassionate and these studies are perceptive in their conception of a socially-constructed self. Yet, ultimately, the concept of self operating in this research is problematic because it centers on a western (especially British and North American) understanding of a unique self as the locus of meaning for human beings. In this perspective, widely held in the United Kingdom, United States, and Canada, Alzheimer's disease robs human beings of their unified, unique, individual selves – which is equated in turn with a loss of personhood. Further, the goal of the restoration of self casts the self as a concrete entity that, like a bodily organ, might be returned to an autonomous, intact state. Implicit in this discourse is the British and North American belief that the ideal, healthy self is an independent self that does not, and should not, require institutionalization, medical care, or other external support. Finally, this model valorizes a self that is both internally and externally consistent, one that does not vary much with circumstances or context – again, a view of self which is not universal, but instead, due to the cultural background of these researchers, is largely limited to British and North American perspectives.

The British and American paradigm of an autonomous self, therefore, is only one of many possible views. Although the neurohistological changes that Alzheimer's disease produces occur similarly in all patients regardless of social context, the radical changes in self that occur in Alzheimer's disease – and our responses to them – are to a large extent culturally variable. Anthropological research has charted substantial differences in the way the effects of Alzheimer's disease and other progressive, degenerative diseases of late life are perceived across cultures (Traphagan, 1998; Long, 1999; Cohen, 1998; Cohen, 1995). Thus, we can and must revise our American view by examining other perspectives.

American insistence upon self-reliance and fixity of self are particularly detrimental to Alzheimer's disease care philosophies. The predominant model of self operating in the United States needs to be revised in order to better accommodate the contingent state of self in Alzheimer's disease proposed in recent scholarship. In order to generate a vision of self in the US that acknowledges a more interdependent, self-in-relation in Alzheimer's disease, we will examine Japanese perceptions of self. A notion of self constituted primarily within social relationships has traditionally been privileged in Japanese culture, with its emphasis on the social over the individual self. Japanese social construction of self thus provides a useful model for exploring how we might conceive of Alzheimer's disease as a condition in which the "individual self" has become subordinated to a "relational self."[6]

Alzheimer's disease foregrounds the fact that the self is largely a cultural construct. Exploring cross-culturally notions of self, both generally and in Alzheimer's disease, affords us insight into different ways of constructing the self, thereby expanding our present conceptions of what is to be valued in human relationships. Revising views of self and of changes that occur in Alzheimer's disease will not only enable us to develop creative, responsible, and responsive care systems, but will also enrich our current perception of how a self is connected to larger social and cultural contexts.

A medical view of Alzheimer's disease and dementia

Alzheimer's disease is the most prevalent dementia in both the United States and Japan. According to 1990 estimates, approximately 994,000 people were affected by senile dementia in Japan, and about 28,000 others had presenile dementia. By 2010, the figure for senile dementia cases is projected to rise to more than two million people in Japan (Kasahara, 1993, p. 76). In the US, an estimated four million individuals are currently experiencing dementia, and dementia is the fourth leading cause of death in adults (University of Michigan Health System Web Site, accessed October 23, 1998).

Dementia is a medical syndrome that is characterized clinically by loss of cognitive abilities in a previously intellectually intact individual. It is different from mental retardation, in which an individual never attains normal intellectual abilities. Dementia is a symptom associated with a number of different illnesses, including structural brain lesions, such as tumors, and metabolic deficiencies, such as thyroid dysfunction. Because senile dementia and Alzheimer's disease have the same neuropathological characteristics, in recent literature, both conditions have been designated dementia of Alzheimer type (Kasahara, 1993, p. 77). The most common cause of dementia is Alzheimer's disease.

Biologically, Alzheimer's disease causes progressive degeneration of nerve cells in specific areas of the brain. These areas include subcortical structures as well as areas of the cortex, including temporal, and less commonly, frontal lobe parietal areas. Other degenerative dementias affect other regions of the brain, including more prominent damage to the frontal lobes.

The pattern of cognitive impairment in Alzheimer's patients is quite variable. Perception, language, memory, and attention can all be affected by cognitive impairments associated with Alzheimer's disease. Those patients in whom the frontal lobe is affected may have particular problems in that they lose initiative, including the ability to plan and monitor their own behavior. Moreover, patients with dementia of Alzheimer type frequently exhibit anisognosia, a condition in which individuals are not at all aware that they are experiencing a disease.

Alzheimer's disease patients are confronted with disparities between their abilities, their self-perceptions, and how others believe they are capable of performing. Thus, due to the nature of the biological damage, its location, and resulting cognitive problems, it is not surprising that patients with Alzheimer's disease have limitations in their ability to perceive and assess themselves. The most significant observation usually made by others about Alzheimer's disease patients is that the self has changed. An inexorable progression toward a total loss of self is commonly cited as the hallmark of Alzheimer's disease, yet, paradoxically, there is no physiological location for the self nor a reliable test for measuring changes in self – though there are methods for measuring both changes in self-perception and cognitive function. Because we have no neuroanatomical means of locating the self, and because it is extremely difficult for patients to communicate abstract ideas about their experience of the disease, it is impossible to objectively gauge the state of an Alzheimer's disease patient's self. Thus, perceptions of changes in self in Alzheimer's disease are necessarily subjective assessments made by others through social interaction with the patient. Studies about the nature of self in Alzheimer's disease have therefore often been limited to theoretical discussions and/or experiments of intentional design drawing upon interviews with, observation of, or literature written by individuals who are considered representative of people with dementia (Sabat and Harré, 1992; Kitwood and Bredin, 1992; Fontana and Smith, 1989; Gubrium, 1988). Below, we discuss some of these studies, the conclusions reached by their authors, as well as the limitations of such research.

What happens to the self in Alzheimer's disease?: conflicting views

As noted above, Alzheimer's disease is often conceptualized as an assault upon the self, a disease in which "[t]he self has slowly unraveled and 'unbecome' a self ..." (Fontana and Smith, 1989, p. 45). This fundamental assumption about the effects of Alzheimer's disease has informed such influential caregiver resources as *The Loss of Self* (Cohen and Eisdorfer, 1986) which states that "[b]oth the victim and the family suffer with the inexorable dissolution of self" (p. 22). This view of the self lost in Alzheimer's raises two significant questions: what is a self that it can be lost through disease, and how is self defined as different from cognitive function?

In the contemporary United States, where there is a strong emphasis on the integrity of the individual, rational thought, moral agency, and other cultural markers of an independent self, this "loss" of self is seen as catastrophic. For Americans, these markers of self are connected with cognitive function, and rationality in particular. To lose cognitive function is to lose a significant aspect of self, as well as fundamental independence. Yet – as we shall see when we turn to conceptions of self in Japan – other cultures often place greater value on social relationships and the responsibilities that exist within communities, rather on than independence or individual needs. Especially in Japan, the relational self is a powerful cultural concept.

This variation in conceptions of self between Japan and the United States is just one example supporting notions of self as sociocultural constructions rather than universal constants. As "healthy" selves vary across cultures, so too changes in self associated with Alzheimer's disease must vary. Thus, there can be no concrete, universal self in Alzheimer's disease, nor a uniform loss of self, that exists across cultures. Further, since we have no objective means of measuring the self, it is problematic to define and chart the self through observable changes in cognitive function, as has often been the case. Recent research supports a revised, variable vision of the self in Alzheimer's disease, challenging the notion of the lost self in Alzheimer's disease, and further demonstrating through various means how self is constructed socially. More specifically, some theorists have endeavored to engender significant improvements in Alzheimer's patient treatment by recognizing personhood, an aspect of the self which they claim is denied when the Alzheimer's self is conceived only through cognitive ability (Kitwood and Bredin, 1992; Sabat and Harré, 1992).

Stephen Post, in his book *The Moral Challenge of Alzheimer Disease* (1995), discusses predominantly negative portrayals of individuals affected by Alzheimer's disease. He identifies such pessimistic views as a partial consequence of the excessive value placed on cognition since the Enlightenment. Post sees American society as overly cognitive: the rational self is valued more than the emotional self; facts become more important than values. As a person with Alzheimer's disease loses cognitive function, he or she becomes less valued because his or her ability to think rationally deteriorates. He notes that in this worldview, paramount in European and American culture, rationality is viewed as the dominant human attribute enabling a sense of self and social connectedness.

Like Post, several researchers have agreed that the equation of cognitive function with selfhood has valorized rationality over other aspects of human experience and led to an adverse view of both Alzheimer's and Alzheimer's disease patients. Further, some scholars have noted that, in order to allow our view of what happens to the self in Alzheimer's disease to reflect the variability of self across cultures, and thus better care for Alzheimer's disease patients, it is necessary to differentiate between self and cognitive ability. Kitwood and Bredin agree with Post that western psychology, with its overemphasis on "hypercognitivism," has too closely linked concepts of personhood and cognitive ability, thus inhibiting efforts to create a humane perspective on dementia (1992, p. 278). Herskovits notes that "in sharp contrast to the current Alzheimer's construct, in which cognitive function is a central and defining characteristic of the self that is especially vulnerable to attack by the disease," several recent theories (Gubrium, 1988; Sabat and Harré, 1992; Fontana and Smith, 1989; Bogdan and Taylor, 1989; Robertson, 1991; Gubrium and Wallace, 1990; Kitwood and Bredin, 1992) have separated "the status or viability of the 'self' ... from cognitive ability" (Herskovits, 1995, p. 159).

The necessity of questioning the nexus between cognition and self prevalent in the United States, the United Kingdom, and Canada is supported by the fact that different, but equally valid models of the self and the self in Alzheimer's disease operate in other cultures. The dominant British and North American model of the self in Alzheimer's disease has been impacted largely by our cultural conceptions of aging and our valorization of rationality. Herskovits argues that the central Alzheimer's construct – that Alzheimer's disease is a destroyer of the self, and therefore an enemy to be conquered – has intensified the already overwhelmingly negative conception of aging in American culture. She locates the source of such pessimistic discourse in both the medical establishment and sociocultural norms which valorize youth. She further notes that although there has been much speculation about how Alzheimer's disease patients experience the disease and changes in self, there have been few attempts to understand their perspective, possibly due to the overwhelming negative characterization and fear of Alzheimer's disease (Herskovits, 1995, pp. 147–148). The predominant American model of self discussed by Herskovits has also been cited as central by British authors (Kitwood and Bredin, 1992; Sabat and Harré, 1992). These models do not, however, represent the culturally and ethnically diverse American and British populations which hold differing views of self, nor the multiplicity of worldviews held in other countries. For instance, youth is not uniformly valorized over old age around the world. Recently, Alzheimer's researchers have begun to investigate cultural conceptions of self and aging in attempts to improve our understanding of the impact of perceptions of self on Alzheimer's patient status and experience (Cohen, 1995; Cohen, 1998).

Although the British and American model that prizes human reason and consequently defines self through cognitive ability has been challenged in recent publications, further cross-cultural research is necessary. Often, emphasis on experimentation and empiricism in the scientific method and our persistent faith in medical science as an objective field has perpetuated our enculturated privileging of human reason. To better understand the self in Alzheimer's disease, we must continue to look beyond emphasis on cognitive experience alone as the vital index of the human condition. As Kitwood and Bredin have noted, "the psychiatry of old age has had an overwhelming tendency to make the brain rather than the personhood of the dementia sufferer its central focus of attention; the inquiry has been technical rather than personal." Further, they speculate that medical and scientific researchers of diseases of aging have been "reluctant to articulate and implement a clear concept of the human subject" because the failure to acknowledge subjectivity allows "psychiatry and psychology to conform to a notion of natural science" (Kitwood and Bredin, 1992, p. 270). As Herskovits has noted, the current Alzheimer's construct in the United States has perpetuated the current medicalized discourse which urgently justifies the need to battle Alzheimer's disease because it is a thief of self (1995, pp. 148–149, 150–152). Military metaphors, such as the casting of Alzheimer's disease as an enemy of self, abound in American conceptions of medical care, and have also emphasized physical aspects of disease over personal effects (Annas 1995, p. 745).

In order to separate conceptions of self from cognition and other empirical measures, we must continue to look to cultures in which the Euro-American medical model has less power. We have chosen to discuss Japanese culture because it is one in which the self, and particularly the aging self, is conceived differently than in American culture. Even though the medical model functioning in Japan has been profoundly affected by Euro-American tradition – especially since the United States' occupation of Japan following World War II – Japanese perceptions of self have historically been less grounded in notions of individual cognition. By looking to Japan and other countries, we can further modify our view of self in Alzheimer's disease, and revise how we care for people experiencing the disease.

"Personhood" and Alzheimer's disease

If personhood revolves largely around self, and self is dependent on cognitive function, then the loss of cognitive function precludes the possibility of self, which in turn severely diminishes recognition of personhood in the Alzheimer's disease patient. Yet, paradoxically, recent scholarship has advocated responsive Alzheimer's disease care that centers on the patient's humanity (Herskovits, 1995). If we cannot recognize personhood in Alzheimer's disease patients, how can we care compassionately for them? The key seems to lie in modifying our assumptions about what constitutes a person, much as we have had to modify our view of what constitutes a self.

It is our view that our attention must focus on humanity not as defined by cognitive function, but rather on a notion of interrelational personhood. Since we have discovered that selves are constructed relationally, we must focus on facilitating a caregiver perspective on the Alzheimer's disease patient which allows for a relational conception of self. Because self is an elusive and shifting concept, we need to redirect our attention away from further, unproductive disputes about the nature of self. Instead we must confront how the Alzheimer's disease patient's subjective experience is shaped through relationships with those around him/her. Thus, the problem of self in Alzheimer's disease can be defined best not as a question of the individual's sense of self, but rather, as an issue of how caregivers negotiate the changes in their relationship to the person affected by Alzheimer's disease. How can caregivers learn to understand

and respond to an individual experiencing the world in a way that is at odds with our American individualistic, independent-minded model of personality and human experience? We can explore this question through recently-published perspectives on the experience of self in Alzheimer's disease and corresponding care philosophies for persons affected by Alzheimer's disease. While we disagree in part with some of the theories of self asserted in this literature, we can use these theories to move toward the goal of caring for Alzheimer's disease patients as persons.

Some researchers have persisted in privileging western notions of cognitive function in their attempts to define personhood in Alzheimer's disease, despite the fact that many researchers agree that the cognitive status of the Alzheimer's disease patient remains elusive. Such a definition of personhood is bound to American notions of rationality and cognitive function as definitive indicators of self, as discussed earlier.

David H. Smith (1992) discusses what he calls the "person-focused view" and cites the criteria for personhood advanced by H. Tristam Englehardt, Jr.: persons "are persons…when they are self-conscious, rational, and in possession of a minimal moral sense" (Englehardt, Jr., 1986, p. 109). Smith observes that at some point in the progression of dementia, the person experiencing symptoms "begins to count as less than, or have a different status than, the rest of us" (p. 47). Smith also contends that "[p]ersonhood hinges on the ability to accept responsibility" (p. 47). Reliance upon others is devalued in Smith's conception of personhood. Despite this claim, we have to recognize that our understanding of the kind of functioning necessary for participation in society can and does vary between cultures. This realization has significant implications for treatment of Alzheimer's disease.

Andrea Fontana and Ronald W. Smith (1989) have theorized that due to the subjective nature of the self in Alzheimer's disease, any aspects of self that are recognized in the patient by the caregiver are merely the result of caregiver compensation for a self that is undeniably absent.

> [W]here once there was a unique individual there is but emptiness. Witnessing … the "unbecoming" of self creates a feeling of emptiness in the caregivers' hearts. Thus, they act as agents for the victim and impute to him or her the last remnants of self … [W]e cannot help but wonder how much of what we have considered to be the last vestiges of the patients' self has not been in fact a process of "filling the gaps" on our part. Perhaps, what is left, after the victims' self "unbecome," are but the scarce remains we have attributed to them.
>
> (Fontana and Smith, 1989, p. 45)

While this perspective recognizes that self is, at least in part, a socially constructed project, the authors have inverted the relationship. They fail to acknowledge that in formulating their theory of the fate of self in Alzheimer's disease, they have been profoundly influenced by the widespread Alzheimer's construct, in which the disease attacks and devours the self. The authors' use of the phrase "unique individual" and the word "victims" to describe the patient's self before and after the onset of Alzheimer's (respectively) proves that they are also subscribing to the central medical metaphors which characterize Alzheimer's as a losing battle in which a self is inevitably, irretrievably lost. Thus the caregiver's expectations concerning the loss of self have already determined that no relational construction of self may take place. The only subjective self allowed a voice in this relationship is that of the caregiver.

This singular self can be contrasted with the relational self – and the possibility of personhood – suggested by Sabat and Harré (1992) and Kitwood and Bredin (1992). Notably, for these theorists, "the *relational self* supersedes the *autonomous self* of classical liberal humanism" (Herskovits, 1995, p. 159). Extending this perspective, we contend that self is largely constructed and constituted within social relationships, thereby enabling Alzheimer's disease patients' personhood through social networks. In this way, the recognition of personhood positively affects the caregiving relationship.

Our concern here is not with the possibility of restoring self to an autonomous, pre-Alzheimer's state, but rather with relationships between Alzheimer's disease patients and their families, friends, and other caregivers. Many researchers have approached quality-of-life issues of Alzheimer's disease through the concept of personhood, especially in literature published in the last ten years. This somewhat amorphous term seems initially difficult to comprehend, especially when applied to someone experiencing Alzheimer's disease. Yet a closer examination reveals that most health care professionals who have discussed personhood as an important focal point for that care of Alzheimer's disease and dementia patients have used the term in a way that complements the understanding of self as defined largely through relationships we have outlined in this chapter.

In much of the recent literature, the term personhood has been used to designate the quality of life experienced by the Alzheimer's disease patient, specifically through personal relationships (Kitwood and Bredin, 1992; Sabat and Harré, 1992). Researchers have differed in their means of measuring and qualifying personhood in Alzheimer's disease, yet most scholars and researchers agree that personhood is what must be maintained or restored in order to allow the Alzheimer's disease patient, who continues to exist as a human self to some degree, to have a continuity of their experience as a person.

Sabat and Harré (1992) have responded to the idea that Alzheimer's disease results in a loss of self, questioning the idea that a disease can directly engender such a loss (pp. 443–444). These authors employ the constructionist theory of the nature of self to explore the possibility of its loss in disease, theorizing that only social aspects of the self are indirectly lost as a result of the disease. They argue that it is not cognitive function, such as memory, that constitutes a "self of personal identity" (p. 447). Concerning personhood and cognitive function, they maintain that one "could dispense with psychological memory…without ceasing to meet the criteria for personhood" (p. 447). For Sabat and Harré, personhood is established through caregiver identification and recognition of indices of the Alzheimer's disease patient's sense of self, such as use of indexical pronouns (e.g., "I" and "me") by the Alzheimer's disease patient (p. 447). Participation of others in the social environment is necessary for recognition of personhood: "social recognition ... will have profound effects upon the ways in which the person's behaviour is viewed and the ways in which the person is then treated by others" (p. 446).

Like Sabat and Harré, Kitwood and Bredin (1992) also see the key aspect of Alzheimer's disease care as keeping the sufferer's personhood intact. They criticize what they consider the dominant model used by care practitioners in residential treatment centers in which the problem of self is situated in the patient. Kitwood and Bredin contend that the dismantling of the personhood of Alzheimer's disease patients emerges out of the patterns of social interaction in which the professional contributes to the problem. These authors consider the reactions of other people to the Alzheimer's disease patient to be critical to the patient's quality of life. In Alzheimer's disease, with the self in flux, it is important to validate the patient's personhood through caregiver relationships in order to enable a socially-constituted self to emerge. In terms of the development of the self, personhood emerges in a social context: it is "provided ... by the presence of others" (p. 275). Some patients who seem to have lost all or nearly all cognitive functions show significant reversal of their impairment when their social relationships are improved, leading to positive changes in "social skill, independence and continence" (p. 278).

Clearly, when caring for people with dementia of Alzheimer's type, we are dealing with people whose selves have become much more contingent, or relationally-defined, than we are comfortable with in our individualistic American worldview. One solution is to learn to value different ways that the self can operate in order to reorient our perspective as caregivers. In Alzheimer's disease, we frequently emphasize that the patient's way of processing reality is what has deteriorated. Shifting the focus to realize that what has been lost is our way of relating to that person allows us to avoid an opposition in which we prize our concept of self over that of the affected person. This opens up the possibility of devising a new way of relating to that person. Consequently, many of those involved with Alzheimer's disease research and care have advocated treatment of persons affect with Alzheimer's disease that recognizes that "humanity is still there" (Gubrium, 1986, p. 93), a recognition of personhood.

Japanese views of self

Despite the common-sense notion that in a "healthy" person the self is a consistent, coherent locus of personality, feelings, and other aspects of human experience, we have observed that the self is considerably less fixed than this dominant model suggests. The primacy of the American notion of a rational and fixed self can be called into question through comparison to Japanese cultural perceptions in which the self is not fundamentally characterized as an autonomous entity. Herskovits (1995) stresses the need for such cross-cultural investigations: "Cultures with relational selves, such as Chinese and Indian communities, would be intriguing locations for comparative research regarding the image of the self and subjectivity in senility or, if the disease construct is locally relevant, in Alzheimer's" (p. 161, note 11). In this section, we explore concepts of self in Japanese culture, and discuss how they can contribute to how we care for, interact with, and empower a relational self in Alzheimer's disease.

As we have been arguing, Alzheimer's disease is a condition that is intimately linked to culturally-defined notions of the self. One traditional way to describe the difference between American and Japanese notions of self has been to do so through the dichotomy of individuality versus relationality.

A common American view of the self conceives it to be something set apart from society: one can assert a sense of self or have rights independent of social rules and institutions. The healthy self is rational, distinct from such irrational demands as those made by one's body, emotions, and spiritual needs. However, in Japan, self has often been defined in terms of networks of social relationships (Doi, 1973; Kondo, 1990; Rosenberger, 1992). This contrasts with the dominant emphasis in the United States on the centrality of the individual self. Although psychological and sociological conceptions of self exist in Japan, the notion of acting together as a community or country seems to be stronger than the way of thinking about society as populated by discrete selves with human rights which predominates in the US. Dependence on others may be considered a weakness in the United States, but dependence on others is seen as acceptable and necessary in Japanese society (Doi, 1973). The dominance of rationality in defining human uniqueness is less evident.

Through interconnected sets of social relationships, then, self in Japan is endowed with significant meaning. One's sense of self is determined in changing contexts of family, co-workers, and larger local and national affiliations. As Rosenberger (1992) points out, "The very word for self in Japanese, *jibun*, implies that self is not an essentiality apart from the social realm. *Jibun* literally means 'self part' – a part of a larger whole that consists of groups and relationships" (Rosenberger, 1992, p. 4).

Lebra (1992) also argues that self, for the Japanese, is contingent upon social context. She points out that Japanese will usually refer to themselves as "teacher" when addressing students, and as "uncle" when an adult male who is a stranger addresses a child, thereby avoiding the use of "I" (p. 111). The terms used for identification of self in these instances function as statements of relationship between speaker and listener rather than as declarations of an autonomous self. Lebra identifies this type of speech as "empathetic identification," a term first used by Suzuki (1986).

The above perspectives on the self support a view of a Japanese sense of self that is based in relationality. This is not to say that there is no inner sense of self, but rather that because of the high-context nature of Japanese culture and society, far more emphasis is placed upon the definition of self in terms of others than in the US. It is important to bear in mind that Japanese people can and do conceive of an independent self, although, because of the importance of social context in Japan, self can be played out in various ways depending on the situation. Thus, conceiving of the Japanese self as constituted solely through relationships represents an unnecessarily extreme view that reifies Japanese culture in much the same way that the ruined self is made the centerpiece of the current Alzheimer's disease construct. Significantly, a view of self expressed only through relationships allows for no concrete, contiguous sense of self, and therefore obviates the need to develop ways of caring for Alzheimer's patients which attempt to recognize the patient's self. This kind of logic makes no inroads toward developing Alzheimer's care regimens which keep personhood intact.

Following such scholars as Rosenberger (1992) and Long (1999), we suggest conceiving of the function of self in Japan as moving along a "continuum of inner/outer, a recognition that self may be differently negotiated in different places" (Long, 1999, p. 2). While other scholars have cited the relational status of self in Japan as evidence that there is no essential self, Long proposes that concepts of an independent self exist in Japanese culture. Her model acknowledges a self that vacillates between *uchi* (inner) and *soto* (outer), and thus emphasizes the fluidity of conceptions of self in Japan, particularly when contrasted with the vision in the United States of a self which is expected to be integrated and reliably fixed, absolute rather than contextually defined.

Distinctions made between normal effects of aging and pathological diseases are another significant difference between Japan and the United States that underscores the social function of self in Japanese culture. For example, Traphagan (1998) has studied how Alzheimer's disease and other neurohistological diseases involving dementia are not feared in Japan as much as is a category of general decline associated with old age known as *boke*. This condition is not feared for the pathological effects more usually associated with diseases of old age, but rather for the anxiety that the elderly experience about burdening their children with daily care responsibilities. Rather than focus on the medical, scientific view of disease, Japanese seem more concerned with the social effects and outcomes of aging.

In attempting to improve Alzheimer's disease care, we can benefit from understanding that self may not be a constant internally unified entity, but rather a changing one. Thus, in treatment of Alzheimer's patients, it is very important to continue to create a context for these individuals in order to preserve a contiguous relational self, despite the severe loss of cognitive function. By exploring Japanese notions of self, both generally and in Alzheimer's disease, we have elicited a different way of conceiving the self, and thereby expanded on our present conceptions of personhood and what is to be valued in human relationships.

Conclusion

The physiological changes produced through Alzheimer's disease have neurohistological similarities in all patients regardless of social context, but the self that appears to be so radically altered is enacted through social relationships and is therefore intimately bound to cultural constructs. Thus, the problem of self in Alzheimer's disease is not ultimately located in the patient's internal sense of self. Rather, the problem centers on how caregivers attempt to understand and respond to the patient's profoundly changed experience of the world, and how to reconcile that altered, dependent self with the view of self valorized by our individualistic, independent-minded American perspective.

Comparisons of Japanese models of self with those operating in the US have supported the claim that self is constructed out of the particularities of time, place, and social context and is therefore contingent, rather than static or fixed. Through recognition of and inquiries into the fluidity of notions of self across cultures, we have to be able to engage with the effects of Alzheimer's disease beyond the hypercognitive model emphasizing the ongoing destruction of self. By challenging the current, pervasively negative constructs of self in Alzheimer's with contentions that the self in Alzheimer's disease must be uncoupled from cognitive ability in order to validate the patient's personhood, we have achieved alternative ways of understanding the self in Alzheimer's disease and thus moved toward the improvement of caregiving practices.

Alzheimer's disease represents a relatively recent and growing challenge to all countries that face the problem of how to care for an aging population. Epidemiologically, Japan and the United States are on the forefront of this aging trend, with an estimated 23 percent of the Japanese population reaching the age of 65 or older by 2015 (Ministry of Health and Welfare, 1991), and the US Bureau of the Census estimating that the population over 80 years old will grow to over six million by the same date (Randall, 1993). As leading economic powers, both countries possess some of the resources necessary to approach the problem systematically. However, in addition to being a financial concern, caring for individuals with Alzheimer's is also a conceptual and sociological issue. Neither country has resolved how Alzheimer's disease should be approached and understood, particularly with regard to how different cultural views of self can impact on care philosophies for Alzheimer's patients. Further cross-cultural comparisons will yield richer theoretical and ethical discussions concerning dementia, as well as sharing of practical information about how to develop better care systems for persons and families affected by the disease. As we care for an increasing elderly population that also grows more diverse, we need to be sensitive to the multiplicity of ways that they have experienced self.

Notes

1 The authors want to acknowledge the help of Lisa J. Robertson in researching and editing this chapter.
2 Throughout this paper we call into question the term "self." For stylistic reasons, subsequent use of this term will be written without quotation marks. However, we want to remind the reader that we use the term advisedly because of its multiple, conflicting connotations.
3 Much of the scholarship on conceptions of self has focused on Alzheimer's disease specifically. However, some scholars have written more generally about the loss of self in dementia, a

condition associated with various diseases. We will confine our remarks here to Alzheimer's disease, although much of what we argue could be applied to other diseases in which dementia is a significant symptom.

4 Kitwood and Bredin (1992) also view the self along a continuum, but their conception concerns ideas of subjectivity and intersubjectivity which puts the self in a fractured state when self is not seen as unified or coherent, as in their view of the state of the self in dementia. See especially pages 276–277.

5 Using this description as a point of departure, Kitwood and Bredin (1992) conclude that the pivotal objective in dementia care is "keeping the sufferer's personhood in being" (p. 269). They assess that the present lack of recognition for personhood in dementia patients can be resolved by "see[ing] personhood in social rather than individual terms" (p. 269). Although Kitwood and Bredin recognize that not all cultures equate personhood with the concept of the individual self, they chart self-development through changes in conceptions of subjectivity and intersubjectivity without discussing varying cultural perceptions of the relevance of this process. Exploring specific cultural differences in the relationship between status of self and personhood, particularly contrasts as significant as those between the United States and Japan, aids us in challenging traditional western models of self – and dementia care – that do not adequately recognize a relational model of personhood.

6 For an extensive discussion of the "relational self," see Shweder, 1991.

References

Annas, G. (1995). Reframing the debate on health care reform by replacing our metaphors. *New England Journal of Medicine, 332*, 744–747.

Bogdan, R., and Taylor, S.J. (1989). Relationships with severely disabled people: The social construction of humanness. *Social Problems, 36*, 135–148.

Cohen, A., and Eisdorfer, C. (1986). *The loss of self: A family resource for the care of Alzheimer's disease and related disorders.* New York: W.W. Norton & Company.

Cohen, L. (1998). *No aging in India: Alzheimer's, the bad family, and other modern things.* Berkeley: University of California Press.

Cohen, L. (1995). Toward an anthropology of senility: Anger, weakness, and Alzheimer's in Banaras, India. *Medical Anthropology Quarterly, 9*, 314–334.

Doi, T. (1973). *The anatomy of dependence.* Tokyo: Kodansha International.

Englehardt, H.T., Jr. (1986). *The foundations of bioethics.* New York: Oxford University Press.

Fontana, A., and Smith, R.W. (1989). Alzheimer's disease victims: The "unbecoming" of self and the normalization of competence. *Sociological Perspectives, 32*, 35–46.

Gubrium, J.F., and Wallace, J.B. (1990). Who theorizes age? *Aging and Society, 10*, 131–149.

Gubrium, J.F. (1988). Incommunicables and poetic documentation in the Alzheimer's disease experience. *Semiotica, 72*, 235–253.

Gubrium, J.F. (1986). *Oldtimers and Alzheimer's: The descriptive organization of senility.* Greenwich, CT: JAI Press.

Herskovits, E. (1995). Struggling over subjectivity: Debates about the "self" and Alzheimer's disease. *Medical Anthropology Quarterly, 9*, 146–164.

Kasahara, H. (1993). How many patients with dementia of the Alzheimer's type are there in Japan? *Asian Medical Journal, 36*, 76–84.

Kitwood, T. (1990). The dialectics of dementia: With particular reference to Alzheimer's disease. *Ageing and Society, 10*, 177–196.

Kitwood, T., and Bredin, K. (1992). Towards a theory of dementia care: Personhood and well-being. *Ageing and Society, 12*, 269–287.

Kondo, D.K. (1990). *Crafting selves: Power, gender, and discourses of identity in a Japanese workplace.* Chicago: University of Chicago Press.

Lebra, T.S. (1992). Self in Japanese culture. In N. Rosenberger (Ed.), *Japanese sense of self* (pp. 105–120). Cambridge: Cambridge University Press.

Long, S.O. (1999). *Shikata ga nai*: Resignation, control, and self-identity in Japan. In S.O. Long (Ed.), *Lives in motion: Composing circles of self and community in Japan*. Ithaca: Cornell East Asia Series.

Ministry of Health and Welfare. (1991). *Health and welfare statistics*. Tokyo: Health and Welfare Statistics Association.

Post, S.G. (1995). *The moral challenge of Alzheimer disease*. Baltimore: Johns Hopkins University Press.

Randall, T. (1993). Demographers ponder the aging of the aged and await unprecedented looming elder boom. *Journal of the American Medical Association, 269*, 2331–2332.

Robertson, A. (1991). The politics of Alzheimer's disease: A case study in apocalyptic demography. In M. Minkler and C.L. Estes (Eds.), *Critical perspectives on aging: The political and moral economy of growing old* (pp. 135–150). Amityville, NY: Baywood Publishing Company.

Rosenberger, N.J. (Ed.) (1992). *Japanese sense of self*. Cambridge: Cambridge University Press.

Sabat, S.R., and Harré, R. (1992). The construction and deconstruction of self in Alzheimer's disease. *Ageing and Society, 12*, 443–461.

Shweder, R.A. (1991). *Thinking through cultures: Expeditions in cultural psychology*. Cambridge, MA: Harvard University Press.

Smith, D.H. (1992). Seeing and knowing dementia. In R.H. Binstock, S.G. Post, and P.J. Whitehouse (Eds.), *Dementia and aging: Ethics, values, and policy choices* (pp. 44–54). Baltimore: Johns Hopkins University Press.

Suzuki, T. (1986). Language and behavior in Japan: The conceptualization of personal relations. In T.S. Lebra and W.P. Lebra (Eds.), *Japanese culture and behavior* (pp. 142–157). Honolulu: University of Hawaii Press.

Traphagan, J.W. (1998). Localizing senility: Illness and agency among older Japanese. *Journal of Cross-Cultural Gerontology, 13*, 177–188.

University of Michigan Health System Web Site. Online. Available HTTP: http://www.med.umich.edu/mismr/alzheimers.html (accessed 10/23/98).

17 Epilogue: downsizing the material self

Late life and long involvements with things

David W. Plath

> How old would you be if you didn't know how old you are?
> Leroy (Satchel) Paige

In this International Year of Older Persons I am three birthdays beyond the keyhole where US society inserts its 65-year-old members categorically into Late Life. As a newcomer to the territory I am low on direct experience, and know the place mainly through hearsay. But I can offer personal testimony on one issue in Late Life that years of reading gerontology journals did not prepare me for: and that is the problem of things.

Material objects. Possessions. Impedimenta. All the detritus that accumulates around us during our decades of "cumbering the earth," a charming nineteenth-century phrase that was applied to the elderly. A modest example: the first day of this year also marked the end of my employment in the university that has been my sheltered workshop for more than three decades. I am obligated to cease cumbering the campus. Which means, in practical terms, that before the year is half over I must vacate the office I have been using for almost twenty years. Which in turn means I must decide what to do with all that stuff *in* the office. Somehow I must dispose of more than a thousand books and reprints, some 200 or so videotapes, and twenty drawers full of files. The figures do not include cartons under the tables and stacked in corners – cartons stuffed with never-got-them-sorted newspaper clippings in English and Japanese, plus a few in languages I do not read such as Thai and German.

If you can't take it all with you, where are you supposed to leave it? The Fourth Age, the focus of this book, is a time of frailty, when most people require caregiving attention, modest or massive, from others. During the Third Age, by contrast, most of us can deal with most of our needs more often than not. For many of us, one of those needs is to downsize the material self, to put it onto a reducing diet, to give away or recycle or discard most of that accumulated stuff. In the ideal Hindu life cycle, Late Life is when one should become a *sannyasin*, leave all of those possessions at home, and retreat alone into the forest to meditate. This may be spiritually admirable, good for one's soul, but morally questionable to the extent that it cumbers one's kin with the burden of one's downsizing. Caregiving in the Fourth Age, then, may be contingent upon how effectively one has downsized during the Third Age.

So day after day I have to make choices. Some books and papers are easy to give away or to discard. But some of my possessions seem to possess me – it is as if they have put guilt trips on me so that I feel obliged to preserve them regardless of my indifference to them. And some are so embedded in my autobiography that if I were to lose them I would mourn the departure of a piece of my self.

I have begun donating most of my professional books to university libraries, and throwing all but a few of my files into the recycling bin. The exceptions are books and files I need for projects not yet completed, or ones that have some personal cachet – e.g. a book that was given me by its author. Sorting through these items is time-consuming and a drain on physical energy but it does not require much mental energy.

The mentally draining category involves all my souvenirs of anthropological pilgrimage. Fieldnotes is the generic term for such items of tangible evidence that one has engaged in anthropology's iconic mode of professional inquiry. In addition to notes in the strict sense the category includes photos, maps, questionnaire protocols, audio and video recordings and all sorts of other artifacts "collected" in situ. In the ideology of the profession the process of "collecting" has transmuted such items into Scientific Data. They should not simply be discarded. Their collector-of-origin is supposed to arrange for their perpetual care – for the possible edification of some future generation. In reality, librarians and curators are unpassionate about providing perpetual care for fieldnotes other than those prepared by a scholar deemed to be of world stature. The excuse of choice these days is that Anything Worth Preserving Can Be Put on The Web. So this second category is one on which I must expend both physical and mental energy.

If that second category is socially significant, a third category is personally so. It involves very little physical energy, at least in my case: there are only a few items, and they can easily be stored or transported. But there is a cost in psychic energy in the form of fear of loss: their survival and my survival are difficult to disentangle. Healthy self-care in the Third Age means not just brushing my teeth, taking my vitamins, and disposing of things that have become a bother; it means husbanding things that have become – borrowing a term from Montaigne – *consubstantial* with me.

Such things are priceless to me in the sense that none of the market mechanisms in the world economy can generate an adequate measure of their value-in-exchange, no auction-sale price is likely to seem equivalent, and no similar item would serve as an acceptable replacement. Their value has to be measured by the calculus of biographical experience, not that of economic goods and services. By their very weight and durability such objects offer evidence that I possess individual weight and biography, that my self is a tangible entity, mortal to be sure but perdurable. Or to use a memorable phrase from

Jules Henry, these objects provide a measure of my "capacity to be missed" (Henry, 1973, p. 22).

Montaigne used the term *consubstantial* to describe his long involvements with the book that was his literary life-work. Twice over a period of seventeen years he radically rewrote and re-edited his *Essays*. But with each successive edition the book grew longer. To cut out anything he had written, said Montaigne, felt almost like cutting off pieces of his own flesh. In words that call to mind the *seikatsu tsuzurikata undō* in Japan 400 years later (similar in purpose but with no known historical link) he explained that he had not just been composing words on a page, he had been composing – putting order and meaning into, we might say – his very life. As he writes in one much-quoted passage:

> Painting myself for others, I have painted my inward self with colors clearer than my original ones. I have no more made my book than my book has made me – a book consubstantial with its author, concerned with my own self, an integral part of my life.
>
> (Montaigne, 1958, p. 504)

Montaigne makes rewriting seem so self-risky that it might need to be rewarded with hazardous-duty pay. By comparison, clearing out the office does not feel like a life-threatening mission. It has been a comfortable place to do my work and to meet with students and colleagues. Losing access to the office is a form of status-degradation, though more symbolic than pragmatic these days when compared with losing free and easy access to the Internet. And office-loss is not even in the same league with the mobility-loss reported by ex-Presidents and executive officers. Interviewed some time after he had left the White House, Harry S. Truman was asked what he missed most by being out of office. What he most mourned, he said, was that he no longer could pick up the telephone and say, "Get Air Force One ready: I'm going to San Francisco for lunch." And *The Wall Street Journal* recently reported (November 3, 1998, p. B20) that chief executive officers of large corporations are beginning to demand lifetime access to the company jet as part of their price for agreeing to retire.

But if I can't retain access to the office there are, nevertheless, items *in* the office that I will go to some effort to retain. Example: on my shelf is a worn copy of *Fortune* magazine for April, 1944, a special issue devoted entirely to Japan. That April issue has become rare enough that if I were to sell my copy it might earn me the price of a gourmet dinner. The issue is of interest to those who study Japan, because the people who produced it seem to have assumed that their readers had extensive knowledge about Japanese society of the prewar and wartime periods. (For years I have intended to write a short essay based on the issue; maybe someone else will take up the challenge).

In addition to its potential market value and scholarly significance, that April issue of *Fortune* has a meaning that is purely personal. It memorializes a micro-mystery, which is that to this day I do not know who gave me that copy of the magazine, or why.

I first saw a copy of that special issue when I was a graduate student. One of my mentors told me to look it up as a way of appreciating the complicated mixtures of fact and fantasy in US images of Japan. Later, as an instructor, I sometimes borrowed the library's copy and passed it around the room while I addressed the question of images and their changes through time. A day or two after one such class session, what is now "my" copy of the magazine turned up unannounced in my office mailbox. No name was inscribed on it. No stamps declared it to be the property of some library or research collection. No note asked for its return. The statute of limitations expired years ago, but no one ever has come forward to confess having perpetrated this deed of generosity. I shared that magazine with two subsequent generations of students. At another university, years earlier, another anonymous benefactor left me a statuette of Ninomiya Sontoku. I used it, too, in the classroom as an emblem of Japanese values on studiousness – sometimes wondering if the donor's more subtle message to me was that *I* should be more studious.

If the building were to burn down before I finish moving out of my office I would be saddened by the loss of a few objects such as that issue of *Fortune*. And of course the loss of some memorable letters from colleagues and friends. But I would risk my life to retrieve only one item from the conflagration: my copy of Ruth Benedict's *The Chrysanthemum and the Sword*.

Not because my copy has any trade-in value. In a used-book fair it might bring in twenty-five cents. The spine is bent, the cover stained, the corners threadbare. Page after page is marred by underlining. Some is in pencil, some in ink (three different colors, each from a different rereading) including old-fashioned fountain-pen ink that has run into the soft paper. In the margins are lines, brackets, asterisks, exclamation points, question marks, and alongside one passage the word *peke* ("mistake") written in childish *hiragana*.

The book has been a blotter soaking up traces of my struggle to understand Japan and to teach about it. Written inside the front cover is "1954, San Diego" and my signature. At the time I was a junior officer in the US Naval Reserve on my way to a post in Yokohama. Reading Benedict en route, along with Clyde Kluckhohn's *Mirror for Man*, tweaked my curiosity about scholarship, enough that some months later I applied for admission to graduate school. Until that time I had vowed never to become an egghead.

That was only the first of several trips across the Pacific that Benedict, in book form, has taken with me. It has been a curious romance. Not that she has traveled with me constantly – but often enough to have earned herself a heap of frequent-flyer miles. I have read her book more times than any other, even more times than any of the books I have written.

Also in the book are marks that I did not make and that I can't always decipher. Those are traces left by students who borrowed the book from me. I regard their marks as interest payments on the loan. Like a worn-down volleyball, my copy of *The Chrysanthemum and the Sword* offers a record of long involvements in an academic version of Geertzian deep play.

The problem of things in Late Life, to shrink-wrap it in a phrase, is a problem of tangible biography. We rely upon things in order to define our individualness and objectify our ever-fragile memories of personal experience. In marvelously varied and wonderfully colored ways – most of which are yet to be studied and shaped into usable scholarly knowledge – our self-awareness is contingent upon our lifecourse baggage. By extension so are our potentialities for further self-knowledge and action.

Samuel Beckett remarked that memory is an instrument of discovery, not just of reference (Beckett, 1931, p. 17). Our lifecourse baggage, as a kind of materialized memory, similarly is not simply an embalming of what once happened: a thing *preserved* becomes a wager, a sustentation, a confession that pleads for life to be allowed to go on happening. This dimension of downsizing may not be obvious in my attachment to a copy of *The Chrysanthemum and the Sword*; it leaps into view in a sequence of episodes that Yasushi Inoue reports in his *Chronicle of my Mother* (1982). Though Inoue is best known as a writer of fiction, the book is a factual – intimate, poignant – portrait of his own mother as she slides into senility after her seventy-fifth year.

Most of the time Mother mentally is back in her childhood. Over and over she talks about events that must have taken place when she was ten years old – long before any family member now alive had been born. There are, however, moments when she is operating on-line, acting in the real-time frames of Now; moments when she is the strong-willed matron her children have known for decades.

Not that she cares about the day-to-day running of the household; she retired from those responsibilities years ago. All she cares about, is obsessed by, is the family's repayment of funeral gifts. These return-gifts are one of the major – and most publically visible – responsibilities of any Lady of the House, and serve as a measure of her career performance in the role.

Japanese society is famous for its high frequency of gift exchanges. Households usually maintain a gift ledger, recording dates and occasions and estimated values for items received and presented. For many life-cycle rites the preferred item is cash, since it makes valuation easy: when your turn comes to repay, you know the appropriate amount to offer. "When she heard that so-and-so was ill she automatically assumed that the person would die," Inoue writes about Mother.

> And she went for the funeral gift ledger to check the amount of cash she would have to give, which corresponded to the amount her family had received from that family in the past on a similar occasion ... The figure was meaningless in any case, for the value of money had changed drastically since the old days and she could not compute the difference without help, but she was not satisfied unless she did that.
>
> (Inoue, 1982, p. 72)

Son-in-law Akio is philosophical. "I suppose receiving funeral gifts and returning the amount received is definitely the most basic aspect in the give-and-take of human relationships," he tells Inoue. "It's spooky; yet I think it's also beautiful.

Epilogue: Downsizing the material self 339

A person is born, marries, has children, and then dies. If life is condensed, perhaps this is all there is" (Inoue, 1982, p. 72).

But daughter Shikako, Akio's wife, has a different interpretation. She hides the gift ledger in a dresser drawer. As she explains to Inoue, "I somehow feel that after we have returned all we owe on funeral gifts, Granny will die. She will then have drawn a line through each gift that has been returned" (Inoue, 1982, p. 74).

Nine thousand miles across the Pacific Ocean, arguing instead from interview data, the authors of one of the best studies ever done on the material self in the United States arrive at a similar conclusion. "If, as we have argued, the self of mature adults tends to be structured around networks of past and present relationships, which are often embodied in concrete objects," write the authors of *The Meaning of Things: Domestic Symbols and the Self*, "then depriving an older person of such objects might involve the destruction of his or her self" (Csikszentmihalyi and Rochberg-Halton, 1981, p. 102).

"Might involve" is the necessary qualifier, in my view: a healthy human self operating in its ordinary milieu seems quite resilient, able to marshal many layers of defenses. That resiliency could be strained, though, by personal crisis or environmental press – by incarceration, for instance, when one is drafted into the military, or sentenced to prison, or relocated into an old folks' home. Military recruits and others taken into Goffmanesque "total institutions" often report the following: when first inducted they felt a sudden, seemingly complete loss of identity. It was triggered when, having already had to strip naked, they were ordered to hand over their wristwatch or finger rings – their last piece of second skin. Thomas Cole and colleagues' Visible Biographies project (see Nguyen, Hill and Cole, Chapter 14, in this volume) is a pioneering attempt to address this problem for nursing home inductees.

There are, to be sure, extreme examples: dramatic instances in which a person seems to have been willing to die rather than surrender an object inseparable from his core of being. I think of the Cambodian journalist Haing Ngor, best known for his starring role in the film "The Killing Fields." Thieves accosted him outside his Los Angeles home late one night, demanding money. Ngor handed them his wallet, but when he refused to part with a gold locket hanging from his neck they shot him dead. The locket contained a photo of his dead wife, the only memento of her that he had been able to take with him when he escaped from his war-wracked homeland.

"The old Americans I studied do not perceive meaning in aging itself," writes Sharon Kaufman in *The Ageless Self*, "Rather, they perceive meaning in being themselves in old age" (Kaufman, 1986, p. 6). In part we perceive who we are by examining reflections coming from all sorts of personal objects. Each of us probably treasures an object, or several objects, that embody our central threads of individual continuity and change – objects that other people are likely to regard as weird if they do not know what the objects mean to us. But as Cole's project suggests and Ngor's death emphasizes, among the most valued personal objects (and perhaps the highest common-denominator objects

Table 17.1 Special objects mentioned at least once by respondents of three different generations

Children (n=79)	percentage mentioned	Parents (n=150)	percentage mentioned	Grandparents (n=86)	percentage mentioned
1. Stereos	45.6	1. Furniture	38.1	1. Photos	37.2
2. TV	36.7	2. Visual art	36.7	2. Furniture	33.7
3. Furniture	32.9	3. Sculpture	26.7	3. Books	25.6
4. Musical inst.	31.6	4. Books	24.0	4. TV	23.3
5. Beds	29.1	5. Musical inst.	22.7	5. Visual art	22.1
6. Pets	24.1	6. Photos	22.0	6. Plates	22.1
7. Miscellaneous	20.3	7. Plants	19.3	7. Sculpture	17.4
8. Sports equip.	17.7	8. Stereos	18.0	8. Applicances	15.1
9. Collectibles	17.7	9. Appliances	17.3	9. Miscellaneous	15.1
10. Books	15.2	10. Miscellaneous	16.7	10. Plants	12.8
11. Vehicles	12.7	11. Plates	14.7	11. Collectibles	11.6
12. Radios	11.4	12. Collectibles	12.0	12. Silverware	10.5
13. Refrigerators	11.4	13. TV	11.3	13. Musical inst.	10.5
14. Stuffed animals	11.4	14. Glass	11.3	14. Weavings	10.5
15. Clothes	10.1	15. Jewelry	11.3	15. Whole room	10.5
16. Photos	10.1				

Source: Csikszentmihalyi and Rochberg-Halton, 1981, p. 85.

Note: Interviews were conducted with 82 families in Chicago and Evanston, IL. Half of the families were upper middle class and half lower middle class. Approximately two-thirds were White, one-third Black, and 3 percent Oriental.

across most societies) are those "mirrors with memories", our personal and family photographs. They offer a strategic point of attack for research on self-care in Late Life as well as research on how caregiving by others might better be tailored to individual needs.

"Perhaps the major icons of continuity in American culture today are photographs," suggest Csikszentmihalyi and Rochberg-Halton on the basis of their interviews with three-generation families in Chicago and Evanston, Illinois. "They seem able to provide a record of one's life, and of the lives of one's ancestors, and can be handed down to one's descendants" (Csikszentmihalyi and Rochberg-Halton, 1981, p. 241). The Illinois study also found that the older we become, the more highly we treasure our family photos: see Table 17.1. Photos were ranked at the bottom of a list of "special objects" mentioned by children; grandparents, on the other hand, ranked photos at the top.

Not that the Late Life self always wants to be contemplating its own face in the photos. Having micro-analyzed dozens of US family albums, Richard Chalfen found that "on-camera participation" (his term for it) tends to diminish as one gets older. Seniors are visible in family albums mainly in shots taken during family reunions, or during birthday and wedding anniversary celebrations, or when relatives or friends have come to visit (Chalfen, 1987, p. 90).

Chalfen's explanation for this is that older people "may not want to be seen in snapshots that show either the natural effects of aging, such as wrinkles, awkward postures, a different smile because of false teeth, or even thick-lensed

Epilogue: Downsizing the material self 341

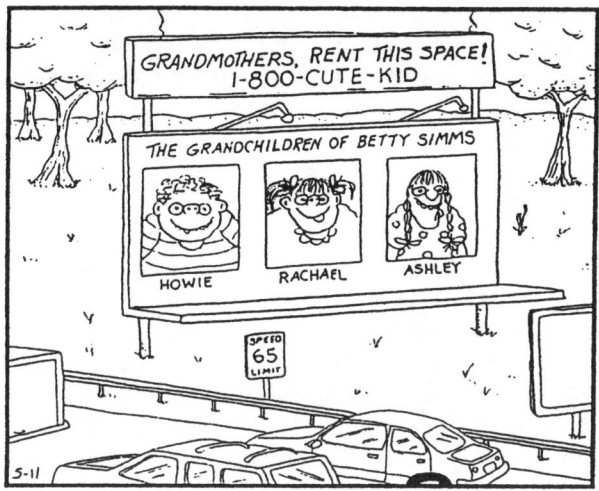

Figure 17.1 Close to home
Source: *Japan Times,* Tokyo edition, May 11, 1997

eyeglasses" (Chalfen, 1987, p. 91). In Late Life such motives may be operating some of the time. But there is a powerful exception. Many seniors actively put themselves in front of camera in order to have memorial portraits made. They engage in a kind of self-taxidermy of one's face as one wants it to be remembered after one has died. This is a superb example of how humans record what did happen (posing for a portrait) in order to encourage things to go on happening – and to continue happening even after we have lost our individual quick of life.

And yet while we continue to draw breath (and have not been done in by nursing home shock) the images we want others to view are most likely to be photographs of our children and grandchildren. The proud grandmother assertively displaying photographs of her grandkids to anyone willing to look, has become a cliché figure in American humor: see Figure 17.1. And you frequent flyers may have learned how risky it is to sit next to one of us geezers during air travel. Laptops and hand-held computers have empowered us, and we can ruin your sleep as we scroll obsessively through dozens of digitized images of our darlings.

Conclusion

Victorian scholars of the self – I think of William James as an example – were as attentive to its material side as they were to its social or psychological ("spiritual" in James' vocabulary) dimensions. "Between what a man calls *me* and what he simply calls *mine,* the line is difficult to draw," wrote James in his *Principles of Psychology:*

> In the widest possible sense, a man's Self is the sum total of all that he can call his, not only his body, and his psychic powers, but his clothes and his house, his wife and his children, his ancestors and friends, his reputation and words, his land and horses and yacht and bank account.
>
> (James, 1890, pp. 291–292)

For a century, however, people in academia have downplayed the importance of the physical objects of selfness. Material things have of course not been totally forgotten, but neither have they been overstudied to the point of diminishing intellectual returns. My own searches have turned up little beyond the studies of Csikszentmihalyi and his collaborators, already mentioned, and those of Lita Furby (1978). To stretch the point so as to be brief: in the twentieth century we have had a powerful urge to regard object-relations as manifestations or reflections or expressions of something else. We take that something else to be a deeper structure or an underlying dynamic of human action, which we with our X-ray vision will proceed to reveal as the real meaning of things.

For a Freudian, then, possessions become the passive targets of "object-cathexes" that spring from primal unconscious drives. For a Meadian (as in the lines I quoted from *The Meaning of Things*) the self "is structured" by human relationships; material things only "reflect" that lower-level structuring activity. In theorizing, objects are given only the role of bridesmaid, invited to enhance the glory of the star of the show. I am suggesting that it may be just as reasonable to reverse these presumed lines of influence or causality: if I am carrying around and displaying a packet of snapshots of my grandchildren I am actively attempting "to structure" my connections with other people and at the same time I am cathecting or depositing some valuation, some meaning, upon my separate existence. "Agency" seems to be the latest term-of-fashion for this process: see Gell, 1998.

Meaning becomes muscular only when we domesticate it, personalize it, frame our own lives with it. Whether this process of personalizing tends to change markedly as people enter upon Late Life is yet another item on the roster of under-investigated issues in human development. As can be seen in Table E1, our long involvements with objects and possessions seem to take a new turn in the Third Age. Many people begin to realign and reassign items in their lifecourse baggage. And many of them seem to be trying to communicate, perhaps now and perhaps only in the retrospect made available to others by one's death, a preferred sense of identity and self-worth. People living obscure lives may in their own ways be doing what Presidents of the United States are said to be doing in their final months in office: seeking The Verdict of History.

If we pay more attention to the meaning of things in Late Life we may perhaps begin to outgrow the limitations of life-review and life-history techniques. Biographical approaches – and I speak as practitioner and enthusiast – are caught in a love/hate relationship with the vagaries of human memory. They are further limited by the semantic carrying capacity of grammatical coding. Experience is not always encoded into stories, and so may not always be retrievable in story form. Proust's multi-volume memories were first triggered by things; he needed years to turn them into stories. Most people are capable of telling stories about their lives but they do not necessarily perceive their lives as being a story or anthology of stories. Lifecourse baggage offers an alternative encoding of personal experience, if we have the wit to discover what things may mean.

"A biography is considered complete if it merely accounts for six or seven selves," wrote Virginia Woolf, "whereas a person may well have as many as a thousand" (quoted in Whittemore, 1989, p. 125). By investigating what things mean to people in older age, and how people care for the self by caring for things, we can begin to broaden the base of our researchable population. We can begin to draw autobiographical evidence from that segment of society anywhere – a sizeable segment, in my estimation – that does not share our academic appetite for Doing a Reading on verbal reports.

And once we have a good collection of evidence from that larger arc of the old-age population we may finally be able to address the fanning-out process that is so much a part of human aging: that the longer we live the more different we become, each of us accumulating a unique package of personal experience – and unique collection of personal things. I offer you the researchable proposition that in Late Life one downsizing does not fit all.

References

Beckett, S. (1931). *Proust*. New York: Grove Press.
Chalfen, R. (1987). *Snapshot versions of life*. Bowling Green, OH: Bowling Green State University Popular Press.
Csikszentmihalyi, M., and Rochberg-Halton, E. (1981). *The meaning of things: Domestic symbols and the self*. Cambridge: Cambridge University Press.
Furby, L. (1978). Possessions: toward a theory of their meaning and function throughout the life cycle. *Life-Span Development and Behavior, 1*, 297–336.
Gell, A. (1998). *Art and agency: An anthropological theory*. Oxford: Oxford University Press.
Henry, J. (1973). *On sham, vulnerability and other forms of self-destruction*. New York: Vintage Books.
Inoue, Y. (1982). *Chronicle of my mother* (J.O. Moy, Trans.). Tokyo: Kodansha International.
James, W. (1890). *The principles of psychology*. New York: Macmillan.
Kaufman, S. (1986). *The ageless self: Sources of meaning in late life*. Madison: University of Wisconsin Press.
Montaigne, M. de. (1958) *The complete essays of Montaigne* (D.M. Frame, Trans.). Stanford, CA: Stanford University Press. (French original published as *Essais*, 1572–1588).
Whittemore, R. (1989). *Whole lives: Shapers of modern biography*. Baltimore: Johns Hopkins University Press.

Glossary

Accountability dilemma Accountability is the expectation that organizations are answerable to those who are associated with their activities. The accountability dilemma is a situation in which an organization's multiple accountabilities conflict, resulting in disturbance or confusion in the organization's daily operations.

Advance directive A medical legal document which allows an individual to declare personal preferences for maintaining or terminating life support in a situation of terminal illness or permanent unconscious state at some time in the future. In the US, two forms of advance directives, living wills and durable powers of attorney for health care (DPAHC), are widely recognized. Living wills in Japan may be used to express similar sentiments but, unlike the US, do not have the status of legal documents.

Boke Japanese colloquial term for confusion or mild senility often associated with a general decline in old age. The assumption that *boke* is a normal part of the aging process helps create the anxiety of many elderly people that they will burden their children with daily care responsibilities.

Coresidence The sharing of a household, here used to refer to an adult child (and family) living in the same household with elderly parents. In the first half of the twentieth century, the *ie* model of the household (see *Ie* below) assumed that the successor child (generally the oldest son) would remain in the household. There are also more recent forms of coresidence, such as a frail parent moving in with an adult child who had previously established an independent household, or *nisedai setai*, where three generations live in two households located in the same building or compound.

Cultural construction A perspective that emphasizes the social attribution of meaning, thus culturally "creating" the understanding and use of an object or idea.

Demographic imperative The necessity of changes in society due to changes in the size and composition of the population. Here, the impact on social and health programs that must be dealt with during the decades of baby boomer retirements 2010–2030.

Geriatric health care facility See *rōjin hoken shisetsu*.

Gold Plan   See Ten Year Strategy To Promote Health Care and Welfare Services for the Elderly.

Hospice care   A multidisciplinary approach to the care of terminally ill individuals that emphasizes quality of life rather than efforts to prolong survival; relief of physical, psychological, and spiritual distress; and bereavement support. Hospice care may be home-based (the emphasis in the US) or institution-based (the emphasis in Japan). In the United States, "hospice" most often refers to a form of end-of-life care that conforms to guidelines for eligibility for Medicare reimbursement.

Ie   Multigenerational stem family that constituted the upper-class ideal during Japan's Tokugawa period (1600–1868) and served as the basis for the family legal code in the first half of the twentieth century. Ideally, an *ie* existed in perpetuity, with one married couple (or surviving spouse) together with their unmarried children in each generation comprising the living members of the household. The cultural preference was for the eldest son to succeed his father as head of the household, and his wife to take on the responsibilities of the adult female role (see also *yome*).

Informal care   Home care or help for the elderly by family members, friends, neighbors, and more recently, voluntary organizations, usually given free of charge.

Jibun   Japanese word for "self," literally translated "self part," recognizing an individual self, but one which is inherently connected to a larger group.

Kaeshi   Literally, "to return" something. It is frequently used to refer to the return of a past favor.

Kaigo Hoken   Long-Term Care Insurance; specifically, a Japanese public insurance program to be implemented in the year 2000 and financed with insurance contributions and general revenue covering both community and institutional care services for older adults based on need for medical care and social services, regardless of income or the availability of informal care.

Kenkō shindan   Japanese term for an annual physical or health maintenance examination.

Life course   The multiple threads of continuity and points of transition over an individual's life shaped by conscious decisions, subjective experiences, the influence of significant others, and the broader culture. In the social sciences, life-course analysis generally focuses on the relationship of individual aging and maturation to the process of change in the family or other groups, and to the events, perceptions and symbols of the particular historical and cultural context.

Life review   A narrative intervention technique by which an individual recollects his or her life history through a dialogue or collaboration between an elderly person and a health care or social service professional. This process of recollection is thought to help preserve a satisfactory self-image and sense of competence and mastery in the elderly person.

Living will   See advance directives.

Long-Term Care Insurance   See *Kaigo Hoken*.

Managed care A system of medical cost-containment utilized by insurance companies and health care organizations in which decisions about medical procedures, tests, treatments, and other services to patients are closely monitored and controlled.

Medicaid Joint US federal and state program administered by states that finances health care services for individuals who are eligible for federal social welfare programs. For elder care, Medicaid has primarily covered costs of institutional care. However, in recent years, medicaid waivers have provided alternatives by permitting Medicaid benefits to be used for care in the home and community instead of solely in nursing homes.

Medicare US publicly-financed insurance for elders financed primarily with payroll taxes. Medicare Part A "Hospital Insurance" covers a broad range of hospital and post-hospital services, but does not cover outpatient prescription drugs nor long-term care. Medicare Part B covers doctors' fees and certain other health services. Both parts are subject to deductibles and coinsurance.

Medigap insurance In the US, health care insurance that can be privately purchased to cover the difference between charges for services and the amount covered by Medicare, which is usually the copayments and deductibles.

Ningen dokku Literally, "human dry dock." Term derived from the practice of completing a thorough examination of a dry-docked ship, used in Japan to refer to the executive physical. It differs from a regular physical in that it usually includes extensive diagnostic testing.

Nonprofit organizations (NPOs) Voluntary organizations which are recognized as not-for-profit corporations in the legal system. The US has a long history of an active nonprofit sector, in part because provision of some services has not been seen as a responsibility of government. Japan has recently enacted a law which recognizes NPO status, but does not include the tax benefits accorded to American nonprofit organizations. (See voluntary organization.)

Nursing home US law distinguishes two categories of residential institutions providing regular nursing care: skilled nursing facilities and intermediate care facilities. Whereas skilled care institutions are eligible for both Medicare and Medicaid reimbursement, intermediate care nursing homes receive payment only from Medicaid or private funds. Japan also has several types of residential care institutions. *Rōjin hoken shisetsu* are considered medical facilities and are covered under the national health insurance system, whereas *tokubetsu yōgo rōjin hōmu* are classified as social welfare institutions. (See *rōjin hoken shisetsu* and *tokubetsu yōgo rōjin hōmu*.)

Opportunity cost The cost incurred by forgoing an alternative use of a resource, in this case the next alternative use of the informal caregiver's time.

Palliative care Similar in goals and intent to "hospice care," but with greater applicability to earlier stages of the disease process, or to any condition where maximizing the quality of life has higher priority than achieving a

Glossary 347

cure. Increasingly, "palliative care" is replacing "hospice" as the more general term because of the close association between "hospice" and the very last stage of life, which is too narrow for the true applicability of "palliative care." (See hospice care.)

Public subsidy Public funding of the gap between the actual cost of a service and private financing.

Respite care Short-term institutional care intended to provide temporary relief from caregiving responsibilities for family caregivers. In Japan, respite care is often called "short stay service."

Rōjin hoken shisetsu Geriatric health care facility; long term institutional care facilities in Japan for elderly suffering from chronic diseases which require skilled care, but not hospitalization, comparable to skilled nursing homes in the US. However, unlike Japanese nursing homes (*tokubetsu yōgo rōjin hōmu*), geriatric health care facilities can be utilized by any older person regardless of their income or the availability of family care. (See nursing home.)

Social construction of self A sociological approach which emphasizes that selves are created through an on-going process of social interaction.

Soto Literally, "outside." Here, it is used to indicate social and emotional distance in contrast to more intimate relationships. (See *uchi*.)

Ten Year Strategy to Promote Health Care and Welfare Services for the Elderly A comprehensive Japanese national policy for elder care, introduced in 1990 and revised in 1994, mandating and expanding such services as home helpers, day care centers, and short stay respite facilities as well as institutional care. This is also known as the Gold Plan.

Terminal illness Illness from which a person is not expected to recover, often defined programmatically as a life expectancy of six months or less.

Third-party payers In US health care, Medicare, Medicaid and private insurance companies who pay to reimburse providers for services delivered to patients. Payers are not health care providers, but pay on behalf of patients.

Tokubetsu yōgo rōjin hōmu Japanese nursing home for seriously impaired elderly who cannot receive the needed care from their family members. Most are currently privately managed but construction is government subsidized. Operating as welfare institutions, most costs are paid publicly except for a patient fee whose amount is determined according to a sliding scale based on financial need.

Uchi Literally, "inside." The word is often used colloquially in Japan to refer interchangeably to oneself and a close-knit group to which one belongs, especially family. Because "uchi" is non-specific, it is used to support the notion that the concept of selfhood in Japan is highly relational and context-dependent.

Universal entitlement Public programs that make services available to a category of people without regard to demonstrated financial need – for example, to all older persons based on age. In contrast, "selective programs" make services available to a limited number of older persons, such as only those below poverty income levels.

Voluntary organizations Groups of people who come together to provide services to benefit the public and which are neither governmental nor for-profit corporations. The types of internal organization, level of political advocacy, and orientation toward services and clients vary widely. Nonprofit organizations are voluntary organizations which have formal legal recognition.

Volunteer One who elects to participate in activities to benefit the public, without obligation to do so. While it is commonly understood that volunteers are not paid, some volunteers (in both the US and Japan) may receive a stipend or wage, or are reimbursed for their expenses.

Yome Literally translated, "bride." In the *ie*, this was the role filled by the daughter-in-law (regardless of her age or length of marriage) who married into the household, and who normatively provided care to elderly parents-in-law. The term continues to be used to refer to a daughter-in-law, usually the wife of the eldest son, regardless of whether the generations coreside, and continues to connote expectations of responsibility for elder care.

Index

Abe Fellowship PrHoogram 1
accountability; dilemma 207, 208–9, 221, 225, 344; multiple 208; of voluntary/nonprofit organizations organizations (NPOs) 207–8
activities; of daily living (ADL) 68, 100–1; political of elderly 73
acute care 72–3
advance directives 173, 176, 177, 344
African American 78n24, 238, 240, 261
age 134; Fourth 334–5; Third 334–5, 342
Ageless Self, The (Kaufman) 339
aging 1, 2–3, 4, 13n4, 19, 277; cultural assumptions about 324, 330; and health promotion 111, 112, 113, 114; in Japan 25, 39, 46, 83, 84, 88, 121–2, 191, 304, 305, 330, 331, 432; in United States 4, 25, 68, 98, 100–1, 104, 108–9, 115–16, 121–2, 324, 331
aging policies 19, 25–6; Japan 6–9, 12, 29, 37–8, 42–9, 82–96, 97n1; Scandinavian model 91–2; social insurance systems 92–3; in United States 7–9, 12, 52–4, 55, 56, 57–8, 61, 64, 73–5, 98–9, 108–9, 115–16
AIDS (acquired immune deficiency syndrome) 182
Aliyah Center (Venice, United States) 293
Alzheimer's Association (United States) 252
Alzheimer's disease 279–86, 308, 309–10, 313, 318–31, 331n3; caring for people with 318–19, 320, 321, 323, 325–6, 327–8, 330, 331; and conceptions of self 318–19, 320, 321, 322–31, 331n2, n3; medical aspects of 321–2, 325, 330; and personhood 320, 323, 325, 327, 328, 332n5; and quality of life 327, 328; *see also* demented elderly; dementia
American Association of Retired Persons (AARP) 73
Area Commissioners (Japan) 195–6
Asai, A. 125
Aum Shinri Kyō 153
authority relations 6
autonomy; preference for 21–2; of self 319, 320–1, 327, 329

Barnard, D. 150
Beckett, S. 338
Benedict, R. 23, 337
bereavement services 168
Berger, J. 299
Bihāra (Buddhist Hospice) 154, 162n7
bioethics 138–9
boke (mild senility) 330, 344
Bortz, W. 140
Bredin, K. 295, 320, 323, 324, 327, 328, 332n5
Buddhism; in Japan 29, 151, 154; perspectives on health care 154, 162n7
Butler, R. 290

Callahan, D. 122, 175–6, 177
Campbell, J. 193
Campbell, R. 275
cancer; in Japan 148, 162n2, n9, 303, 309, 314; in United States 182, 314
cardiovascular disease (CVD) 111, 112–13
care; acute 72–3; for Alzheimer's disease patients 318–19, 320, 321, 323, 325–6, 327–8, 330, 331; chronic 114, 122; community based 45, 48, 89, 90, 91, 95–6, 97n5, 198–202, 204n12, 245; for demented elderly 275–9, 280,

286–7, 295, 304, 308–16, 318, 332n5; end-of-life 146, 147, 157, 158, 161, 172–3, 176–7, 180–5; 'futile' 69; individualized 289, 291, 299; informal 68, 100, 107, 108–9, 242–4, 310, 345; institutional 29–30, 43, 44, 47–8, 49, 68, 89, 90, 95, 100, 233; long-term 73–4, 291; meaning of 11, 225; palliative 149, 157, 172, 178, 179, 184, 346–7; private 45; respite 47, 245, 257, 265–6, 266, 347; self 319; *see also* home-based care; hospice care; hospital care; intensive care
caregivers; family members 29, 50, 87, 232, 233, 236, 239, 250, 252–5, 257–61, 265, 283, 304, 306, 308–9, 312; informal 108; male 248–60, 264–6; non-relatives 242–4, 310, 313; professional 5, 9–10, 45, 48, 109, 277, 278, 286, 291–2; role of 251, 252, 255, 257–8, 266; support groups for 264
caregiving 1–3, 10–11; cultural assumptions about 249, 251, 253, 255, 259, 267; economic value of 108–9; experience of 11, 108, 242–3, 254–5, 257–8, 260, 264, 266, 268; gender aspects of 5–6, 11, 50, 248–51, 250, 255, 256, 257–8, 260, 266–7; policies 7–9, 29–30, 74, 248, 259, 260–8; research on 2, 10–11, 13n2, 121, 184, 185, 209–21, 232, 250, 251–68, 277, 290–1, 340; skills needed for 255–6, 278–9, 286; *see also* family caregiving
Cassell, E.J. 175
catastrophic medical insurance 72–3, 149
Chalfen, R. 340
charitable organizations 226
Chihara, S. 147
choices, open-ended 22
Christianity, in Japan 153–4
chronic care 114, 122
chronic diseases *see* terminal illnesses
Chronicle of my Mother (Inoue) 338–9
Chrysanthemum and the Sword, The (Benedict) 337, 338
citizens, role of 225
citizens' mutual aid groups (Japan) 198–9, 202, 203n6, 204n9
cognitive abilities, and personhood 321–2, 323–4, 327, 331
Cohen, C.A. 314
Cohler, B. 290
Cole, T. 290, 339

communication styles 256
community based care 45, 48, 97n5, 245; in Japan 89, 90, 91, 95–6, 198–202, 204n12; *see also* home-based care
community bonds, in Japan 313
community center for the elderly (*rōjin fukushi sentā*) 38
Community Welfare Commissioners (Japan) 196
compression of morbidity 110, 111–13, 114, 115
Constitution (Japan) 194–5
consubstantial 335–6
Cooper, J. 99
Cooper, T. 207
coresidence 11, 20–1, 33, 85–7, 89, 90, 238–9, 244–5, 344
costs; of hospice care 150, 156, 157, 159, 162n5, 184; of medical care 4, 137, 141; opportunity 346; of respite care 266
counseling skills 279
coverage; of health insurances 35; by pension schemes 34
Csikszentmihalyi, M. 340, 342
cultural assumptions 19; about aging 324, 330; about caregiving 249, 251, 253, 255, 259, 267; about self 319, 320–1, 323–5, 328–9, 330–1, 332n5; shaping policies 8, 249
cultural construction 344
culture; American 121–2, 173, 249, 321, 323; influencing health care 124, 175; Japanese 121–2, 146, 150–1, 162n6, 249, 321, 325, 329–30, 338–9; Western 28, 33, 323–5

Danis, M. 176
daughters 232, 236, 239, 308–9, 312
daughters-in-law 29, 50, 87, 232, 233, 239, 304, 306, 348
day care centers, adult 47
death; acceptance of 174–8, 183; in Japan 148, 151–4, 161, 162n2; suffering 180; in United States 172–80, 183–5; *see also* dying; end-of-life care; euthanasia; hospice care; palliative care
decision-making; by demented elderly 303, 311–12, 313–14, 315–16; end-of-life 125–6, 138–9, 140, 147, 177
definitional ceremonies, in life review 292–3, 294–5

Index 351

demented elderly; attitudes of family members 306–13; caring for 275–9, 286–7, 295, 304, 308–16, 318, 332n5; creativity of 12, 275–6, 279, 282, 283, 284–6; decision-making by 303, 311–12, 313–14, 315–16; in Japan 276–7, 278, 279–86, 287–8, 303, 304, 305–16, 321; problem behaviors 286; psychological well-being 277, 278, 280, 283–4, 286–7; quality of life 286; support groups 283–4; in United States 313, 321; *see also* Alzheimer's disease
dementia 12, 252, 275, 277–8, 279–83, 287, 297, 321, 331n3; creativity of people with 12, 275–6, 279, 282, 283, 284–6, 287, 288; disclosure of diagnosis 303, 307, 308, 310, 313, 314, 316; research on 313, 320, 322, 323–7, 330
demographic changes *see* aging
demographic imperative 98, 344
Diagnosis Related Groups (DRGs) 77n19, n20
disclosure of diagnosis; to family members 303, 307, 308, 310, 313; to patients 155, 158, 159, 162n8, 286, 303, 307, 308, 310, 311, 313, 314, 316
divorce, in Japan 237, 244
do-not-resuscitate (DNR) orders 138
Dore, R.P. 312
Downie, R.S. 279
durable powers of attorney for health care (DPAHC, United States) 344
dying; at home 161, 173; control of 176–8; medicalization of 5, 162n1, 180; preparations for 151–3; prolonged 140, 174; *see also* death; end-of-life care; euthanasia

Edel, L. 300
Edwards, M. 208
Edwards, W.E. 303
effectiveness, of life-sustaining treatments 129–30
emperor system, Japan 192
end-of-life; care 146, 147, 157, 158, 161, 172–3, 176–7, 180–5; decision-making 125–6, 138–9, 140, 147, 177; *see also* death; dying; hospice care; palliative care
Englehardt, H.T., Jr. 326
Essays (Montaigne) 336
ethnographic methods 293

euthanasia 177

families; living arrangements 231, 234–5, 237, 238–44, 246, 252, 304, 305; role in hospice care 155–6, 159; *see also* coresidence
family caregiving 2, 4, 10–11, 13n10, 94, 148, 231, 238, 244, 246, 248–9, 251, 267–8; burdens of 256–7, 283, 311; conflicts resulting from 253–4; daughters 232, 236, 239, 308–9, 312; daughters-in-law 29, 50, 87, 232, 233, 239, 304, 306, 348; in Japan 11, 28–9, 38, 49–50, 85–9, 95, 96, 97n9, 161, 162n11, 199, 223, 232–3, 237–8, 241, 245, 253–4, 255–60, 283, 303, 306, 308–12; policies on 259, 260–8; role of men 248–62, 264–7; role of women 5, 28, 49–50, 88, 95, 180, 199, 232, 249, 255, 257, 267; skills needed for 225–6, 265, 278–9; sons 250, 253–4, 258, 260, 265; spouses 232, 250, 252–4, 255, 257, 259, 261, 265, 283, 304; in United States 100, 108, 180, 181, 231–2, 234, 235–6, 239–40, 245, 250, 252–4, 255–60; use of formal services 260; *see also* respite care
family factors, in life-sustaining treatments 135–7, 138–9, 140–1
family systems; East Asian 28; Japanese 85–6, 203n5, 237, 303, 312
fascism in Japan 192
fee-for-service financing (FFS) 61, 67–8, 76n4, 149
fertility rates 4, 13n6
FFS *see* fee-for-service financing
financial security 259, 261, 267
Fontana, A. 326
Food Stamp Act (United States, 1964) 60
Forest, K.B. 231
formal care *see* institutional care
Fortune 336–7
Foundation for the Prevention of Dementia (Japan) 277
Fourth Age 334–5
frailty among the elderly 23–4, 96, 334
Fries, J.F. 110, 112
Fukaura, A. 138
fukushi kōsha (welfare-oriented public corporations) 201
Fundamental Law on Policies for the Aging Society (*Kōrei Shakai Taisaku Kihon Hō*, 1995) 39
Furby, L. 342

Furukawa, J. 197, 198, 204n10
'futile' care 69
gender aspects, of caregiving 5–6, 11, 50, 248–51, 250, 255, 256, 257–8, 260, 266–7
gender equality 259; Japan 29, 33, 49–50, 88, 95, 96, 256
gender systems 250
gender-responsive policies 249, 259, 260–2
geriatric health care facilities (*rōjin hoken shisetsu*) 42–4, 50n2, 347
Germany, social policies 82, 92, 93–4
gerontology; preventative 111; research on 12
GHQ (general headquarters of the allied powers, Japan) 192–3, 194, 196
gift exchanges, Japan 338–9
Gold Plan (*Gōrudo Puran*, 1990 and 1994) 46–8, 49, 90–2, 96, 97n6, 193, 245, 345
Great Hanshin Earthquake (1994) 200, 206, 227
grieving process 168, 179, 180, 296
growth capacity among elderly 289, 291
guardianship procedures in Japan 315, 316

habitus 19
Hagestad, G. 23
haiku (short poems) 286
Harré, R. 327–8
Hashimoto, R. 90, 92
Hashimoto, A. 8, 223, 232
health care; access to 72, 75, 78n23, n24; Buddhist perspectives on 154, 162n7; Christian perspectives on 153–6; cultural influences on 121–2, 124, 146, 150–1, 162n6, 173, 175, 249, 321, 323–5, 325, 329–30, 338–9; for the elderly 65, 68–9, 70, 72, 99, 109–10; preventative 110, 113, 115; rationing of 5, 122
Health Care for the Elderly Law (*Rōjin Hoken Hō*, 1982) 36, 40–1, 149
health care expenditures 4–5, 112; in Japan 121, 122; in United States 62, 63, 67–70, 72, 75, 76n7, 77n16, n17, n18, 78n25, 107, 114, 121, 122
health care policies, Japan 147, 157, 160, 161
health care systems; in Japan 86, 88–9, 146–7, 149–50; national 62; in United States 53–4, 57, 61–75, 75n2, n3, 76n4, n5, n6, n8, n9, 77n15, 78n23, n24, 98, 110, 123, 184–5; universal 62–3
health checks 40, 123, 345, 346
Health Insurance for the Aged Act (United States, 1965) 64
health insurances; coverage 35, 149; for the elderly 64, 71–2, 76n9; Japan 35–6, 40–1, 89, 149, 159; private 61–2; public 35–6, 40–1, 61, 76n8, 77n15; United States 72–3, 106; *see also* long-term care insurances (LTCI); Medicaid; Medicare
health maintenance organizations (HMOs, United States) 61, 70, 78n21, 110
health promotion 112, 115; and aging 111, 112, 113, 114; United States 110–11
Henry, J. 336
Herskovits, E. 324, 325, 329
High, D.M. 313
home-based; care 47, 48, 87, 97n9, 198–9, 202, 203n7, 209–10, 233, 265, 306, 311; hospice care 149, 159–61, 165–6, 181
homelessness, United States 59–60, 217
Hori, K. 198
hospice care 9, 65, 69, 146, 179–80, 345, 347; costs of 150, 156, 157, 159, 162n5, 184; educational goals 157; eligibility for 158–9, 161, 167; family role 155–6, 159; home-based 149, 159–61, 165–6, 181; ideals of 150–5, 157, 159, 161, 177; in Japan 146–7, 148–61, 162n4, n5, 304; links with Christianity 153; nurses 156, 183; patients 155, 164–5; physicians 156, 157, 182–3; private rooms 157, 159, 161; quality assurance 168–9; in United States 179, 180–4; volunteers 148, 168; *see also* death; dying; end-of-life care; palliative care
hospice philosophy 146, 147, 148, 155, 157, 179, 182, 183
hospital care in Japan 88–9, 148, 149, 233, 304, 306
households; in Japan 4, 20, 85–6; in United States 4, 23; *see also* families, living arrangements
housing policies; in Japan 44, 89, 245–6; in United States 58–60, 74, 246
Hulme, D. 208

ie (multigenerational stem family) 238–9, 345

Index 353

Individual Retirement Accounts (IRAs, United States) 108
individualized care 289, 291, 299
indoor relief *see* institutional care
informal care 68, 107, 108–9, 242–4, 310, 345; *see also* family caregiving; home-based care
informed consent 148, 155
Inoue, Y. 338–9
institutional care 29–30, 43, 44, 47–8, 49, 68, 89, 90, 95, 100, 233; *see also* hospice care; hospital care; nursing homes
instrumental activities of daily living (IADL) 68
intensive care 125
interdiction order (Japan) 315
interest groups, old age 49, 97n3, 219, 283
intergenerational justice 6
Internal Revenue Service (IRS, United States) 211
Ishida, T. 191–2, 196

Jaffe, D.J. 11
James, W. 341–2
Japan 336; aging 4, 25, 32, 39, 46, 49, 83, 84, 88, 121–2, 191, 304, 305, 330, 331; aging policies 6–9, 12, 29, 37–8, 42–9, 82–96, 97n1; Buddhism 29, 151, 154; cancer 148, 162n2, n9, 303, 309, 314; Christianity 153–4; community based care 89, 90, 91, 95–6, 198–202, 204n12; community bonds 313; conceptions about United States 7; Confucian heritage 83; coresidence 11, 20–1, 33, 85–7, 89, 90, 344; culture 121–2, 146, 150–1, 162n6, 249, 325, 329–30, 338–9; daughters 308–9, 312; daughters-in-law 29, 50, 87, 232, 233, 239, 304, 306, 348; death 148, 151–4, 161, 162n2; demented elderly 276–7, 278, 279–86, 287–8, 303, 304, 305–16, 321; divorce 237; emperor system 192; family caregiving 11, 28–9, 38, 49–50, 85–9, 95, 96, 97n9, 161, 162n11, 199, 223, 232–3, 237–8, 241, 245, 253–4, 255–60, 283, 303, 306, 308–12; family system 85–6, 203n5, 237, 303, 312; fascism 192; gender equality 29, 33, 49–50, 88, 95, 96, 256; gift exchanges 338–9; guardianship procedures 315; health care expenditures 121, 122; health care policies 147, 157, 160, 161; health care system 86, 88–9, 146–7, 149–50; health insurances 35–6, 40–1, 89, 149, 159; home-based care 149, 198–9, 202, 203n7, 209, 233, 306, 311; hospice care 146–7, 148–61, 162n4, n5, 304; hospital care 88–9, 148, 149, 233, 304, 306; households 4, 20, 85–6; housing policies 44, 89, 245–6; informal care 243–4, 310; institutional care 89, 90, 95, 233; life course trajectories 24; long-term care insurances 82, 92–6, 160, 200–1, 233, 263, 265, 345; medical technology 123–4, 148; nursing homes 43, 87, 89, 233, 304, 306, 311, 314, 315; palliative care 149, 157; paternalistic system 192, 193, 196; pensions 31–2, 34–5, 41–2, 84, 85, 261; physicians 125, 132–3, 138–9, 146–7, 148, 155, 156, 157, 160, 162n3; political divisions 28; poverty 284; respite care 245, 265–6; sense of security 20–1, 26, 232–3; sense of self 328–30; social policies 28–32, 34–49, 82–3, 96, 97n2, 191–203, 203n2, n3, 213, 245, 259, 262–3, 315; socio-economic developments 3–6, 28–9, 32–3, 84, 86; suicide rates 7, 13n8; voluntary/nonprofit organizations (NPOs) 10, 49, 206, 209, 211–12, 214–16, 221, 222, 223, 224, 226–7; volunteers 195–6, 198–202, 203n4, n8, 206, 211, 212–16, 221, 222, 223, 224, 226–7; war efforts 30–1; Western cultural influences 28, 33
Japan Socialist Party (JSP) 90
Japanese Association of Hospice and Palliative Care Units 147, 158–9, 166–9
Japanese language 307, 329
Jewish elderly 292–3
jibun (self) 329, 345
Johnson, M.M.S. 292
justice, intergenerational 6
Jutsukyū Kisoku (Relief Order, 1874) 29–30

Kahana, E. 10–11
kaigo fukushi-shi 45
Kaigo Hoken Hō (Long-Term Care Insurance Law, 1997) 8, 82, 93–6, 160, 193, 200–1, 233, 263, 265, 345
Kaigo no Shakaika o Susumeru Ichimannin Shimin Iinkai (Ten Thousand Citizens' Association for the Promotion of

354 *Index*

Socialization of the Care of the Elderly and Impaired) 49
Kastenbaum, R. 177
Kaufman, S. 25, 339
Kearney, M. 178
kenkō shindan (annual physical examination) 123, 345
Kennedy, J.F. 57
Kichuchi, M. 122
Killick, J. 276
Kitwood, T. 295, 320, 323, 324, 327, 328, 332n5
Kōbe earthquake *see* Great Hanshin Earthquake (1994)
Kobrin, F.E. 238
kōreika shakai mondai (aging-society problem) 84, 88
Kōreika Shakai o Yokusuru Josei no Kai (Women's Association for the Realization of Better Aging Society) 49
Kōrei Shakai Taisaku Kihon Hō, 1995 (Fundamental Law on Policies for the Aging Society) 39
Kramer, J.H. 314
Kutza, E.A. 55
Kyūgo Hō (Public Relief Law, 1932) 30

labor policies 261–2, 267
late life 334, 340–1
Lear, M.W. 175
Leary, T. 177–8
Lebra, T.S. 24, 329
legal concerns; in caring for demented elderly 315–16; of life-sustaining treatments 137
Liberal Democratic Party (LDP, Japan) 84, 90
Lieberman, M.A. 314
life course; analysis 12, 23, 345; baggage 334–43; trajectories 23–5
life expectancy 4, 13n5; United States 68, 100
life review 12, 280–3, 285, 289–90, 291–2, 342–3, 345; definitional ceremonies 292–3, 294–5; ethnographic methods 293; life story interviews 293–4, 296, 297–8; narrative 290, 293; storyboard 289, 290, 294, 295, 298–9; visual material 294, 298–9
life story interviews 293–4
life-sustaining treatments 121, 124, 140–1; costs 137, 141; effectiveness of 129–30; family factors 135–7, 138–9, 140–1; legal concerns 137; patients' preferences 123, 132–3, 139, 140–1, 173, 175, 176; physicians' approach 124–41; research on 124–40, 176; United States 123
Livelihood Protection Law *see Seikatsu Hogo Hō* (Livelihood Protection Law, 1946 and 1950)
living arrangements, of families 231, 234–5, 237, 238–44, 246, 252, 304, 305
living wills 173, 344
Long, S.O. 125, 147, 153, 330
long-term care (LTC) 73–4, 82, 94, 95–6, 99, 100, 103, 106–7, 204n10, 263, 267, 291
long-term care insurances (LTCI) 8–9, 47, 49–50, 72, 73, 74, 78n26, 345; Japan 8, 82, 92–6, 160, 200–1, 233, 263, 265, 345; United States 103, 104, 105, 106–8
Loss of Self, The (Cohen and Eisdorfer) 322
LTCI *see* long-term care insurances
Lynn, J. 174

Maeda, D. 194
Maguire, C.P. 313
managed care 61, 68, 70, 110, 111, 139, 184, 346
March, J.G. 8–9
material self, downsizing of 334–43
Medicaid (United States, 1965) 57, 64, 65–6, 71, 72, 75, 77n14, 103, 106, 263, 346; waivers 233, 245
medical insurances *see* health insurances
medical technology 69, 121, 122–3, 175, 180; Japan 123–4, 148; United States 123
Medical Trust Accounts (MTAs, United States) 108
medicalization of dying 5, 162n1, 180
Medicare Catastrophic Coverage Act (MCCA, 1988) 73
Medicare (United States, 1965) 57, 64, 65, 66, 67, 70–1, 72, 75, 76n10, 77n11, 78n21, 103, 104, 106, 180–1, 263, 346; hospice benefit 180; HMO 61, 68, 70, 110
Medigap insurance plans 66, 346
Meiji era (Japan, 1868–1912) 29, 192
memory 338; loss of 283–4; procedural 287
men; as family caregivers 248–62, 264–7; *see also* sons; spouses

Miller, E.M. 11
Ministry of Health and Welfare (Japan) 149–50, 156, 158, 192
Minobe, R. 84
Moen, P.H. 231
Montaigne, M. de 335, 336
Moral Challenge of Alzheimer Disease, The (Post) 323
morbidity compression 110, 111–13, 114, 115
multiple accountabilities 208
Myerhoff, B.G. 292–3

narrative 290, 293
National Association of Welfare Institutions for the Elderly (Japan) 37
national health care systems 62
National Health Insurance Law for the Self-Employed (*Kokumin Kenkō Hoken Hō*, 1958) 35–6, 40, 41
National Hospice Organization (United States) 181
National Institutes of Health (NIH, United States) 185
National Pension Insurance System (*Kokumin Nenkin Seido*, 1985) 41–2
National Registration System of Trained Careworkers 45
National Retirement Pension Insurance Law for Self-Employed People (*Kokumin Nenkin Hō*, 1959) 34–5, 42
National Retirement Pension Insurance Program for the Employees of Private Firms (*Kōsei Nenkin Hoken*) 31
National Social Welfare Council (Japan) 194, 199
needs, in old age 23–6, 46, 49, 55, 68, 75, 100, 104
network, of resources 22–3, 312
Neugarten, B.L. 25
'New Deal' Program (United States) 52, 55, 193
Ngor, H. 339
nin'i dantai (arbitrarily established organizations) 199–200
ningen dokku ('human dry dock') 123, 346
nisedai setai (two-generation household) 20, 344
Nishio, M. 200
Nonprofit Organization Act (Japan, 1998) 200, 201–2, 206, 227
nonprofit organizations (NPOs)/voluntary organizations 10, 199–200, 202, 206–9, 211, 346, 348; accountability of 207–8; advocatory activities 208, 221, 222–4; board members 207–8, 211, 216, 218, 219, 220; financial performance 215, 218, 222; in Japan 10, 206, 211–12, 214–16, 221, 222, 223, 224, 226–7; leadership of 215, 217, 220; legal status 206, 211, 214, 215, 216, 219, 225, 227; outreach activities 214; service providers 208–9, 215–16, 221–3; in United States 206–7, 209–10, 211, 216–20, 221, 222, 223–4, 225–6
Novack, D.H. 314
nurses; in hospice care 156, 183; patient ratio 150, 156
nursing homes 43, 48, 87, 346; adjustment to life in 289, 293, 295, 296, 298; admission to 314; caregivers 291–2; in Japan 43, 87, 89, 233, 304, 306, 311, 314, 315; residents 289–300, 304; in United States 100, 101, 103–4, 105, 252, 289–300

Okamitsu, N. 93, 97n8
Old Age Assistance program (OAA, United Sates, 1935) 56
Old Age Insurance program (OAI, United States, 1935) 56
old age security 20, 26; contingency approach 21–3, 26, 232; protective approach 20–1, 26, 232
Old Age and Survivors Disability Insurance program (OASDI, United States, 1956) 56, 57
Old Age and Survivors Insurance program (OASI, United States, 1939) 56, 64
old-age interest groups 49, 73, 97n3, 283
Olsen, J.P. 8–9
Omori, W. 200
ontological security 20
opportunity costs 346
Ory, M.G. 99
outreach activities 214

pain control 147, 152, 153, 154, 167–8, 173, 177
palliative care 149, 157, 172, 178, 179, 184, 346–7; *see also* end-of-life care; hospice care
Patient Self-Determination Act (United States, 1991) 123
patients; age 134; in hospice care 155, 164–5; information about diagnosis 155, 158, 159, 162n8, 286, 303, 307,

308, 310, 311, 313, 314, 316; preferences in life-sustaining treatments 123, 132–3, 139, 140–1, 173, 175, 176; relationship with physicians 146–7, 148, 155
pensions 267; financing of 6; in Japan 31–2, 34–5, 41–2, 84, 85, 261; in United States 56, 74
personhood 320; in Alzheimer's disease 320, 323, 325, 327, 328, 332n5; criteria for 326; relationship with cognitive abilities 323–4, 325, 326, 327; relationship with self 319; restoring of 320, 332n5
photographs 335, 339, 340
physicians 9, 121; approach to life-sustaining treatments 124–41; in hospice care 156, 157, 182–3; in Japan 125, 132–3, 138–9, 146–7, 148, 155, 156, 157, 160, 162n3; lack of trust in 148, 162n3; payments 70; relationship with patients 146–7, 148, 155; role in hospice care 156, 157; in United States 132, 133, 138–9, 175, 182–3, 314
Pietrukowicz, M.A. 292
Plath, D. 24
pokkuri (sudden death) 151
policies; on aging 6–9, 12, 19, 25–6, 28, 37–8, 42–9, 52–4, 55, 56, 57–8, 61, 82–96, 97n1, 98, 248; on caregiving 7–9, 29–30, 74, 248, 259, 260–8; gender-responsive 249, 259, 260–2; on health care 147, 157, 160, 161; on housing 44, 58–60, 74, 89, 245–6; shaped by cultural assumptions 8, 249; on working practices 261–2, 267; *see also* social policies
policy makers 231, 244, 268
Policy Statement on the 'Society of Longevity' (*Chōju Shakai Taisaku Taikō*, 1986) 39
political activities of elderly 73
Post, S.G. 323
poverty; in Japan 284; in United States 59–60, 217, 261
powers of attorney 316, 344
preventive; gerontology 111, 286; health care 110, 113, 115
private care 45
private health insurances 61–2
procedural memory 287
professional caregivers 5, 9–10, 45, 48, 109, 277, 278, 286, 291–2

prospective payment system (PPS) 67, 70, 77n19, n20
psychological approach, in caring for people with dementia 275, 277, 279–88
psychological well-being 277, 278, 280, 283–4, 286–7, 290, 295, 296
public health insurances; in Japan 35–6, 40–1; in United States 61, 76n8, 77n15
Public Relief Law *see Kyūgo Hō* (Public Relief Law, 1932)
public subsidies 347
Putnam, T. 224

quality; of care 168–9, 315; of life 133–4, 140, 286, 327, 328
quasi-incompetence order (Japan) 315

Randall, F. 279
rationality, valued by Western culture 323, 329
rationing of health care 5, 122
Relief Order *see Jutsukyū Kisoku* (Relief Order, 1874); *Kyūgo Hō* (Public Relief Law, 1932)
relocation of workers 4
reminiscence; in nursing homes 290; in treating dementia 280–3
research; on caregiving 2, 10–11, 13n2, 121, 184, 185, 209–21, 232, 250, 251–68, 277, 290–1, 340; comparative 121; on dementia 313, 320, 322, 323–7, 330; on dying 174; on the elderly 10, 234, 250; in gerontology 12; on life-sustaining treatments 124–40, 176; qualitative 132; *see also* ethonographic methods
resource network 22–3
Resource-Based Relative Value Scale (RBRVS) 70–1, 78n22
respite care 47, 245, 257, 265–6, 347
retirement 334–6; benefits 40, 42, 52, 74; system 56
Rice, K. 313
Riley, M.W. 99
Rochberg-Halton, E. 340, 342
rōgo mondai (aging problem) 84
Rōjin Hoken Hō (Health Care for the Elderly Law) 36, 40–1, 149
rōjin hoken shisetsu (geriatric health care facilities) 42–4, 347
rōjin mondai (old-people problem) 84–5, 86–8
Roosevelt, F.D. 55

Rosenberger, N.J. 329, 330

Sabat, S.R. 327–8
St Christopher's Hospice (United Kingdom) 147, 179
Saunders, C. 147, 179
Scandinavian model for aging policies 91–2
security; contingency approach 21–3, 26, 232; diffused 23; financial 259, 261, 267; notions of 19–20; in old age 20; ontological 20; protective approach 20–1, 26, 232; structured 23
Sehgal, A. 176
Seikatsu Hogo Hō (Livelihood Protection Law, 1946 and 1950) 30
Seirei Hospice (Japan) 147, 156, 160, 163–6
Seirei Mikatagahara Hospital (Japan) 149
selective programs 347–8
self; in Alzheimer's disease 318–19, 320, 321, 322–31, 331n2, n3; autonomous construction of 319, 320–1, 327, 329; conceptions of 318–19, 328, 331n2, n3, 332n4; continuity of 12; cultural perceptions of 319, 320–1, 323–5, 328–9, 330–1, 332n5; in Japan 328–30; material 334–43; measurement of 322, 323, 328; recreation of 295; relational 319, 320, 321, 323, 325, 327, 328, 329–30, 332n6, 342; relationship with personhood 319; restoring of 320, 327; social construction of 319, 321, 326, 328, 347; in United States 330, 339; *see also* personhood
sheltered housing programs 44
Shindō, M. 198
Showa era (Japan, 1926–1989) 192
'Silver Housing Project' (Japan) 44
Siu, A.L. 99
skilled nursing facility 65, 104
skills needed for caregiving 225–6, 265, 278–9
Smith, D.H. 326
Smith, R.W. 326
social insurance systems 92–3
social policies; benefit entitlements 55, 92, 93; in Germany 82, 92, 93–4; in Japan 28–32, 34–49, 82–3, 96, 97n2, 191–203, 203n2, n3, 213, 245, 259, 262–3, 315; reform 197–8, 203; in United States 52–64, 74–5, 75n1, 245, 262, 263–4; *see also* aging policies;
health care policies; housing policies; pensions
Social Security Act (United States, 1935) 55–6, 64
social welfare *see* social policies
social welfare corporations 194–5, 202
social welfare councils 194, 196
sons, in family caregiving 250, 253–4, 258, 260, 265
Sōshiki (*The Funeral*, film) 153
soto (outside) 330, 347
spouses, in family caregiving 232, 250, 252–4, 255, 257, 259, 261, 265, 283, 304
Stephens, G.G. 175
storyboards 289, 290, 294, 295
suffering 150, 152, 154, 176, 178, 184
suicide rates 7, 13n8
Supplemental Security Income program (SSI, United States, 1972) 57–8
support groups 252, 283
SUPPORT Principal Investigators 141
Suzuki, S. 149
Suzuki, T. 329

Taisho era (Japan, 1912–1926) 192, 195
Tamiya, T. 154, 162n7
Tanaka, N. 201
Tax Equity and Fiscal Responsibility Act (TEFRA, United States, 1982) 70, 77n19
Ten Year Strategy to Promote Health Care and Welfare Services for the Elderly *see* Gold Plan (Japan)
terminal illnesses 113–14, 122, 158–9, 174, 177, 180, 347; *see also* AIDS; cancer
The Wall Street Journal 336
Third Age 334–5, 342
third-party payers 67, 77n16, 347
Thomas, W.H. 291
three-generation households 20, 344
Tobin, J.J. 6
tokubetsu yōgo rōjin hōmu (nursing homes) 43, 87, 304, 306, 347
Tokugawa era (1603–1868, Japan) 29
trained care workers 45
Traphagan, J.W. 330
Truman, H.S. 336

uchi (inside) 330, 347
United States; aging 4, 25, 68, 98, 100–1, 104, 108–9, 115–16,

121–2, 324, 331; aging policies 7–9, 12, 52–4, 55, 56, 57–8, 61, 64, 73–5, 98–9, 108–9, 115–16; cancer 182, 314; chronic care 114; conceptions about Japan 6, 337; culture 121–2, 173, 249, 321, 323; daughters 232, 236, 239; death 172–80, 183–5; demented elderly 313, 321; end-of-life care 172–3, 180–5; family caregiving 11, 100, 108, 180, 181, 231–2; great depression of 1930s 55; health care expenditures 62, 63, 67–70, 72, 75, 76n7, 77n16, n17, n18, 78n25, 107, 114, 121, 122; health care system 53–4, 57, 61–75, 75n2, n3, 76n4, n5, n6, n8, n9, 77n15, 78n23, n24, 98, 110, 123, 184–5; health insurances 61, 72–3, 76n8, 77n15, 106; health promotion 110–11; home-based care 210, 265; homelessness 59–60, 217; hospice care 179, 180–4; households 4, 23; housing policies 58–60, 74, 246; informal care 100, 107, 108, 242–3; institutional care 100, 233; life course trajectories 25; life expectancy 68; life-sustaining treatments 121; long-term care 99, 100, 103, 106–7, 263; long-term care insurances 103, 104, 105, 106–8; medical technology 123; nursing homes 100, 101, 103–4, 105, 289–300; palliative care 172; pensions 56, 74; physicians 132, 133, 138–9, 175, 182–3, 314; poverty 59–60, 217, 261; preventive health care 110; respite care 265–6; sense of security 21–3, 26, 232–3; sense of self 330, 339; social policies 52–64, 74–5, 75n1, 245, 262, 263–4; socio-economic developments 3–6, 56, 99, 102–3; voluntary/nonprofit organizations (NPOs) 206–7, 209–10, 211, 225–6; volunteers 206, 211, 216–18, 220, 223–6
universal entitlements 347–8
universal health care systems 62–3

user charges 159, 161, 214

Visible Lives project (United States) 289–300, 339
visual material in life review 294
Vita, A.J. 114
voluntary/nonprofit organizations (NPOs) 10, 199–202, 206–7, 211, 346, 348; accountability of 207–8; advocacy activities 208, 221, 222–4; board members 207–8, 211, 216, 218, 219, 220; financial performance 215, 218, 222; in Japan 10, 206, 209, 211–12, 214, 221, 222, 223, 224, 226–7; leadership of 215, 217, 220; legal status 206, 211, 214, 215, 216, 219, 225, 227; outreach activities 214; service providers 208–9, 215–16, 221–3; in United States 206–7, 209–10, 211, 216–20, 221, 222, 223–6
volunteers 10, 209, 211, 225, 348; in hospice care 148, 168; in Japan 195–6, 198–202, 203n4, n8, 206, 211, 212–16, 221, 222, 223, 224; payment of 211, 212, 222; role of women 199; training of 216; in United States 206, 211, 216–18, 220, 223–6
voucher system 95
vulnerability expectations 23–4, 26

Warner, N. 313
Welfare for the Elderly Law (*Rōjin Fukushi Hō*, 1963) 37, 40, 45
well-being, psychological 277, 278, 280, 283–4, 286–7, 290, 295, 296
Western culture 28, 33, 323–5, 329
WHO *see* World Health Organization (WHO)
women; as family caregivers 5, 28, 49–50, 88, 95, 180, 199, 232, 249, 255, 257, 267; participation in labor force 4, 5, 33, 244, 259, 260; volunteers 199; *see also* daughters; daughters-in-law; spouses
workers, relocation of 4
workplace policies, family-friendly 261–2, 267
World Health Organization (WHO) 179
Writing Lives (Edel) 300

yasuraka na shi (peaceful death) 152
Yodogawa Christian Hospital (Japan) 149
yogo rōjin hōmu (old people's homes) 87
yome (bride, daughter-in-law) 232, 348
yūryō (paid) volunteers 211

zaikai (finance world) 41, 50n1